Chronic Pain
Management for
Physical Therapists

Chronic Pain Management for Physical Therapists

Edited by

Harriët Wittink, M.S., P.T., O.C.S.

Clinical Instructor in Anesthesia/Pain Management, Tufts University School of Medicine, Boston; Clinical Specialist, New England Medical Center Pain Management Program, Boston

Theresa Hoskins Michel, M.S., P.T., C.C.S.

Assistant Professor of Physical Therapy, Post-Professional Program in Physical Therapy, MGH Institute of Health Professions, Boston; Physical Therapy Clinical Associate, Physical Therapy Services, Massachusetts General Hospital, Boston

With a foreword by

Daniel B. Carr, M.D., F.A.B.P.M.

Saltonstall Professor of Pain Research, Vice-Chairman for Research, and Medical Director, New England Medical Center Pain Management Program, Department of Anesthesiology, Boston; Professor of Anesthesiology and Medicine, Tufts University School of Medicine, Boston

Butterworth–Heinemann
Boston   Oxford   Johannesburg   Melbourne   New Delhi   Singapore

Butterworth–Heinemann supports the efforts of American Forests and the Global ReLeaf program in its campaign for the betterment of trees, forests, and our environment.

Cover Artwork: "Headache" by John Crowley
© Novartis (Sandoz Pharmaceuticals)

Library of Congress Cataloging-in-Publication Data
Chronic pain management for physical therapists / edited by Harriët Wittink, Theresa Hoskins Michel ; with a foreword by Daniel B. Carr.
    p.   cm.
   Includes bibliographical references and index.
   ISBN 0-7506-9740-7
   1. Chronic pain--Physical therapy.   I. Wittink, Harriët.
  II. Hoskins Michel, Theresa.
   [DNLM: 1. Pain--therapy. 2. Chronic Disease--therapy.
  3. Physical Therapy--methods.   WL 704 C5583 1997]
  RB127.C496   1997
  616'.0472--dc21
  DNLM/DLC
  for Library of Congress   97-4332
                                           CIP

British Library Cataloguing-in-Publication Data
A catalogue record for this book is available from the British Library.

The publisher offers special discounts on bulk orders of this book.
For information, please contact:
Manager of Special Sales
Butterworth–Heinemann
313 Washington Street
Newton, MA 02158-1626
Tel: 617-928-2500
Fax: 617-928-2620

For information on all Butterworth–Heinemann medical publications available, contact our World Wide Web home page at: http://www.bh.com/med

10 9 8 7 6 5 4 3 2 1

Printed in the United States of America

*To Ray Maciewicz, who gave me a place to belong,
and who continues to teach and challenge me*

H.W.

*To all my students, former, present, and future, who
help me evolve, challenge me, stimulate me, and
far surpass my highest dreams for them*

T.H.M.

Contents

APPENDIXES

Contributing Authors

Joanna R. Allan, M.Ed., R.P.T., L.M.H.C.
Physical Therapist and Biofeedback Therapist, Pain and Headache Management Center, Health South Rehabilitation Hospital, Sarasota, Florida

Gerald M. Aronoff, M.D., F.A.B.P.M., F.A.A.D.E.P.
Assistant Clinical Professor of Psychiatry, Tufts University School of Medicine, Boston; Director, Mid-Atlantic Center for Pain Medicine, Presbyterian-Orthopaedic Hospital, Charlotte, North Carolina

Lisa Janice Cohen, M.S., P.T., O.C.S.
Assistant Academic Coordinator of Clinical Education, Graduate Programs in Physical Therapy, MGH Institute of Health Professions, Boston; Physical Therapist, New England Medical Center Pain Management Program, Boston

Scott M. Fishman, M.D.
Instructor in Anesthesia, Harvard Medical School, Boston; Codirector, Massachusetts General Hospital Pain Center, Department of Anesthesia, Massachusetts General Hospital, Boston

Rosemary Goodall, P.T.
Physical Therapist, Department of Physical Therapy, Mid-Atlantic Center for Pain Medicine, Presbyterian-Orthopaedic Hospital, Charlotte, North Carolina

Ed Green, P.T.
Physical Therapist, Department of Physical Therapy, Mid-Atlantic Center for Pain Medicine, Presbyterian-Orthopaedic Hospital, Charlotte, North Carolina

Ronald J. Kulich, Ph.D.
Assistant Professor of Anesthesia, Tufts University School of Medicine, Boston; Clinical Director, New England Medical Center Pain Management Program, Boston; Clinical Instructor, Tufts University Dental School, Boston

Margaret Layden, P.T.
Physical Therapist, Department of Physical Therapy, Mid-Atlantic Center for Pain Medicine, Presbyterian-Orthopaedic Hospital, Charlotte, North Carolina

Raymond Maciewicz, M.D., Ph.D., F.A.B.P.M.
Associate Professor of Dentistry and Medical Director, Gelb Craniomandibular Pain Center, Tufts University Dental School, Boston

Theresa Hoskins Michel, M.S., P.T., C.C.S.
Assistant Professor of Physical Therapy, Post-Professional Program in Physical Therapy, MGH Institute of Health Professions, Boston; Physical Therapy Clinical Associate, Physical Therapy Services, Massachusetts General Hospital, Boston

Andrew W. Sukiennik, M.D.
Assistant Professor of Anesthesiology, Tufts University School of Medicine, Boston; Director, New England Medical Center Pain Management Program, Boston

Alan Witkower, Ed.D.
Clinical Instructor in Psychology (Psychiatry), Harvard Medical School, Boston; Assistant Director of Outpatient Pain Services, Spaulding Neighborhood Rehabilitation Center, Medford, Massachusetts

Harriët Wittink, M.S., P.T., O.C.S.
Clinical Instructor in Anesthesia/Pain Management, Tufts University School of Medicine, Boston; Clinical Specialist, New England Medical Center Pain Management Program, Boston

Melissa Wolff, M.S., P.T., A.T.C.
Adjunct Faculty, Health Programs Department, Walters State Community College, Morristown, Tennessee; Senior Physical Therapist, Department of Rehabilitation Services, University of Tennessee Medical Center at Knoxville

Foreword

Chronic pain exacts an economic toll of tens of billions of dollars a year in the United States alone and a human toll of suffering that cannot be calculated. Specialists who practice pain management on a daily basis believe it obvious that patients with chronic pain have universally developed secondary problems due to disuse, asymmetries, and muscle imbalances. Most commonly, chronic pain patients become deconditioned while enduring their chronic pain problem, regardless of its specific pathology. This deconditioning can take the form not simply of loss of muscle mass and strength but also of reduced flexibility, range of motion, and functional capacity. These losses may lead to new patterns of pain, which has been evident since the earliest origins of recorded medical practice. The ancient Greeks placed great emphasis on physical means to restore patients to full health and had a highly developed practice to achieve this end. Even earlier, a variety of medicinals were used and supplemented by nondrug therapies such as immobilization, counterstimulation, and acupuncture or its primitive equivalent, therapeutic tattooing. Today, the International Association for the Study of Pain (IASP) has endorsed a multidisciplinary approach to chronic pain. This approach, by definition, involves not only medical therapy or injections but also the use of behavioral and physical modalities. No facility may term itself a comprehensive, multidisciplinary pain management center in the absence of on-site expertise in physical therapy or rehabilitation. The IASP, which recommends worldwide standards for pain management facilities, reached this position based on current international consensus among a select group of experts in pain management.

The IASP Task Force on Professional Education has published a core curriculum for professional education in pain, the second edition of which became available in 1995. The recommendations made by this erudite group of pain professionals have been followed by the editors of this book, making it the first volume for physical therapists to help meet the needs of a comprehensive pain curriculum.

Chronic Pain Management for Physical Therapists reflects state-of-the-art, current-day practice. It is a particular pleasure for me to note that its multi-disciplinary authorship is uniquely Bostonian in character, chiefly derived from the New England Medical Center and Massachusetts General Hospital; the MGH Institute of Health Professions, which seeks to educate leaders in the fields of physical therapy, nursing, and communications disorders; and affiliated medical schools—the Tufts University School of Medicine and Harvard Medical School. Most of the authors have at one time or another worked in the multidisciplinary functional restoration of individual patients under their shared collaborative management. This volume therefore speaks eloquently of the importance of shared goals and a collaborative spirit to the success of any pain management program. Because of these shared goals and the importance—recognized for more than 2,000 years—of physical therapy and rehabilitation of patients with pain, I believe that this volume warrants a place on the bookshelves not only of physical therapists but also of physicians and other allied health professionals who frequently manage patients with chronic pain.

Amid an ongoing profusion of books on all aspects of pain assessment and management, this volume stands out as truly innovative. This is the first book to cover, comprehensively, the complex topic of chronic pain management from the physical therapist's point of view. As such, it will immediately fill a void as a textbook for the education of physical therapists dealing with this increasingly important problem. By studying this book, particularly the chapters on functional status and physical therapy, health professionals who are not also physical therapists will learn much. Ultimately, all patients will benefit.

Daniel B. Carr, M.D.

Preface

This book was written for students in physical therapy; their teachers; and practicing physical therapists, physical therapy assistants, and other health care providers interested in the role of physical therapy in the management of patients with chronic pain.

Although pain management has been a specialty for a number of health care providers for many years, the same is not true for physical therapists, as judged by the absence of American Physical Therapy Association board certification in pain management and the under-representation of physical therapists in professional pain organizations. Few physical therapy curricula offer instruction in pain management, despite the fact that our patients' most common complaint is pain.

Fortunately, more physical therapists are joining professional pain organizations. The International Association for the Study of Pain (IASP) reports that their physical therapy membership has increased from 70 members in 1994 to 124 members in 1995 worldwide (IASP Bulletin 1995).* This growing membership indicates an increasing interest and participation of physical therapists in the pain field.

The IASP published a proposed pain curriculum for students in occupational therapy or physical therapy in 1994 (see Appendix I). We strove to include most of the components of that course outline in this book, and it is our hope that pain management courses will be an integral part of physical therapy education in the future.

This book has been an experience in friendship and collaboration among very dedicated workers in the field of pain management. Without their sacrifice and generosity, we could never have made such a complete effort to cover the guidelines of the IASP. We sincerely thank all of our contributors as well as our colleagues and coworkers who contributed in meaningful, but less tangible ways. To our patients, who challenge, stimulate, and therefore teach us, we want to express gratitude.

*IASP Bulletin Jan/Feb 1995.

We owe an enormous debt of gratitude to our friends and colleagues in the pain field. To Ray Maciewicz and Judith Spross, who got us there in the first place; Heinrich Wurm, who had the vision for our interdisciplinary pain program; Ron Kulich, Andrew Sukiennik, and Dan Carr, who are team members and friends, and with whom working is a daily pleasure; Alan Witkower, who keeps us sane; Lisa Cohen and Deborah Rochman, who share our passion for the rehabilitation of pain patients; Martin Acquadro, Suzanne LaCrosse, Gerry Aronoff, Alyssa LeBel, Jim Rainville, David Keith, Steve Scrivani, Salah Salman, Noshir Mehta and his staff; and all of the others who have taught us what we know and made us feel part of a family, thank you!

H.W.
T.H.M.

1   Chronic Pain Concepts and Definitions

Melissa Wolff, Harriët Wittink,
and Theresa Hoskins Michel

A person with chronic pain is referred to you. You cringe. You have the sinking feeling that the patient will challenge, drain, frustrate, and perhaps anger you. You wish the patient would go somewhere else. Perhaps you could refer him or her to the pain clinic down the street. You wonder how therapists there can work with patients with chronic pain, and you wish for the hundredth time that chronic pain patients would not come to you. Does this sound familiar? We all have treated patients with chronic pain, and we know that the usual approaches will probably be unsuccessful. This book is written with the understanding that information about pain is increasing and changing on a daily basis, and it aims to ease tension, decrease anxiety, and give the reader information and techniques to provide effective care for patients with chronic pain.

Think about different pain experiences you may have had—a toothache, headache, fracture, or surgery. How would you describe the pain to an empathetic listener? Is your throat scratchy, burning, or tight? Is your fracture site throbbing, aching, or torturously painful? How do you know your listener really understands what it means to you to have this pain? Does your listener know you missed your child's performance at school because of the surgery? Is your listener aware that this is the fourth time you have had debilitating headache in 4 months and that you are worried about keeping your job?

Consider other types of pain. You argue with your parents. You slam down the phone and are angry and hurt. Your stomach is in knots, and you have a headache. Are you in pain? You certainly are. You attend the funeral of a friend. You feel empty and sad. Would you describe the experience as painful? You probably would.

Pain involves both sensation and emotion. Physical pains are linked with emotional responses, and emotional pains are linked with physical responses. Chronic pain involves a complex interconnection of multiple factors that we explore in this chapter and book. It is important to recognize that tissue damage is not the only source of pain and that it is impossible to separate the functions of the mind and the body when treating pain. No two people will describe pain in the same way or have exactly the same pain experience.

Models of Pain

Multicomponent views of pain are a recent development. Before the 1960s, the mind and body were seen as distinctly separate. Descartes envisioned the human organism as being divided into the mind and body. He considered the nerves to be tubes that connected the brain to the nerve endings in the skin and other tissues. This was known as the *specificity theory*. Pain was considered a reflex response to a physical stimulus (Descartes 1644). If the stimulus was known, the pain was predictable and explainable. Using this paradigm, cutting the pathway for pain should eliminate the pain. This model did not explain phenomena such as phantom pain and recurrent pain after nerve resection, however. This traditional biomedical model assumed that all pain was a symptom of an underlying cause. Once the cause was found and fixed, the patient should be relieved of pain. If the cause of pain was not found, the patient was thought to be lying or crazy. Unfortunately, these beliefs often still influence treatment for those with intractable pain.

The Gate-Control Theory

In 1965, Melzack and Wall published a new theory on pain mechanisms called the gate-control theory (Melzack and Wall 1965). They proposed that noxious stimuli reaching the spinal cord could be suppressed by non-noxious information converging on the same level. These non-noxious stimuli could come from the periphery or descend from the brain and close the gate to the noxious stimuli. This theory meant that pain would no longer be regarded as merely a physical sensation from a noxious stimulus. The experience of pain could be modulated consciously by mental, emotional, and sensory mechanisms. Physical therapists rely heavily on this theory when trying to decrease pain. Applying modalities such as transcutaneous electrical nerve stimulation, performing a massage, engaging the patient in conversation as a distraction, and educating the patient about his or her condition are ways that the gate-control theory is used.

Biopsychosocial Models

The gate-control theory formed the physiologic basis of the biopsychosocial model of medicine. The biopsychosocial model views pain as an interaction of biological, psychological, and social phenomena. This model recognizes that the person who "reports pain and is observed to be suffering, or reports suffering is not imagining pain" (Fordyce 1995).

Nolan's Model
Nolan (1990) describes five different and linked components in the experience of pain: physiologic, perceptual, affective, cognitive, and behavioral

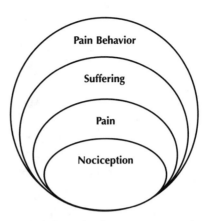

FIGURE 1.1 *A schematic diagram for the components of pain. Only pain behavior is measurable and observable. (Redrawn with permission from JD Loeser. Chronic Low Back Pain. New York: Raven, 1982;145.)*

components. The *physiologic* component that is the tissue source of the pain experience is known as *nociception* and is a result of an abnormality in the tissue. Much of physical therapy is directed at correcting the physiologic damage associated with pain. Chronic pain patients may not benefit from these techniques because the physiologic component is often not the major source of the pain experience.

The *perceptual* component of pain reflects the individual's perception of the quality, location, severity, and duration of the pain stimulus. This differs from the *affective* component, which is influenced by psychological factors. Positive and negative emotions such as fear, grief, anxiety, hostility, joy, relief, and relaxation will affect the overall pain experience and response to intervention. The *cognitive* component, which also can positively or negatively affect outcome, is based on what the patient knows and believes about his or her pain. These beliefs are influenced by culture, past personal experience, acquired knowledge, and the experiences of others with whom the individual is familiar. These influences all interact to complement rehabilitation efforts or obstruct them.

The *behavioral* component, which is the manner the patient expresses pain to others through communication and behavior, is a blend of the other components. It is expressed in the smiling face of a person recovering from successful cancer surgery or in the scowling face and slumped posture of a person suffering from headaches. The behavioral component is the part most immediately visible to the observer. It is influenced by a complex history unique to the individual.

Loeser's Model

A similar model of pain with four components was developed by Loeser (1982) and is outlined in Figure 1.1. The first component, *nociception*, is the detection of tissue damage, which activates a specific set of receptors in the A delta and C fiber range, with *pain* being the subsequent cognitive recognition of the nociceptive stimulus carried by the peripheral and central nervous

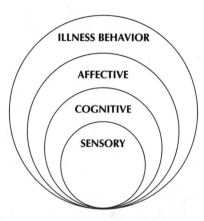

SOCIAL ENVIRONMENT

ILLNESS BEHAVIOR

AFFECTIVE

COGNITIVE

SENSORY

FIGURE 1.2   *A cross-sectional analysis of the clinical presentation and assessment of low back pain and disability in one point in time. (Reprinted from G Waddell, M Newton, I Henderson, et al. Fear-Avoidance Reliefs Questionnaire [FARQ] and the role of fear-avoidance beliefs in chronic low back pain and disability. Pain 1993;52:164 with kind permission of Elsevier Science—NL, Sara Burgerhartstraat 25, 1055 KV Amsterdam, The Netherlands.)*

system. *Suffering,* the second component, is the negative affective response brought about by pain, depression, fear, or other events in the patient's emotional life. As with the Nolan model above, the outward and comprehensive manifestation of the pain event is the *pain behavior* (Loeser and Egan 1989). Like other behaviors, it is influenced by cultural background and environmental consequences (Loeser and Fordyce 1983) and is communication or action by the patient that the observer interprets as suggesting nociception has occurred. Verbal and nonverbal behaviors such as taking medication, refusing to go to work, and going to doctors are all included in this category. Another common pain behavior is fear avoidance, which is the avoidance of activities because of fear of reinjury and physical harm.

The relationship between components is not fixed and can vary among individuals and stages of the patient's life. Consider the example of a finger fracture. The suffering for a concert pianist with this injury may be extreme, whereas a high school football player with the same injury may not suffer at all. The nociception is the same for both and the awareness of the pain may be similar, but the suffering and pain behaviors are likely to be extremely different.

Waddell's Model

Waddell expanded on Loeser's model to develop a model emphasizing illness rather than disease (Figure 1.2). The term *illness* refers to the internal, subjective experience of an individual who is aware that personal well-being has been jeopardized and to how that person perceives and responds to that experience. *Distress* is an emotional disturbance caused by stress and characterized by a variable combination of anxiety, increased bodily awareness, and depression (Waddell et al. 1984). Distress is largely secondary to the physical disorder (illness) and becomes better or worse, depending on the success or failure of treatment. Distress arising from unrelated causes may aggravate or perpetuate physical pain. *Illness behavior* can be assessed clinically as "observable and potentially measurable actions and conduct [that] express and communicate the individual's own perception of disturbed health," such as guarding, rubbing, sighing, and grimacing (Waddell et al. 1984). This is similar to the pain behavior described previously in Loeser's model. *Illness behavior* is defined as the lack of physical and social functioning, disrupting normal life.

Leventhal et al. (1980) developed a definition of illness behavior that focuses on the individual's perception and interpretation of his or her symptoms. They outlined the following four components: (1) the individual's awareness and labeling of sensations, (2) the individual's assumptions regarding the etiology of sensations, (3) the individual's anticipation of the consequences of the sensations, and (4) the individual's estimate of the duration of the symptoms.

The term *abnormal illness behavior* refers to inappropriate descriptions of symptoms and inappropriate responses to examination within the context of the clinical interview and examination. Symptoms and responses to examination may be inappropriate or nonorganic in the limited sense that they do not fit the usual clinical presentation of physical disease. These symptoms and responses have been shown to be statistically and clinically separable from the normally accepted symptoms and signs of physical disease and to be more closely related to affective and cognitive disturbances (Waddell et al. 1989).

The definition of *suffering* includes distress. Suffering is "distress brought about by the actual or perceived impending threat to the integrity or continued existence of the whole person" (Cassell 1991).

It is interesting to note that definitions of pain and suffering include mention of both actual and perceived events. Failure to attend to the suffering component may promote or prolong suffering itself (Cassell 1991).

Disablement Models

Disability, as defined by Nagi (1991), is a pattern of behavior that emerges over long periods of time during which the individual experiences functional limitations to such a degree that he or she cannot be overcome to create some semblance of "normal" role and task performance. This is the description of the *sick role*. People with chronic pain often present themselves in these sick roles with chronic illness behavior and chronic disability that is increasingly dissociated from the physical problem. There may be scant evidence of remaining nociceptive stimulus; however, the memory has been established, and emotional distress, depression, disease conviction, and adaptation to chronic pain and disability occurs. Chronic pain becomes a self-sustaining condition that is resistant to traditional medical management. Physical treatment directed at a hypothetical but unidentified and possibly nonexistent nociceptive source is not only unsuccessful, but also potentially damaging (Waddell 1987).

Physical therapists are familiar with the concepts of disease, impairment, functional limitations, and disability. The assumption is made that pathologic states lead to impairments, and impairments lead to functional limitations, which in turn lead to disabilities. This basic scheme is consistent in three major, published disablement models: the Nagi Scheme (1965); the International Classification of Impairments, Disabilities, and Handicaps (ICIDH) (Wood 1980), which adds the category of handicap after disability; and the National Advisory Board on Medical Rehabilitation Research (1992), which uses the term *societal limitation* instead of handicap.

These three major schemes are discussed and compared by Jette (1994). He emphasizes that the value to the clinician of describing restrictions in a patient's performance in terms of such schemes lies in the ability to identify the extent to which disabilities are a result of social and physical environmental factors, instead of factors within the individual. Some performance problems seen in patients with chronic pain may be best managed by environmental modifications rather than hands-on therapy. Jette provides the example of a rigid work environment, which can be a barrier that increases disablement in a patient. Working with employers to help patients may improve the productivity of certain patients with chronic pain. The basic definitions of these schemes based on the ICIDH model are as follows (Cole and Edgerton 1990):

> **Disease or disorder** "Something abnormal occurs within the individual; this may be present at birth or acquired later. A chain of causal circumstances, the 'etiology,' gives rise to changes in the structure or function of the body, the 'pathology.' Pathologic changes may or may not make themselves evident; when they do they are described as 'symptoms and signs.' These features are the components of the medical model of disease."
>
> **Impairment** "An abnormality of structure, function, or both at the organ level. At this stage of the model, an affected individual becomes aware of the pathology or, in behavioral terms, becomes aware that he or she is unhealthy. Subclasses of impairment include disfigurement and intellectual, psychological, language, aural, visceral, skeletal, and sensory abnormalities."
>
> **Disability** "Restriction or lack of ability to perform an activity in a manner considered normal, a disability is a disturbance manifested in the performance of daily tasks. Disabilities are the functional consequences of impairments. Principal subclasses of disabilities are concerned with behavior, communication, personal care, locomotion, body disposition, dexterity, and particular skills."
>
> **Handicap** "A disadvantage resulting from an impairment or a disability, a handicap limits or prevents the fulfillment of a role that is normal (depending on age, sex, and social and cultural factors) for the affected individual. Handicaps largely reflect societal attitudes toward people with disabilities and impairments. Handicaps include physical dependency, lack of mobility, and economic dependency."

Nagi (1991) recognized a need for a concept that bridged the presence of an impairment and an individual's disability. He therefore proposed the concept of functional limitation, in which the process of disease leads to impairment, and constructed the following model:

active pathology → impairment → functional limitation → disability

In Nagi's model, *impairment* is a loss or abnormality of an anatomic, physiologic, mental or emotional nature. *Functional limitation* includes impairments set on the individual's ability to perform the task and obligations of his or her usual roles and normal daily activities. These include roles within the family, peer group, community, work and other interaction settings as well as activities involved in self-care. Whereas *impairment* refers to the tissues, organs, and systems, *functional limitation* refers to the whole person. Not all impairments lead to functional limitation or directly to disability (e.g., shoulder trauma [pathology] that leads to shoulder pain [impairment] can result in difficulty reaching overhead [functional limitation], which is disabling for a school teacher who needs to write on a blackboard but not for a typist whose work does not include overhead reaching). *Disability* is defined as patterns of behavior that emerge over long periods of time during which an individual experiences functional limitations to such a degree that he or she cannot create some semblance of "normal" overall role performance or to such a degree that an individual's overall behavior is less than adequate to meet the expectations normal for one's age and sex as well as one's social and cultural environment. It refers to social rather than organismic functioning.

Nagi recognized that disability also includes the individual's definition of the situation and reactions and the definition of the situation by others and their reactions and expectations (family, friends, associates, employers and organizations and professions that provide services and benefits). According to Nagi, this model is most appropriate for injuries and diseases that have identifiable onsets and for those that have stable residuals—this model may not be suitable for chronic illnesses. Although implied, the model does not account well for the behavioral response of patients to their impairments and for the consequences of their behavioral responses having an impact on impairments, physical functioning, and disability. A person's response to an impairment may be more disabling than the impairment itself. Disability may be related more to patient beliefs and fears than to actual inability to perform socially accepted roles.

The model seemingly assumes a linear relationship between these domains. From the perspective of a disease model, chronic pain dysfunction appears to be a disparate set of signs and symptoms, many of them (e.g., sleep disturbance, depression, and psychosocial disability) not pathognomonic to a particular disease (Dworkin et al. 1992). Unfortunately, based on this model, many physical therapists continue to believe that treating pain will result in increased physical functioning and decreased disability. This may be true for some patient groups, but it does not fit the chronic pain population. A poor correlation exists between subjective pain ratings and the patient's ability to perform functional activities (Waddell 1987, Rainville et al. 1992). Waddell et al. (1984) showed, for instance, that the amount of treatment received by patients with back pain was more influenced by their distress and illness behavior than by the actual physical disease.

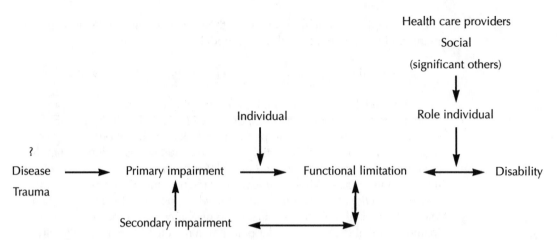

FIGURE 1.3   *Wittink's proposed integration of Nagi's (1991) disablement model and biopsychosocial models of pain (unpublished data 1996).*

Wittink (unpublished data 1996) attempted to integrate the disablement model proposed by Nagi with the biopsychosocial models previously described with the goals of maintaining a conceptual model (Nagi 1991) widely used within the physical therapy community and adapting it to models existing in pain management (Figure 1.3).

In Wittink's pain model, disease (e.g., diabetes), trauma (e.g., work-related injuries), and unknown factors (e.g., fibromyalgia) can lead to pain, which becomes a primary impairment of the individual.

Wittink's pain model includes the following elements:

Primary impairment   A loss or abnormality of an anatomic, physiologic, mental, or emotional nature as a *direct* result of disease, trauma, or unknown factors of which a dominant symptom is pain.

Individual response   The patient's response to the primary impairment(s) that results from the patient's belief system (cultural background, religion, age, race, sex, childhood experiences, etc.) and influences subsequent behaviors. These behaviors are collectively called "illness behavior." Fear of pain (Vlaeyen et al. 1995), fear-avoidance behavior (Fordyce et al. 1981, Waddell et al. 1993), and fear of movement/(re)injury (Vlaeyen et al. 1995) are illness behaviors and can lead to functional limitations and secondary impairments.

Functional limitation   See definition by Nagi (1991).

Secondary impairments   Impairments caused by the patient's response to pain. Long-lasting avoidance of activities has detrimental consequences both physically (loss of range of motion, aerobic fitness, muscle strength, and endurance) and psychologically (see Chapter 9). Secondary impairments may further limit the patient's ability to function and may contribute to the pain experience. An ongoing cycle may develop increasing patient distress and suffering. Secondary impairments are common in chronic pain syndrome patients.

Role individual   The patient's belief system as it pertains to role performance; this belief system includes family, work and social roles. This belief system is influenced by significant others, social factors, and health care providers, all of whom may reinforce or decrease illness behaviors, functional limitation and disability by how they respond to the patient.

Significant others   Partners, friends, and the patient's children, who do not respond to the pain the patient *feels*, but to how the patient *expresses* himself or herself. They respond to the patient's illness behavior and inability to "do things"—that is, to functional limitations and disability.

Social influences   Outside factors over which the patient may not have control, such as environmental and occupational factors, employer attitudes, and litigation. One factor is fear of work-related activities (Waddell et al. 1993, Vlaeyen et al. 1995).

Health care providers   All health care providers the patient comes in contact with (e.g., physicians, physical and occupational therapists, chiropractors, osteopaths). Recommendations by health care providers can have a powerful influence on patient functional limitation and disability. Catchlove and Cohen (1982) state that not insisting on a return to work acknowledges the patient's view of himself or herself as "regressed, dependent, and incapable." Patients demonstrated a better return-to-work rate when they were instructed to do so either during or after treatment compared with a control group for whom return to work was not a component of therapy.

Disability   See definition by Nagi (1991).

This model is consistent with evaluation and treatment approaches used by physical therapists who specialize in pain management. Evaluation includes, aside from physical assessment, an assessment of the patient's illness behavior; fear of pain and movement, functional limitations, and disability. In cooperation with the psychologist, the physical therapist can formulate a good sense of the patient's belief systems, which helps direct treatment. Included in treatment are behavioral methods, such as decreasing fear of injury and physical activity by quota-based progressive exercise programs, education on hurt versus harm, performance-contingent rewards, as well as setting of functional goals. Models of pain treatment are further discussed in Chapter 12.

Definitions and Classifications of Pain

The various models of pain provide a basis for understanding of chronic pain. They reinforce that pain is a complex, subjective, perceptual phenomenon with uniquely personal dimensions. McCaffery and Beebe (1989) defined pain as "whatever the experiencing person says it is, existing whenever he says it does." The consensus definition of pain developed by the International Association for the Study of Pain is "an unpleasant sensory *and* emotional experience associated with actual *or* potential tissue damage, *or* described in terms of such damage" (Merskey and Bogduk 1994). Both of these definitions emphasize that pain does not have to be seen on an x-ray, by magnetic resonance imaging (MRI), or in lab tests to be considered a true experience of pain.

Other terms that are useful in understanding chronic pain are the following:

Allodynia Condition in which a normally nonpainful stimulus is perceived as painful

Hyperalgesia Increased perceived intensity of a "normally" painful stimulus

Hypoalgesia Decreased response to a normally painful stimulus

Central pain (pain located in the central nervous system) and neuropathic pain (pain due to disease or injury to the nerve) are types of pain initiated or caused by a lesion or dysfunction in the nervous system. An example of central pain is pain from a thalamic infarct. Possible causes of neuropathic pain are traction on a nerve, ischemia, and sympathetic dysfunction. Summation, or progressive aggregation of perceived pain with repeated application of an identical stimulus, is typical in neuropathic pain patients (Fields 1991).

Two terms that are key in understanding the experience of chronic pain patients are *pain threshold* and *pain tolerance*. Pain threshold refers to the lowest level at which a stimulus is recognized as painful by the person experiencing the stimulus (Merskey and Bogduk 1994). The pain threshold seems to be more dependent on physiologic factors than pain tolerance (Merskey and Spear 1967). Pain tolerance, however, has a wider variation and is influenced by the individual's personality, belief system, and past painful experiences. It is the greatest level of pain a person is prepared to endure (Merskey and Bogduk 1994). Pain tolerance varies greatly among individuals and within a person. On days that are already frustrating, an irritation that may seem minor on other days can become a major disturbance. Pain threshold may vary only slightly in an individual, whereas pain tolerance can change significantly within one person from situation to situation.

Pain is also divided into the categories of chronic and acute pain (Table 1.1). Some individuals experience pain that does not fit into either of these categories perfectly, however. Further distinctions between the various pain states include acute, subacute, recurrent acute, ongoing acute, chronic, and chronic pain syndrome (Crue and Pinsky, 1984). The distinguishing characteristics of these pain states are summarized in Table 1.2.

Additional Information on Chronic Pain—Differentiating Between Chronic Pain and Chronic Pain Syndrome Patients

Understanding these different types of chronic pain requires a comprehensive understanding of pain mechanisms. The physiologic basis of peripheral and central pain are described in detail in Chapter 2. At a basic level, chronic pain is a phenomenon of the central nervous system. Whether it is

TABLE 1.1   Major differences between the two categories of pain

Acute pain	Chronic pain
1. Pain is a symptom	1. Pain is a disease
2. Well-defined time of onset	2. Ill-defined time of onset
3. Pathology is often identifiable	3. Pathology often unidentifiable
4. Objective signs of autonomic activity	4. Absent or adapted autonomic nervous system activity
5. Response to tissue injury	5. Response to peripheral and/or central changes in somatosensory pathways
6. Has a biological function	6. Unknown biological function
7. Often relieved by treatment directed at pain	7. Does not respond to treatment directed at pain
8. Usually responsive to medication	8. Less responsive to medication
9. Associated with anxiety	9. Associated with depression, hopelessness, weight loss, libido loss, disturbances, helplessness
10. Primarily involves the individual	10. Involves the individual, family, social network, lifestyle
11. Works well in the medical model	11. Does not work well in the medical model

SOURCE: Adapted from MS Wolff. Chronic Pain—Assessment of Physical Therapists' Knowledge and Attitudes. Boston: Massachusetts General Hospital Institute of Health Professions, 1989. Thesis.

an increase in sympathetic receptor activity (Perl 1993), pain caused by a primary lesion or dysfunction in the central or peripheral nervous system (Merskey and Bogduk 1994), or distortion of non-noxious peripheral input (Crue and Pinsky 1984), chronic pain often is not amenable to standard therapeutic modalities and rehabilitation efforts. This is why physical therapists find successful treatment for chronic pain to be so elusive.

Pain that persists beyond presumed nociceptive input associated with normal tissue healing time can be considered chronic. In chronic pain, the sympathetic and neuroendocrine responses characteristic of acute pain become habituated so that the central nervous system becomes accustomed to the idea of being in pain. It is almost as if the brain develops a memory for pain, much like the skill of learning to ride a bicycle is never unlearned. The same may be true of chronic pain. A pattern is established in the central nervous system of a person with chronic pain that is difficult, if not impossible, to erase; therefore, the person persists in the belief that pain is present.

In chronic pain and chronic pain syndrome, it becomes less clear what the underlying physical disorder is. There may indeed be very little objective evidence of any remaining nociceptive stimulus. Even if the cause of the pain is known, as is the case with painful peripheral neuropathy in diabetic, acquired immunodeficiency syndrome (AIDS), or multiple sclerosis patients, to date no treatment is available to cure the pain. It is helpful to

TABLE 1.2   Distinguishing characteristics of acute and chronic pain states

Pain state	Characteristic
Acute pain (e.g., pain resulting from fractures, ruptures, avulsions, blockages, burns, etc.)	Up to a few days' duration Mild or severe Cause known or unknown Presumed nociceptive input
Subacute pain (e.g., postoperative pain, postfracture pain)	A few days' to a few months' duration
Recurrent acute pain (e.g., pain from sickle cell crises, rheumatoid arthritis, migraines)	Recurrent nociceptive input from underlying chronic pathologic process
Ongoing acute pain (e.g., pain from uncontrolled malignant neoplastic disease)	Continued nociceptive input
Chronic pain (e.g., sympathetically maintained pain, intractable low back pain, headache)	Non-neoplastic Usually more than 6 months' duration No known nociceptive input Pain often made more severe by any type of subsequent sensory input Seemingly adequate adaptation to functioning in the life process by the patient
Chronic pain syndrome (e.g., sympathetically maintained pain, intractable low back pain, headache)	Chronic pain(s) with poor adaptation to the life process by the patients Pain becomes the central focus of the patient's existence

SOURCE: Adapted from BL Crue, JJ Pinsky. An approach to chronic pain of non-malignant origin. Postgrad Med J 1984;60:858.

think in terms of functional impairment when deciding how to approach treatment. This will help differentiate between chronic pain and chronic pain syndrome patients.

Chronic Pain Patients

Chronic pain patients tend to function despite their pain. They often work and fulfill their social roles. Their quality of life may be impaired due to their pain, and they may not function at the level they wish to; however, they do not regard their pain as disabling. In these patients, the relationship between pain, tissue damage, and the degree of functional impairment is proportional. Abnormal illness behavior is usually not present.

Case Example
The patient is a 35-year-old woman complaining of chronic headaches that have been ongoing for a year. Her headaches are present in the morning and increase in intensity through the day. She works full-time as

a secretary, which involves much work at a computer, and has a part-time job as a security guard at night. She is married and has two children, ages 10 and 8. Household duties are shared with her husband. She believes her headaches interfere with her concentration at work. She also feels more tired and has had difficulty with her second job. At night, she has trouble falling asleep due to the pain in her head and neck.

On examination, she presents with forward head and poor posture. She has normal cervical range of motion (ROM), normal upper extremity strength, reflexes, and sensation. Her pectoralis, sternocleidomastoid, and suboccipital muscles are short, and her cervical extensors, neck flexors, serratus, and middle and lower trapezius are weak. Palpation of her suboccipital muscles reproduced her headache, as did testing of C0–C1 and C1–C2 joint mobility, which was limited. In this case, the patient had chronic pain, but a relationship could be established between her pain and objective findings.

Therapy is directed at restoring normal muscle balance, cervical joint mobility and posture. This resulted in decreased intensity, frequency, and duration of her headaches and improved sleep and job performance.

Case Example
The patient is a 62-year-old female with nonpulmonary sarcoidosis. She complains of severe bilateral lower leg pain. She is retired and performs all her household duties, but at a slower rate than she previously did. She cooks and shops independently and maintains a productive social life with her husband, children, and grandchildren. On examination, she presents with 0/5 strength of her foot dorsiflexors and a slight plantar flexion contracture of both ankles. Hamstrings and gastrocnemius length are significantly decreased. Her gait is abnormal, with short step length and absent knee flexion.

A light touch to her lower legs provokes an unpleasant tingling sensation. Knee and ankle jerks are absent bilaterally. She is diagnosed with painful peripheral neuropathy due to her sarcoidosis. She has an abnormal gait due to bilateral footdrop, causing myofascial pain in addition to her painful peripheral neuropathy.

In this case, the patient has a progressive disease for which there is no cure. Medications are marginally helpful. She has impairments that could be addressed, however. Ankle-foot orthoses for her footdrop help her walk better and, in combination with stretching her tight muscles, eliminate her myofascial pain.

Case Example
The patient is a 50-year-old male who injured his wrist while skiing. Four months later, he had a surgical lunotriquetral arthrodesis and immediately developed unrelenting pain in his hand. His fingers were swollen, discolored, and painful when touched. He rigorously performed his ROM exercises, and though he regained use of his fingers and wrist, pain persisted with use and light touch. Eight weeks after surgery, he was seen by an anesthesiologist for a course of stellate ganglion blocks (see Chapter 10). This was combined with ongoing ROM and strengthening exercises. The

blocks were successful in reducing tactile pain and vascular symptoms. The patient pursued his exercise program and resumed his premorbid activity level.

Chronic Pain Syndrome Patients

Chronic pain syndrome is a complex, multidimensional problem. The Office of Disabilities of the Social Security Administration uses the following criteria to establish a diagnosis of chronic pain syndrome: (1) intractable pain of more than 6 months' duration; (2) marked alteration in behavior with depression or anxiety; (3) marked restriction in daily activities; (4) excessive use of medication and frequent use of medical services; (5) no clear relationship to organic disorder; and (6) history of multiple, nonproductive tests, treatment, and surgeries (Kulich and Baker, in press).

In the chronic pain syndrome patient, chronic pain, chronic disability, and chronic illness behavior become increasingly dissociated from the initial physical problem. Instead, chronic pain and disability are associated more with emotional distress, depression, disease conviction, and adaptation to chronic invalidity (Waddell 1987). This process is discussed further in Chapter 11. In chronic pain syndrome patients, there is no clear relationship between pain and tissue damage and the degree of functional impairment (Vaseduvan 1992, Waddell et al. 1992, Waddell et al. 1993, Rainville et al. 1992). Waddell et al. (1992) showed that severity of pain accounted for only 10% of the variance of physical impairment and disability, and Main and Waddell (1991) showed that a larger proportion of the variance in disability in activities of daily living could be explained better by examining a combination of severity of pain, psychological distress, and illness behavior than by severity of pain alone.

Chronic pain syndrome patients have low activity levels compared with their prepain levels and those of normal controls. Patients are often instructed by their health care providers to "stop when it hurts" or to "let pain be your guide" and thus limit their activity levels. These low activity levels, however, are not always associated with significant physical limitations or with reduction in chronic pain. Patients have often tried to resume normal activity, only to experience an increase in their pain. Fear of pain plays a central role in the lives of chronic pain syndrome patients. They learn to anticipate the painful consequences of engaging in activity and avoid these activities, as they are afraid they will harm themselves by becoming more active. This fear-avoidance behavior (Fordyce et al. 1981) results in a downward spiral of further limitation of activity and increased deconditioning. Vlaeyen et al. (1995) have written about and studied a cognitive-behavioral model of fear of movement/(re)injury (Figure 1.4). This model incorporates a biological component (physical injury), a psychological component (cognitive processes), and a social component (disability).

Pain behavior, such as limping, grimacing, restricting movement, and avoidance of physical activities, also contributes to impairments and functional limitations independent of the initial physical problem. These behaviors persist when they are rewarded in some manner by increased attention

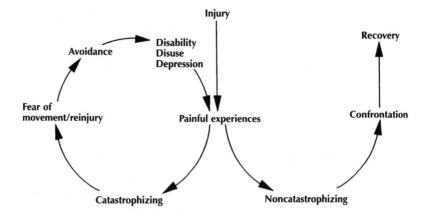

FIGURE 1.4   *Cognitive-behavioral model of fear of movement/(re)injury. (Reprinted from J Vlaeyen, A Kale-Snijders, R Boeven, H van Eek. Fear of movement/(re)injury in chronic low back pain and its relation to behavioral performance. Pain 1995;62:368 with kind permission of Elsevier Science—NL, Sara Burgerhartstraat 25, 1055 KV Amsterdam, The Netherlands.)*

from friends or family, reinforcement from health care providers, or avoidance of disliked activities such as work.

Case Example

The patient is a 54-year-old woman who injured her back 10 months ago while performing a heavy lift at work. X-rays and MRI of her back are negative for pathology. She reports that "everything" makes her back pain worse and that there is nothing she can do to ease her pain. She is unable to lift, carry, bend, walk more than 15 minutes, or sit longer than 10 minutes without significant increase in her pain. She is most comfortable lying down. Her total down time (time sleeping and lying down) is 21 hours per day. Her husband and children perform the housework and the grocery shopping. She occasionally cooks but finds it nearly impossible to stand for the length of time required. She frequently shifts position during the interview, occasionally standing up and rubbing her back. The interview is punctuated with tearful statements such as "I really try, but I can't do it. Nothing has meaning for me. I used to be so healthy, if I have to live like this, I'd rather die."

On physical examination, she is able to bend forward 10%. All other movements are reported to be painful and are restricted by 75%. Hip ROM is painful in all directions and flexion is limited to 70 degrees due to pain. Manual muscle test of the lower extremities is 4/5 throughout. Straight-leg raising tests are negative, and sensation and reflexes are normal. She has no palpable spasm of the back muscles.

Obviously, this patient is overwhelmed by her pain and believes she has no control over it or over her ability to function. Although she has many impairments, none of them indicates an identifiable physical problem or source of pain. She is more likely to be experiencing secondary conditions generated by her abnormal illness behavior. She is treated with a functional restoration program (see Chapter 6) with cognitive behavioral therapy (see Chapter 9) and eventually is able to return to work and resume her role within the family.

Some patients have features of chronic pain syndrome despite their apparent lack of disability and illness, as shown in the following case:

Case Example

The patient is a 35-year-old male complaining of neck, right shoulder, back, and bilateral hip pain. He also complains of numbness bilaterally in his legs when he lies down and occasional numbness in his entire right arm. Pain onset occurred 2 years ago after a motor vehicle accident in which his vehicle was rear-ended. X-ray and MRI findings were normal. Electromyogram findings of both upper and lower extremities were normal. Computed tomography findings of his brain were normal. He had three separate courses of physical therapy in the past 2 years, including ice, ultrasound, stretching, and Nautilus exercise. He reports being mostly pain-free after these treatments but is unable to continue exercising on his own. He has experienced increased pain in the past 2 weeks. He works full-time, owns his own business, and spends most of his working hours driving his car. He is married and has seven children. He is able to do almost everything despite his pain, with the exception of house maintenance and yard work. He strongly desires to be pain free and is unsatisfied with the advice of the neurosurgeon who told him to "live with the pain." He reports feelings of helplessness, hopelessness, anxiety, and difficulty sleeping. He is afraid he will become wheelchair-bound because of his pain and will be unable to take care of his family.

Physical examination reveals normal ROM of his lumbar and cervical spine and normal strength, sensation, and reflexes in his upper and lower extremities. He has myofascial tenderness in his neck and shoulders. His intervertebral motion of the cervical and lumbar spine is normal. Nerve tension tests are negative.

This patient appears to be functioning well, has no objective signs, and yet continues to catastrophize about his pain. He feels unable to control his pain and is somatically focused. He is referred to behavioral medicine and an independent health club exercise program and is given instructions in independent pain management techniques.

The pain behavior of chronic pain syndrome patients is sometimes confused with *malingering*. Malingering is the conscious and purposeful faking of a symptom such as pain for some gain, usually financial (Turk et al. 1983). It is important to realize that true malingering is very rare, probably occurring in less than 5% of patients (Leavitt and Sweet 1986). When the physical therapist understands the concepts of central nervous system changes and the integration of emotional, cultural, social, and psychological factors in the production of pain, it is evident how difficult it is to willfully fake pain.

When in doubt about malingering, the physical therapist should err in favor of the patient.

Social, Cultural, and Psychological Aspects of Pain

It is important to emphasize that the way a person experiences pain is a function of the interrelationship between his or her sociocultural, psychological, and physiologic conditions. Sociocultural factors are those that relate to group interactions in the family, workplace, and community. Cultural factors pertain to beliefs, values, and customs that are transmitted from one generation to another (Jacox 1977). Psychological factors are those that relate to the mental processes of the individual, including personality characteristics, emotional states, and cognitive processes.

Social Aspects of Pain

Social factors may influence the emotional and cognitive states of the individual, making them more vulnerable to illness and pain. Retrospective and prospective large-scale studies demonstrate a high incidence of lower back pain in blue-collar workers (De Girolamo 1991, Masset and Malchaire 1994). Their work is physically demanding, and they tend to be in subordinate positions and dissatisfied with their jobs (Westrin et al. 1972). Job dissatisfaction is a significant risk factor for the onset of lower back pain (Bigos et al. 1991, Skovron et al. 1994). Industrial injury claims for back injuries have risen steadily since 1981 and comprise nearly 32% of total claims in the United States (Hager 1995). Migraine prevalence is also higher in the lower socioeconomic groups and may be a circumstance associated with low income, such as poor diet, poor medical care, or stress (Silberstein and Lipton 1996).

The 1989 National Health interview study (Lipton et al. 1993) provided evidence that gender differences exist in orofacial pain. Although the prevalence of back pain is slightly correlated with age or sex in the adult population, temporomandibular joint (TMJ) pain and headache have a lower prevalence after the age of 65 and a higher prevalence among females (Von Korff et al. 1988).

Cultural Aspects of Pain

Cultural background has an effect on pain perception. For instance, Hardy et al. (1952) found that radiant heat, described by Jewish and Italian people as painful, was described as warm by Northern Europeans. Zborowski (1952) described open complaining and support seeking by Jewish and Italian people, but the underlying attitudes about pain of the two groups were different. Jewish people were more concerned about the cause and meaning of the pain, whereas Italian people were concerned with obtaining immediate relief. Zola (1966) found that Irish and Italian people differed significantly in their perception of pain. Italians complained of more symptoms in more parts of the body with greater degrees of bodily dysfunction. Furthermore,

Italians were most concerned if the symptoms interfered with their social lives, whereas Irish and Anglo-Saxon people were most concerned if their pain interfered with work. Zola noted that Irish people handle their trouble by denial, whereas Italian people handle trouble by dramatization. These coping techniques are reflected in the way people of each culture communicate about their illness. None of these studies should be interpreted as derogatory toward a certain culture. Instead, they are attempts to describe characteristic differences in cultures without judging those characteristics.

Bates et al. (1993) investigated individuals from six different ethnic groups for reports of pain intensity. The individuals were similar in age, gender, income, and medical characteristics. The best predictors of pain intensity variations seemed to be ethnic group and locus of control (LOC) style. LOC is related to patients' beliefs about their sense of control over their pain. Patients with an internal LOC believe that they have a good deal of control over their pain, whereas those with an external LOC tend to believe that the health care provider can "fix" their problem and that they should relinquish control and responsibility to the doctor. Eighty percent of Hispanics in the study by Bates et al. were found to have an external LOC, whereas only 10% of Poles did. The Hispanic group reported the highest pain intensity, followed by Italians. The Polish group reported the lowest pain intensity.

Sanders et al. (1992) found important cross-cultural differences in self-perceived level of dysfunction among patients with chronic lower back pain. Sanders compared individuals from the United States, Japan, Mexico, Colombia, Italy, and New Zealand. Sanders found that lower back pain patients from Mexico and New Zealand had significantly fewer physical findings than other lower back pain groups did and that Americans were the most dysfunctional in psychosocial, recreational, and occupational areas.

These studies reinforce the principle that people with similar learning experiences (culture) are likely to show similar pain perception, expression, and response patterns. These culturally acquired patterns may influence the neurophysiologic processing of nociceptive information as well as the psychological, behavioral, and verbal responses to pain (Bates et al. 1993). Zborowski (1952) points out that any cultural differences do tend to disappear over time in cosmopolitan societies and that other factors, such as educational background and occupation, may have an effect on pain behavior (French 1994).

Psychological Aspects of Pain

The relationship between psychological status and the expression of pain is complex and poorly understood (Romano and Turner 1985). In a study of preschool children, Zuckerman et al. (1987) found the prevalence of recurrent headaches and abdominal pain in children whose mothers were psychologically distressed to be more than twice that in children whose mothers reported few psychological symptoms.

Dworkin et al. (1990) found that those reporting pain at two sites had a five-fold increase in the occurrence of major depression compared with those with no pain, and those with three or more pain sites an eight-fold increase in risk for major depression relative to those with no pain. Number of pain sites proved to be a stronger predictor of major depression risk than the severity or persistence of the pain condition. The prevalence of major depression in patients with chronic back pain is approximately three to four times greater than that reported in the general population (Sullivan et al. 1992). Depression is a common concomitant of all chronic pain (Romano and Turner 1985; Magni et al. 1993).

Anxiety, depression, and other psychological states can produce pain themselves and influence the intensity of pain from other causes. People who are anxious are more sensitive to pain than calm people (Kent 1986). The anticipation of pain and uncertainty regarding its cause tend to raise anxiety, which then increases perceived intensity of pain (Bond 1984). Patients' beliefs about pain and treatment and their perception of disability are powerful predictors of the level of functioning they will achieve. Patients who believe they can control their pain avoid catastrophizing, and those who believe they are not severely disabled show greater improvement (Shutty et al. 1990). Gottlieb (1986) presented findings that showed that dysfunctional beliefs about chronic pain (e.g., "I try not to do as much when I have pain") successfully discriminated 83% of positive versus negative treatment outcomes in an outpatient program. Similarly, Dolce (1987) reported that pain patients' ratings of their concern about engaging in various treatment activities (e.g., exercise) were negatively associated with treatment outcome in an inpatient program.

A study of chronic lower back pain patients found a complex interaction among the psychosocial factors of life adversity, coping, and social support (Klapow et al. 1995). Keefe and Dolan (1986) found that back pain patients exhibited higher levels of motor pain behaviors, were less active, and used more pain medications than TMJ pain patients. Both back pain and TMJ pain patients had high levels of psychological distress, but back pain patients were more likely to use attention diversion, praying, and hoping as coping strategies. Evaluation and treatment of patients' belief and coping systems is extraordinarily important in this population and is further discussed in Chapter 9.

Epidemiologic Scope of the Problem of Pain

Pain is a major health problem in the United States. In a 1987 study, Bonica estimated that approximately 30% of the population of economically developed countries suffered from chronic pain (Fordyce 1995). Fifty million Americans are partially or totally disabled for a few days or a few weeks by chronic pain (Fordyce 1995). Forty-five percent of all Americans seek care for persistent pain at some point in their lives (American Pain Society 1994). Back pain is the second leading symptomatic reason for visits to physician's offices in the United States (Cypress 1983). In 1993, 11.7 million individuals were impaired, and 5.3 million individuals were disabled due to lower back pain (Chan et al. 1993). Most studies have found that 70–90% of the total cost of lower back pain relates to those with either temporary or permanent disability (Frymoyer and Cats-Baril 1991; Webster and Snook 1994; Spitzer et al. 1987). In 1990, the direct and indirect cost of back pain was estimated

to be $75–100 billion (Frymoyer and Cats-Baril 1991). The greater the dura-
tion of disabling lower back pain, the greater the probability of permanent
disability (Waddell 1992). In the interval from the inception of the Social
Security disability income program in 1957 through 1975, the average number of awards for the diagnostically questionable diagnosis of disc disease,
using 3-year averages, increased 2,680% (Fordyce 1995).

In 1992, migraine headaches accounted for substantial morbidity, resulting in an estimated 3 million days spent bedridden each month and lost
labor costs ranging from $6.5 to $17 billion (Osterhaus et al. 1992).
Estimated annual lost work days per 1,000 persons is 820 for tension-type
headache, almost triple that in migraine (270) (Silberstein and Lipton 1996).

Between 1 and 1.5 million Americans are thought to be infected with the
human immunodeficiency virus. Common problems encountered are generalized deconditioning and neurologic dysfunction, including painful neuropathies. In a sample of AIDS patients studied, 35% of patients had
uncontrolled pain (O'Connell and Levinson 1991). Reports of prevalence
vary between 50% and 60% in hospice patients and hospital inpatients, with
somewhat higher rates (68%) among patients cared for at home. Among
patients whose death is imminent (few days to a few weeks), 97% experienced uncontrolled pain (O'Neill and Sherrard 1993).

Magni et al. (1993) reported the frequency of chronic musculoskeletal
pain in the National Health and Nutrition Epidemiologic follow-up study to
be 32.8%. The group comprised significantly more females, older people,
and those with lower incomes.

Attitudes and Beliefs of Physical Therapists

Health professionals expect visual signs of pain and a physical cause of pain.
Both patients and health care providers tend to downplay or altogether
ignore the interrelationship of the emotional, cognitive, and physical aspects
of pain. The patient and the professional are both affected by their own culture, age, sex, personal pain history, beliefs, and expectations. The patient
may expect to be cured without active participation. The rewards for an
external locus of control combine well with the traditional acute biomedical
model. A passive, "good" patient does not complain, tells health professionals what they want to hear, and gets better. The pain is relieved by the professional's best efforts, and if it is not relieved the fault lies with the patient,
not with the professional. Should a patient be so unfortunate as to experience pain relief by "placebo," the pain is obviously not real. Furthermore,
the problems of a patient who has a lifestyle or attitude different from the
mainstream are often considered illegitimate. A drug abuser may be punished and receive less medication and treatment due to his or her lifestyle. A
sickle cell crisis is seen as less painful when it is the third, fourth, or tenth
occurrence. The patient is expected to become accustomed to the pain, and
pain is often assessed through the eyes of an individual who experiences and
reacts to pain differently.

Expanding on these ideas, McCaffery has written about misconceptions
that hamper pain assessment (McCaffery 1995). Though her work relates to

TABLE 1.3   Common myths of pain

1. Pain authority: health team versus family or patient
   Myth   The patient is malingering, trying to fool you, or lying.
   Correction   Believe the patient.
2. Acute pain model versus adaptation
   Myth   It is always possible to see that someone is in pain.
   Correction   Physiologic and behavioral adaptation occur.
                  Lack of expression does not mean lack of pain.
                  The ability to sleep does not mean that one has no pain.
3. Known physical cause of pain versus unknown cause
   Myth   Pain in the absence of a known organic cause is a symptom of
                    psychological problems.
   Correction   Most pain is a combination of physical and emotional stimuli.
                  The cause of pain cannot always be determined by today's assess-
                    ment techniques. (An inaccurate or incomplete diagnosis was
                    recorded in 66.7% of patients with chronic pain at a diagnostic
                    center [Hendler and Kozikowski 1993].)
4. Labels and biases versus care without biases
   Myth   The care provided to people in pain is the same regardless of the
                    clinician's personal values, preferences, or painful experiences.
   Correction   Recognize your own biases and guard against them when treating
                    pain.
5. Pain threshold: uniform versus variable
   Myth   Everyone perceives the same intensity of pain from the same stimuli.
   Correction   Personal physiologic differences, plus factors that contribute to
                    higher or lower endorphin levels, will affect the pain threshold.
6. Pain tolerance: high versus low
   Myth   Experience with pain habituates a person to it.
   Correction   Increased pain experience will likely make one more fearful.
                  Expectations that pain will not be controlled will affect tolerance.
7. Pain relief from placebos
   Myth   A placebo response is proof that the pain is not real.
   Correction   Placebo responses are not well understood and can be powerful.
                  (35% of patients will experience pain relief from placebo
                    [Goodwin et al. 1979].)
8. Control of analgesia
   Myth   The health care team controls the patient's pain.
   Correction   The patient should be given the opportunity to assist in pain control.

SOURCE: Modified from M McCaffery. Pain: assessment and intervention in clinical practice.
Course syllabus, spring 1995.

people with acute and cancer pain, the misconceptions apply to chronic
pain as well. Table 1.3, which is adapted from McCaffery, explores the
myths about pain and the correct professional behavior required to dispel
these myths.

There are many problems in pain assessment and treatment that relate to
the knowledge and beliefs of those responsible for pain management. There is
a lack of formal education for health professionals regarding pain management, particularly in the area of chronic pain management. Inappropriate use
of currently available knowledge also occurs (Wolff et al. 1991). Physical
therapists are not alone in having insufficient educational and attitudinal

preparation for working with patients with chronic pain. Nurses and physicians also have been found to not understand basic concepts of pain management (Myers 1985, Bonica 1978a, Bonica 1978b). Editorials in journals have lamented the insufficient number of hours applied to pain education and propose a curriculum for medical students that would increase exposure to pain theories and management (Liebeskind and Melzack 1988, Pilowsky 1988).

The correlation between insufficient knowledge and antiquated attitudes is detrimental to quality patient care. Inappropriate attitudes result in less than adequate pain management (Halfens et al. 1990, Hauck 1986, Myers 1985, Wolff et al. 1991). These studies strongly suggest the need for expanded education of health professionals concerning basic mechanisms of pain, pain assessment, and pain management. Positive attitudes about pain control also need to be taught and fostered in both patients and health professionals.

Conclusion

There is much that is still not known about pain, making the task of managing chronic pain patients and chronic pain syndrome patients a daunting one for physical therapists. "Mismanagement of intractable pain has tragic and costly consequences: disability, depression, overuse of diagnostic services and procedures, hospitalizations, and surgery, and overuse of inappropriate medications" (American Pain Society, 1994). The complexity of nociceptive transmission and transformation into pain perception is still incompletely understood. One of the most important things to remember in treating patients with pain is that pain is a subjective experience and that the patient's experience should be respected.

References

American Pain Society. The Facts on Intractable Pain. Skokie, IL: American Pain Society, 1994.

Bates M, Edwards W, Anderson K. Ethnocultural influences on variation in chronic pain perception. Pain 1993;52:101.

Bigos SJ, Battie MC, Spengler DM, et al. A prospective study of work perceptions and psychosocial factors affecting the report of back injury. Spine 1991;16:1.

Bond MR. Pain: Its Nature, Analysis and Treatment (2nd ed). London: Churchill Livingstone, 1984.

Bonica JJ. Importance of the Problem. In S Anderson, M Bond, M Mehta, M Swerdlow (eds), Chronic Non-Cancer Pain. Lancaster: MTP, 1978a;13.

Bonica JJ. Cancer pain: a major national health problem. Cancer Nurs 1978b;1:313.

Cassell EJ. Recognizing suffering. Hastings Cent Rep 1991;21:24.

Catchlove R, Cohen K. Effect of a directive return to work approach in the treatment of workman's compensation patients with chronic pain. Pain 1982;14:181.

Chan C, Goldman S, Ilstrup D, et al. The pain drawing and Waddell's non-organic physical signs in chronic low back pain. Spine 1993;18:1717.

Cole TM, Edgerton VR. Report of the Task Force on Medical Rehabilitation Research. Hunt Valley, Maryland: Task Force on Medical Rehabilitation Research, 1990;29.

Crue BL, Pinsky JJ. An approach to chronic pain of non-malignant origin. Postgrad Med J 1984;60:858.

Cypress BK. Characteristics of physician visits for back symptoms: a national perspective. Am J Public Health 1983;73:389.

De Girolamo G. Epidemiology and social costs of low back pain and fibromyalgia. Clin J Pain 1991;7(suppl 1):S1.

Descartes R. "L'Homme." In M Foster (ed) (transl), Lectures on the History of Physiology During the 16th, 17th and 18th Centuries. Cambridge: Cambridge University Press, 1901.

Dolce JJ. Self-efficacy and disability beliefs in behavioral treatment of pain. Behav Res Ther 1987;25:289.

Dworkin SF, Von Korff M, LeResche L. Multiple pains and psychiatric disturbance: an epidemiologic investigation. Arch Gen Psychiatry 1990;47:239.

Dworkin SF, Von Korff M, LeResche L. Epidemiologic studies of chronic pain: a dynamic-ecologic perspective. Ann Behav Med 1992;14:3.

Fields H. Pain Syndromes in Neurology. Oxford: Butterworth–Heinemann, 1991;15.

Fordyce WE. Back Pain in the Workplace. In WE Fordyce (ed), Management of Disability in Non-Specific Conditions. Seattle: IASP, 1995;5,17.

Fordyce WE, McMahon R, Rainwater G, et al. Pain complaint—exercise performance relationships in chronic pain. Pain 1981;10:311.

French S. The Psychology and Sociology of Pain. In P Wells, V Frampton, D Bowsher (eds), Pain Management by Physical Therapy. Oxford: Butterworth–Heinemann, 1994;17.

Frymoyer JW, Cats-Baril W. An overview of the incidences and cost of low back pain. Orthop Clin N Am 1991;22:263.

Goodwin JS, Goodwin JM, Vogel AA. Knowledge and use of placebos by house officers and nurses. Ann Intern Med 1979;91:106.

Gottlieb BS. Predicting outcome in pain programs: a matter of cognition. Paper presented at the annual convention of the American Psychological Association. Washington DC, 1986.

Hager WD. Workers Compensation Back Claim Study. Boca Raton, FL: National Council on Compensation Insurance, 1993;1.

Halfens R, Evers G, Abu-Saad H. Determinants of pain assessment by nurses. Int J Nurs Stud 1990;27:43.

Hardy JD, Wolff HG, Goodell H. Pain Sensations and Reactions. New York: Williams & Wilkins, 1952.

Hauck SL. Pain: problem for the person with cancer. Cancer Nurs 1986;9:66.

Hendler NH, Kozikowski J. Overlooked physical diagnoses in chronic pain patients involved in litigation. Psychosomatics 1993;34:494.

Jacox A. Sociocultural and Psychological Aspects of Pain. In A Jacox (ed),

Pain Source Book for Nurses and Other Health Professionals. Boston: Little, Brown 1977;57.

Jette A. Physical disablement concepts for physical therapy research and practice. Phys Ther 1994;74:380.

Keefe FJ, Dolan E. Pain behavior and pain coping strategies in low back pain and myofascial pain dysfunction syndrome patients. Pain 1986;24:49.

Kent G. Effect of pre-appointment inquiries on dental patients post-appointment rating of pain. Br J Med Psychol 1986;59:97.

Klapow JC, Slater MA, Patterson TL, et al. Psychosocial factors discriminate multidimensional clinical groups of chronic low back pain patients. Pain 1995;62:349.

Kulich RJ, Baker B. Psychological Evaluation in the Management of Chronic Pain and Disability. In PP Raj, G Aronoff, RP Pawl (eds), Current Review of Pain (2nd ed) (in press).

Leavitt F, Sweet JJ. Characteristics and frequency of malingering among patients with low back pain. Pain 1986;25:357.

Leventhal H, Meyer D, Narenz D. The Common Sense Representation of Illness Danger. In S Rachman (ed), Medical Psychology (Vol 2). New York: Pergamon, 1980;7.

Liebeskind JC, Melzack R. The international pain foundation: meeting a need for education in pain management. J Pain Symptom Manage 1988;3:131.

Lipton J, Ship J, Larach-Robinson D. Estimated prevalence of and distribution of reported orofacial pain in the United States. J Am Dent Assoc 1993;124:115.

Loeser JD. Concepts of Pain. In M Stanton-Hicks, R Boaz (eds), Chronic Low Back Pain. New York: Raven, 1982;146.

Loeser JD, Egan KJ. History and Organization of the University of Washington Pain Center. In JD Loeser, KT Egan (eds), Managing the Chronic Pain Patient. New York: Raven, 1989;2.

Loeser JD, Fordyce WE. Chronic Pain. In JE Carr, HA Dengerink (eds), Behavioral Medicine in the Practice of Medicine. New York: Elsevier 1983;331.

Main CJ, Waddell G. A comparison of cognitive measures in low back pain: statistical structure and clinical validity at initial assessment. Pain 1991;46:287.

Magni G, Marchetti M, Moreschi C, et al. Chronic musculoskeletal pain and depressive symptoms in the National Health and Nutrition Examination. I. Epidemiologic follow-up study. Pain 1993;53:163.

Masset D, Malchaire J. Low back pain. Epidemiologic aspects and work-related factors in the steel industry. Spine 1994;19:143.

McCaffery M, Beebe A. Pain: Clinical Manual for Nursing Practice. St. Louis: Mosby, 1989;7.

McCaffery M. Pain: assessment and intervention in clinical practice. Course syllabus, Spring 1995.

Melzack R, Wall PD. Pain mechanisms: a new theory. Science 1965; 150:971.

Merskey H, Spear FG. The concept of pain. J Psychosom Res 1967;11:59.

Merskey H, Bogduk N. Classification of Chronic Pain (2nd ed). Seattle: IASP, 1994.

Myers JS. Cancer pain: assessment of nurses' knowledge and attitudes. Oncol Nurs Forum 1985;12:62.

Nagi S. Disability Concepts Revisited: Implications for Prevention. In AM Pope, AR Tarlov (eds), Disability in America. Toward a National Agenda for Prevention. Washington, DC: National Academy Press, 1991;309.

National Advisory Board on Medical Rehabilitation Research, Draft V. Report and Plan for Medical Rehabilitation Research. Bethesda, MD: National Institutes of Health, 1992.

Nolan MF. Pain: the experience and its expression. Clin Manage 1990;10:22.

O'Connell PG, Levinson SF. Experience with rehabilitation in the acquired immunodeficiency syndrome. Am J Phys Med Rehabil 1991;70:195.

O'Neill WM, Sherrard JS. Pain in human immunodeficiency virus disease: a review. Pain 1993;54:3.

Osterhaus JT, Gutterman DL, Plachetka JR. Healthcare resource use and labor costs of migraine headache in the US. Pharmacoeconomics 1992;2:67.

Perl E. Causalgia: sympathetically-aggravated chronic pain from damaged nerves. International Association for the Study of Pain Clinical Updates 1993;1:1.

Pilowsky I. An outline curriculum on pain for medical schools. Pain 1988;33:1.

Rainville J, Ahern D, Phalen L, et al. The association of pain with physical activities in chronic low back pain. Spine 1992;17:1060.

Romano JM, Turner JA. Chronic pain and depression: does the evidence support a relationship? Psychol Bull 1985;97:18.

Sanders SH, Brena SF, Spier CJ, et al. Chronic low back pain patients around the world: cross-cultural similarities and differences. Clin J Pain 1992;8:317.

Shutty MS Jr, DeGood DE, Tuttle DH. Chronic pain patients' beliefs about their pain and treatment outcomes. Arch Phys Med Rehabil 1990;71:128.

Silberstein SD, Lipton RB. Headache and epidemiology, emphasis on migraine. Neurol Clin 1996;14:421.

Skovron ML, Szapalski M, Nordin M, et al. Sociocultural factors and back pain. A population based study in Belgian adults. Spine 1994;19:129.

Spitzer WO, LeBlanc FF, Dupuis M. Scientific approach to the assessment and management of activity related spinal disorders. Spine 1987;12:S1.

Sullivan MJL, Reesor K, Mikail S, Fisher R. The treatment of depression in chronic low back pain: review and recommendations. Pain 1992;50:5.

Turk DC, Meichenbaum D, Genest M. Pain and Behavioral Medicine: A Cognitive-Behavioral Perspective. New York: Guilford, 1983.

Vasudevan S. Impairment, Disability and Functional Capacity Assessment. In DC Turk, R Melzack (eds), Handbook of Pain Assessment. New York: Guilford, 1992.

Vlaeyen JWS, Kole-Snijders AMJ, Boeren RGB, et al. Fear of movement/(re)injury in chronic low back pain and its relation to behavioral performance. Pain 1995;62:363.

Von Korff M, Dworkin SF, LeResche L, Kruger A. Epidemiology of Temporomandibular Disorders. II. TMD Pain Compared to Other Common Pain Sites. In R Dubner, GF Gebhart, MR Bond (eds), Pain Research and Clinical Management. Amsterdam: Elsevier, 1988;506.

Waddell G. A new clinical model for the treatment of low back pain. Spine 1987;12:623.

Waddell G. Biopsychosocial analysis of low back pain. Baillieres Clin Rheumatol 1992;6:523.

Waddell G, Birchner M, Finlayson D, Main CJ. Symptoms and signs: physical disease or illness behavior? BMJ 1984;298:739.

Waddell G, Pilowski I, Bond M. Clinical assessment and interpretation of abnormal illness behavior in low back pain. Pain 1989;39:41.

Waddell G, Somerville D, Henderson I, Newton M. Objective clinical evaluation of physical impairment in chronic low back pain. Spine 1992;17:617.

Waddell G, Newton M, Henderson I, et al. A fear avoidance beliefs questionnaire and the role of fear avoidance beliefs in chronic low back pain and disability. Pain 1993;52:157.

Webster BS, Snook SH. The cost of 1989 workers' compensation low back pain claims. Spine 1994;19:1111.

Westrin C, Hirsch C, Lindegard B. The personality of the back pain patient. Clin Orthop 1972;87:209.

Wolff MS, Michel TH, Krebs DE, et al. Chronic pain—assessment of orthopedic physical therapists' knowledge and attitudes. Phys Ther 1991;71:207.

Wood PHN. The language of disablement: a glossary relating to disease and its consequences. Int Rehab Med 1980;2:86.

Zborowski M. Cultural components in responses to pain. J Soc Iss 1952;8:16.

Zola IK. Culture and symptoms—an analysis of patient's presenting complaints. Am Sociol Rev 1966;66:615.

Zuckerman B, Stevenson J, Baily V. Stomach aches and headaches in a community sample of preschool children. Pediatrics 1987;79:677.

2   Physiology of Pain

Raymond Maciewicz and Harriët Wittink

Pain is a highly variable experience that involves perception more than sensation. For example, some athletes and dancers may suffer significant injury during competition or performance but not experience pain until much later. Other athletes and nonathletes may complain bitterly of chronic pain with little or no evidence of anatomic pathology. These observations suggest that a person's physical state, past experience, and anticipation all contribute strongly to the interpretation of an event as painful (Nathan 1985).

Although clinical pain often begins with the activation of peripheral nerve fibers that relay nociceptive information, this sensory message can be modified at many levels of the nervous system, greatly affecting the individual's final perception of that information. This chapter reviews some of the major pathways and processes involved in transmission and modification of the complex experience of pain.

The three major components of the nociceptive pathways are (1) nociceptors and their associated peripheral nerve fibers; (2) the central nociceptive or pain pathways, including the dorsal horn and the ascending pathways, the spinothalamic tract, and the spinoreticulothalamic system with connections to the thalamus, hypothalamus, limbic system, and sensory cortex; and (3) the descending pain inhibitory pathways running from the midbrain via the brain stem and medulla to the dorsal horn at all levels of the spinal cord (Thompson 1994). Communication between these pathways occurs through neurotransmission.

Physiology of Nerves and Neurotransmission

Neurons rely on electrical and chemical signals to communicate. Generally, electrical signals are intraneural. Chemical transmission is used for communication between neurons and involves neurotransmitters and peptides. All neurotransmitters share the following characteristics:

1. They are synthesized in the neuron in which they are stored.
2. They are stored in the vesicles of the neuron.
3. They are released with a nerve impulse.
4. They bind with and activate a certain receptor.
5. There is a means by which they can be inactivated.

A variety of substances act as neurotransmitters, including the following monoamines: dopamine (DA), serotonin (5-HT), norepinephrine (NE), and acetylcholine (ACh). The amino acid glutamate acts as an excitatory neurotransmitter and gamma-aminobutyric acid (GABA) acts as an inhibitory neurotransmitter. Glycine is found mostly in the spinal cord, where it is inhibitory, and is found in small amounts in the cerebral cortex, where it is excitatory.

Certain peptides, such as substance P, enkephalins, and beta endorphins, are capable of acting as neurotransmitters but do not have all of the characteristics listed above.

Release of Neurotransmitters

When an action potential moves down an axon and enters the presynaptic terminal of the axon, the opening of voltage-dependent Ca^{++} channels allows the influx of Ca^{++} ions, which initiate release of neurotransmitters from the neuron's vesicles. Neurotransmitters are released in small packets called quanta. The amount of Ca^{++} released will determine the number of quanta of transmitter that are released. The released transmitter then diffuses across the synapse, during which a substantial delay, called the synaptic delay, occurs. Next, the transmitter binds to postsynaptic and presynaptic receptors. Receptors located in presynaptic terminals are called autoreceptors. Changes in the membrane excitability in the postsynaptic neuron occur due to changes in neuron metabolism, which causes depolarization or hyperpolarization (Gilman and Newman 1992).

A single neuron of the central nervous system may receive thousands of signals from other neurons and will thus have receptors for many types of neurotransmitters. Because of this structure, the neuron receives a continuous barrage of inhibitory and excitatory synaptic signals. Each neuron must evaluate all the impulses it is receiving on a moment-to-moment basis and decides whether there is enough excitation to generate a nerve impulse. If there is, the neuron will send nerve impulses down its axon. A few hundredths of a second later, the neuron may stop sending impulses.

Removal of Neurotransmitters

A receptor cannot respond to a second nerve impulse until the transmitter released by the first impulse is removed from both the synaptic cleft and the receptor. Transmitter molecules are easily unattached from the receptor site. Once the transmitter has left the receptor site, it is removed from the synaptic cleft in one of two ways. Some transmitters are broken down into smaller molecules by an enzyme in the synaptic membrane. Other transmitters leave the cleft by re-entering the presynaptic terminal and binding to receptor sites at this terminal. After it is removed, the transmitter is then taken inside the terminal. This process is called reuptake. After reuptake, the transmitter either re-enters a vesicle so it can be used again or is destroyed by an enzyme within the presynaptic terminal. Some drugs can inhibit the reuptake of certain transmitter substances.

Receptors

Receptors are subdivided into families based on their biochemistry, and each family may have subtypes. 5-HT receptors, for example, have three families ($5\text{-}HT_1$, $5\text{-}HT_2$, and $5\text{-}HT_3$) and four subtypes (A, B, C, and D). Thus, receptors are classified as $5\text{-}HT_{1A}$, $5\text{-}HT_{1B}$, etc. These classifications are important when discussing medications, their interaction with receptor sites, and side effects.

The number of receptor sites is not fixed. The number of receptors of the pre- and postsynaptic terminal can either increase (upregulation) or decrease (downregulation) in response to stimulation by the neurotransmitter. For example, the number of ACh receptor sites in muscles increases with denervation of the muscle. This up- and downregulation of receptor sites plays an important role in developing tolerance to certain medications.

Peripheral Mechanisms of Pain and Inflammation

An extensive plexus of free nerve endings in skin, muscle, and internal organs activates small myelinated (A delta fibers) and unmyelinated (C fibers) peripheral sensory axons in the presence of strong sensory input and tissue injury (Nathan 1985).

Nociceptors are receptors responding to stimuli that can cause tissue damage. They are abundant in the skin and the musculoskeletal system. These free nerve endings are the termination of the myelinated A delta and unmyelinated C fibers. The A delta fibers respond mainly to mechanical and thermal stimulation, although they also respond to some pharmacologic agents. Some myelinated afferents have receptors that respond only to intense noxious mechanical stimuli and are thus called high-threshold mechanoreceptors. Because C fibers respond to chemical, thermal, and mechanical stimuli, they are known as polymodal nociceptors. Nociceptors have a higher threshold for activation than the receptors that signal touch, warmth, and cold (A beta fibers) and are able to record the stimulus intensity by correspondingly increasing their firing rate, unlike the A beta fibers. The A delta fibers mainly serve discriminative functions in nociception, their discharge causing the first localized, sharp pain, which possibly produces the withdrawal reflex (also called the flexion reflex). The C fibers give rise to the secondary, aching or burning pain (Lundeberg 1995). The nociceptors can be activated by local hypoxia, leading to a local decrease of pH and injury or inflammation. Tissue injury results in hyperalgesia, the perceptual companion of inflammation (Raj 1996). Tissue-damaging stimuli produce effects that spread beyond the site where they are applied.

Any intense stimulus applied to normal skin will elicit a "triple response" consisting of a red flush at the site of stimulation, a surrounding red flare due to arterial dilation, and local edema due to increased vascular permeability

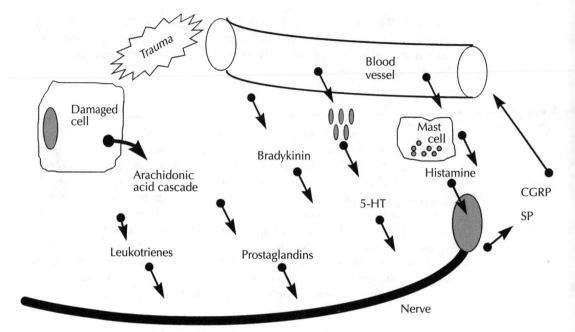

FIGURE 2.1 *Peripheral mechanisms of pain. (CGRP = calcitonin gene–related polypeptide; SP = substance P; 5-HT = serotonin.)*

(Lewis 1942). Many factors contribute to this inflammatory response. Damaged tissue itself activates the arachidonic cascade, resulting in local release of a variety of inflammatory mediators, including prostaglandins and leukotrienes, which can directly activate nociceptive fibers. Increased vascular permeability at the site of injury results in extravasation of plasma proteins and fluid (local edema), resulting in activation of kinin pathways, with local formation of bradykinin, a substance that strongly excites polymodal nociceptors (Hargreaves et al. 1995).

Factors associated with pain and inflammation also arise from local inflammatory cells (mast cells, etc.) that are present in tissue and accumulate at the site of trauma. Degranulation of inflammatory cells results in the local release of histamine, 5-HT, and other factors that increase local swelling and sensitize nociceptors.

Factors released from small-caliber nerve fibers, including peptides such as substance P and calcitonin gene–related polypeptide (CGRP), also appear to play important roles in the generation of the inflammatory response. Several of these substances activate free nerve endings and may contribute to the long-lasting hypersensitivity that usually accompanies an intense stimulus (Figure 2.1).

Another way to enhance nociceptive input from the periphery is by sensitization of nociceptors from repeated noxious stimuli. Perl (1968) demonstrated that polymodal afferent fibers display enhanced sensitivity, lowered threshold to stimulation, and enhanced excitation with repetitive input.

The fact that polymodal nociceptors respond strongly to many of the chemical mediators of inflammation probably explains their relatively non-specific response to any stimulus of sufficient noxious intensity. Although such fibers with high thresholds and polymodal responses are probably good candidates to signal the presence of a potentially tissue-damaging stimulus, they most likely are too nonspecific to convey much of the sensory-discriminative aspects of pain. Nociceptors with more specialized response properties and non-nociceptive sensory afferents are clearly important in shaping the sensory qualities of the noxious stimulus for sensory perception.

It is important to note that physiologic studies in humans confirm that slowly conducting peripheral axons code for pain. Microelectrode studies in normal subjects show that stimulation of individual, slowly conducting sensory axons (Torebjork 1996) evokes a report of pain that is referred to the peripheral cutaneous receptive field supplied by that fiber. This observation demonstrates that under certain conditions single axons can transmit activity that is interpreted as pain by the brain.

Pain Due to Peripheral Nerve Injury

The marked sensitivity of the peripheral nociceptive system is necessary to avoid tissue injury. In diseases that cause nerve injury such as diabetes or herpes zoster infection, however, peripheral afferents may continue to discharge even when the stimulus is absent; such neuropathic pain can occur in the absence of frank tissue injury (since the damage is in the nerve itself) and, in some cases, may persist indefinitely (Maciewicz et al. 1985).

Acute injury to peripheral nerve rarely produces clinical pain, as cutting or compressing the trunk of an undamaged nerve produces only a brief discharge in the severed axons (Bennett 1993). Within a few days after trauma to a peripheral nerve, however, burning pain and mechanical sensitivity can develop at the site of injury; the injury to the nerve is associated with paresthesias in the distribution of the affected nerve. The regenerating tip of a cut peripheral nerve contains numerous small-diameter sprouts that develop a spontaneous discharge, possibly caused by increased ionic permeability in the sprout. If the path for regeneration is blocked, a neuroma forms. Sprouts within a neuroma are sensitive to mechanical stimulation (Tinel's sign), and excitation may occur and be sustained by electrical "cross-talk" between bare axons in close apposition. Similar changes may also occur with chronic compression of nerve in the absence of actual transection. The abnormal activity in such chronically damaged axons is a potential source of clinical pain after nerve injury (Figure 2.2).

Although normal axons exhibit little chemical sensitivity, after experimental nerve injury in rats, the regenerating axon sprouts become sensitive to local or intravenous catecholamines (Wall et al. 1979, Wall and Gutnick 1974); this effect appears to be mediated by alpha-adrenergic receptors on the regenerating fibers. The source of this catecholamine response is uncertain. Many peripheral nerves, however, contain large numbers of unmyelinated, postganglionic, sympathetic efferent fibers that use NE as a neurotransmitter. In damaged nerves, abnormal coupling may occur between these efferent

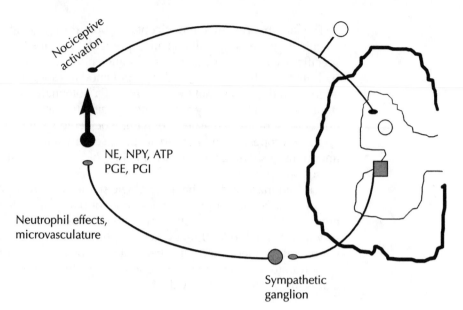

FIGURE 2.2
Sympathetic interactions. (ATP = adenosine triphosphate; NE = norepinephrine; NPY = neuropeptide Y; PGE = prostaglandin E; PGI = prostaglandin I.)

NE, NPY, ATP
PGE, PGI

Nociceptive activation

Neutrophil effects, microvasculature

Sympathetic ganglion

sympathetic fibers and cutaneous afferents, providing a potential source of chronic sensory activation that is catecholamine dependent. The concept of such an abnormal interaction between sympathetic efferents and nociceptive primary afferents is consistent with the observation that stimulating the sympathetic chain supplying efferents to a neuroma produces a discharge in afferent fibers coming out of the neuroma. This abnormal interaction between the sympathetic system and cutaneous afferents may underlie some forms of neuropathic pain that are associated with autonomic dysfunction after nerve injury and may explain some of the clinical features of sympathetic dystrophy (Sweet and Poletti 1985).

Spinal Mechanisms of Nociception

At the entrance of the dorsal roots into the spinal cord, fine myelinated and unmyelinated afferents are located lateral to the large-diameter cutaneous fibers. The fine afferents travel in the dorsal root entry zone for one or two segments and then enter the laminated structure of the dorsal horn, terminating principally in the superficial layers. Small myelinated afferents end in lamina I and V; unmyelinated afferents terminate throughout lamina II (Loh and Nathan 1978). An additional input from small-caliber afferents appears to end in the lateral aspect of lamina V. Many of the fine afferents terminating in these regions contain neuropeptides, including substance P, CGRP, cholecystokinin, and somatostatin. Although the primary excitatory neurotransmitter in most sensory afferent fibers is probably glutamate or another amino acid, there is strong evidence that neuropeptides play an important role in modulating sensory transmission in these afferents (Hokfelt et al. 1983).

Substance P is released from the spinal cord after high-intensity sciatic nerve stimulation, and there is a relatively selective excitation of dorsal horn nociceptive neurons by substance P (Henry 1976). Depletion of substance P with capsaicin is associated with a decreased aversive response in animals to certain types of noxious stimuli, and there is also a marked decrease in substance P terminal staining in the dorsal horn in patients and animals with congenital neuropathy and decreased sensitivity to pain (Pearson et al. 1983). The peptide cholecystokinin is also present in many fine afferents in the dorsal horn and may also be important in pain sensation, although there are still many gaps in our understanding of the roles such neuropeptides may actually play.

Cells important in the processing of nociceptive information are located in several laminae of the dorsal horn. The output neurons are located principally in lamina I and V. Lamina I (the marginal zone of the dorsal horn) consists of a thin sheet of large, high-threshold cells that dorsally cap the spinal gray. Many of the neurons in this region respond exclusively to high-intensity noxious stimulation and are therefore termed *nociceptive-specific cells*. Cells in lamina V, however, appear to receive convergent input from both rapidly conducting A beta axons that code for light touch and more slowly conducting A delta and C nociceptive afferents. Because they receive diverse input, these wide dynamic range neurons respond to moderate mechanical or thermal stimuli and steadily increase their discharge frequency as the stimulus intensity reaches the noxious range (Iggo et al. 1985). Both nociceptive-specific and wide dynamic range neurons are likely important for normal nociception.

An important feature of these dorsal horn nociceptive neurons is the convergence of deep afferents on the same cells that receive cutaneous inputs. Most clinically relevant pain involves deep tissues rather than the skin only. There does not appear to be a major ascending projection that carries exclusively visceral information, however. Instead, nociceptive afferents arising from the gastrointestinal tract, deep tissues, or muscle appear to converge on relay cells with cutaneous receptive fields. The convergence of deep and cutaneous afferents onto the same cells is likely to account for the clinical phenomenon of referred pain (Cervero 1985). There are many common clinical examples of this, including cardiac pain referred to the left shoulder, vascular head pain referred to the forehead, and renal pain referred to the perineum. The curious referral patterns of some myofascial trigger points may also be explained similarly (Figure 2.3).

Lamina II (the substantia gelatinosa) of dorsal horn receives the bulk of unmyelinated dorsal root afferents, and in the inner part of lamina II these unmyelinated afferents overlap with small myelinated afferents as well. Although a small number of cells in this region have long projections that reach the brain, most substantia gelatinosa cells appear to make local connections at the segment level or interconnections with adjacent segments. Because lamina II receives major input from unmyelinated afferents, it is clearly in a prime position to act as a relay for input from small afferents within the dorsal horn. There is a high density of peptide-containing neurons in lamina II. Such cells are in a good position to shape the response properties of neurons that then relay to the brain stem and thalamus,

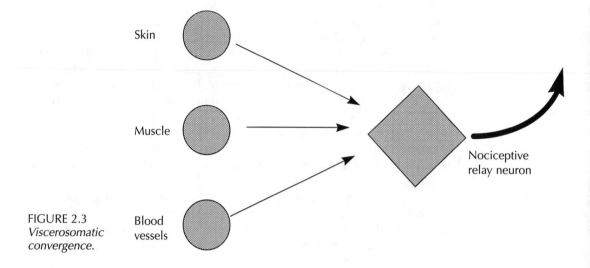

FIGURE 2.3
*Viscerosomatic
convergence.*

Skin

Muscle

Blood
vessels

Nociceptive
relay neuron

although there is still no clear consensus concerning the way this occurs
(Cervero and Iggo 1980).

Changes in Dorsal Horn Due to Pain

Activation of peripheral nociceptors or trauma to peripheral sensory nerves
can result in changes not only at the site of injury, but also within the dorsal
horn of the spinal cord; these central effects may be important in the development of chronic pain and hypersensitivity after an acute event. There is
increasing evidence that the response of pain-relaying spinal cord neurons is
highly plastic and that long-term changes in excitability and receptive field
properties can be induced by noxious stimulation or peripheral trauma.

Lesions of peripheral nerve distal to the dorsal root ganglion can induce a
spectrum of changes not only at the site of damage, but also at the spinal
cord (Dubner 1993). Degeneration of small afferents and their terminations
in dorsal horn can occur with peripheral nerve lesions. This degeneration
may be accompanied by a loss of neuropeptides (substance P, somatostatin,
cholecystokinin) contained in these afferents (Figure 2.4).

Physiologic studies also show that peripheral nerve lesions may cause a
decrease or loss of normal presynaptic and postsynaptic mechanisms of inhibition of fine afferent terminations in dorsal horn. Peripheral nerve lesions
may therefore induce changes in the spinal relay, causing it to become more
sensitive to potentially nociceptive inputs. These central effects may be
important for the development of neuropathic pain (Devor and Wall 1981,
Woolf and Wall 1982, Basbaum and Wall 1976, Wall and Devor 1981).

Lesions between dorsal root ganglia and the spinal cord also cause significant changes in dorsal horn and more central pain pathways. These changes
may be a source of neuropathic pain associated with deafferentation. This condition has been studied experimentally in animals with multiple-level dorsal
rhizotomies and in animals with partial injury to the sciatic nerve (Bennett and
Xie 1988a, 1988b). After dorsal rhizotomy, neurons within the experimentally

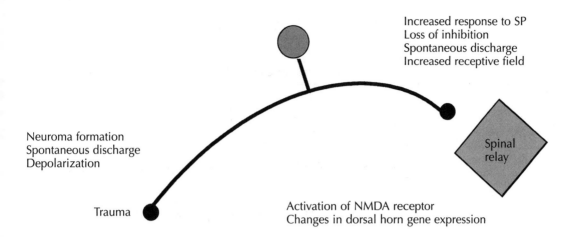

Increased response to SP
Loss of inhibition
Spontaneous discharge
Increased receptive field

Neuroma formation
Spontaneous discharge
Depolarization

Spinal
relay

Trauma

Activation of NMDA receptor
Changes in dorsal horn gene expression

FIGURE 2.4   *Peripheral trauma can evoke changes in pain transmission centrally. (NMDA = N-methyl-D-aspartate; SP = substance P.)*

deafferented dorsal horn develop a spontaneous, irregular hyperactivity, and sensory receptive fields, when present, are abnormal or reorganized. After a few months, abnormal activity can also be recorded at the level of the thalamus, evidence that the abnormal central discharge that may correlate with deafferentation pain is, over time, transmitted further centrally.

Within the trigeminal system, even an endodontal pulpectomy performed on a cat (a common root canal procedure) can result in long-term changes in excitability and reorganization of dorsal horn receptive fields, emphasizing the extent and sensitivity of these changes.

There is additional evidence that central changes may be associated with some forms of chronic neuropathic pain in humans. Tasker (1984) has shown that stimulation of the anterolateral columns of the spinal cord in patients with deafferentation pain can produce contralateral burning sensations, a finding not seen in patients with nociceptive pain. At the level of the thalamus, medial thalamic and medial midbrain stimulation again results in contralateral burning that may reproduce the patient's clinical pain. The central changes in neuropathic pain may even extend to the cerebral cortex. Electrical stimulation of the appropriate parts of the somatosensory cortex is reported to elicit pain in patients with clinical pain of neuropathic origin, whereas stimulation of somatotopically adjacent cortical regions not associated with the site of clinical pain produces only localized paresthesias. These findings are evidence that damage at one level in the somatosensory system can induce changes in the remaining central pathways that may be responsible for continued clinical pain of neuropathic origin. Therapies that are directed only at peripheral nerve or the spinal segment initially involved in producing the pain syndrome may therefore be ineffective.

There is evidence that glutamate receptors in spinal dorsal horn may play an important role in these physiologic changes induced by peripheral trauma or nerve injury. As noted above, glutamate may be a transmitter in primary nociceptive afferents. Within the dorsal horn, nociceptive activation of one

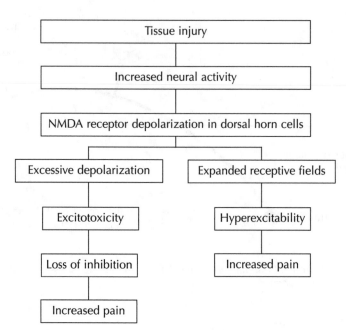

FIGURE 2.5
Potential series of events in central sensitization after peripheral activation. (NMDA = N-methyl-D-aspartate.)

class of glutamate receptors, the *N*-methyl-D-aspartate (NMDA) receptors, causes prolonged depolarization and repetitive discharges in dorsal horn cells. Even in the setting of relatively minor trauma, such as a partial sciatic nerve injury, there is evidence that the abnormal excitation in dorsal horn caused by the trauma is associated with anatomic damage and physiologic change in postsynaptic neurons. These neurotoxic effects may be one cause of long-lasting central changes that underlie some forms of neuropathic pain discussed in the section on pain due to peripheral nerve injury. Experiments have shown that drugs that block NMDA receptors appear to prevent the development of neuropathic pain experimentally, supporting the view that these receptors are important in the genesis of neuropathic pain (Figure 2.5).

Supraspinal Levels

Most of the nociceptive information relayed from dorsal horn to the brain travels in a crossed pathway in the ventrolateral quadrant of the spinal cord (the spinothalamic tract). Spinal cells that join the spinothalamic tract are located primarily in laminae I, IV, and V, with smaller numbers found in laminae II and III. Their axons cross the midline and often travel as much as two segment levels before entering the contralateral lateral column (Willis 1985). There they join with other afferent fiber systems to form a mixed ascending projection within the ventrolateral column. At each successive spinal level, new fibers join the spinothalamic tract, pushing the axons from caudal segments laterally. At supraspinal levels, afferents from the spinothalamic tract terminate heavily in a variety of brain stem and thalamic nuclei. Mehler et al. (1960) propose that spinothalamic afferents can be divided into two groups: those in the neospinothalamic tract, which carries sensory-discrimi-

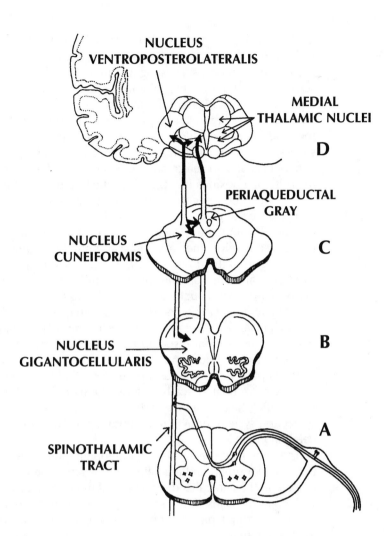

NUCLEUS
VENTROPOSTEROLATERALIS

MEDIAL
THALAMIC NUCLEI

D

PERIAQUEDUCTAL
GRAY

NUCLEUS
CUNEIFORMIS

C

NUCLEUS
GIGANTOCELLULARIS

B

A

SPINOTHALAMIC
TRACT

FIGURE 2.6
*Ascending pain
pathways.
A. Dorsal horn.
B. Brain stem.
C. Midbrain.
D. Thalamus.*

native information about pain directly to the thalamus, and those in the phylogenetically more primitive paleospinothalamic (or spinoreticulothalamic) tract, which terminates largely in a variety of brain stem nuclei (Figure 2.6). This more diffuse paleospinothalamic system may mediate many of the autonomic and affective reactions to pain. As many as one-half of the fibers in the spinothalamic tract never reach the thalamus at all, ending instead in the reticular formation of the brain stem. These spinoreticular fibers terminate on both sides of the caudal brain stem, ending principally in the nucleus gigantocellularis. Many terminations also occur in more rostral sites, including the midbrain reticular formation and the hypothalamus.

Thalamic Level

Spinothalamic fibers that are likely to be important in bringing painful sensations to conscious perception terminate directly in the thalamus. The three thalamic regions engaged by the spinothalamic tract (the ventroposterolateral nucleus [VPL], the posterior-group nuclei, and the medial thalamic nuclei) differ from one another in their anatomic relations and the response properties of their neurons, suggesting that they have different functional roles in sensation. Within the VPL, spinothalamic afferents terminate in a somatotopic fashion that overlaps the major terminal field of the lemniscal system, which relays light touch and joint sensation. The orderly arrangement of endings and the convergence of light touch and pain information within the VPL suggest that this nucleus may be involved in defining the sensory-discriminative aspects of pain sensation, including the coding of location, nature, and intensity of a noxious input. Cells in the VPL project principally into the primary somatosensory cortex, supporting this view.

The posterior-group nuclei of the thalamus also receive major input from the spinothalamic tract (Mehler et al. 1960). Like the VPL, the posterior group also receives medial lemniscal input, but in this region, fibers ascending from the dorsal column nuclei contribute only minor input relative to the amount from the spinothalamic tract. A majority of neurons in the posterior group nuclei are responsive to potentially painful stimuli and have bilateral receptive fields with no somatotopic organization. Many such neurons have wide dynamic range response properties. Cells in the medial thalamus have similar response properties. Some perifascicular neurons respond to innocuous inputs, but the majority have very large somatosensory receptive fields that respond preferentially to potentially painful stimuli and are not topographically ordered (Dong et al. 1978). The posterior-group and medial thalamic nuclei, which also have a rather diffuse subcortical projection system, project in a nontopographic manner to most parts of the cerebral cortex.

The wide receptive fields and nontopographic arrangement of afferents in the posterior group and medial thalamus are evidence that these areas participate in the generalized activation of the forebrain, which is associated with pain. It has also been shown that lesions of the posterior thalamus in animals attenuate pain responses. In humans, such lesions are also reported to relieve pain (Mark et al. 1960), and electrical stimulation of these structures elicits contralateral sensations of burning pain. Considering the multiple sources of diffuse input to these thalamic nuclei and their reciprocal connections with limbic forebrain structures, it is possible that lesions that effectively relieve clinical pain may do so by disrupting the affective component of the pain response.

Normal perception of pain includes both sensory-discriminative attributes, which pinpoint the presence and location of an intense stimulus, and affective components, such as the fear, alerting, and autonomic effects associated with pain. Within the thalamus, these functions appear to be partially separated; the sensory-discriminative aspects of pain may be relayed through the VPL, whereas the affective components are transmitted through the medial thalamus and posterior-group nuclei.

The original work of Mark and coworkers (1960) further supported the idea that clinical pain was represented in two ways in the human thalamus. In their studies, lesions placed in the medial thalamus in pain patients often relieved the suffering associated with painful lesions while leaving sensation apparently intact; lesions placed in VPL, on the other hand, reduced somatosensory discrimination but had little effect on the patient's report of pain.

Brain Stem Control of Nociceptive Transmission

The experience of pain is extremely variable. Physiologic factors, psychological characteristics, and past experience all have an impact on the perception of pain. Therefore, it is not surprising that the brain contains powerful endogenous systems that gate the flow of nociceptive information from the dorsal horn through to the level of conscious perception. Although there are multiple points where pain perception can be modulated, the most extensively studied system originates in the midbrain periaqueductal gray (PAG) region.

Reynolds (1969) showed that electrical stimulation of the PAG region produces analgesia in animals without other evidence of behavioral disruption; similar effects are reported in humans. The analgesia evoked by stimulation of the PAG region is at least partly due to inhibition of the somatosensory responses of spinal dorsal horn cells (Carstens et al. 1979). PAG stimulation selectively inhibits the responses of dorsal horn neurons to a variety of nociceptive stimuli, with relatively little effect on non-noxious responses.

The PAG region may also be an important site for the central analgesic actions of opioid analgesics. Microinjections of morphine into the PAG produce analgesic effects similar to those produced by PAG electrical stimulation (Yeung et al. 1977), and the analgesic effects of PAG stimulation can be partially reversed by the opioid-antagonist naloxone. These effects are most likely mediated by the high density of opioid binding sites found throughout the PAG, although enkephalin-containing neurons and opioid receptors that are likely to be important in analgesia are also densely localized at other sites in the superficial dorsal horn and the nucleus raphe magnus (RM).

The inhibitory effect of PAG stimulation on dorsal horn cells is somewhat surprising, since only a small number of PAG neurons project directly into the spinal dorsal horn. In contrast, there is a very large projection from the PAG to the medullary nucleus RM and the adjacent medial reticular nuclei (Abols and Basbaum 1981). Many RM cells, in turn, have descending projections to spinal dorsal horn, where they collateralize and terminate in laminae I, II, and V, evidence that the descending pathway important for PAG-induced analgesia relays in nuclei of the medial medulla before reaching trigeminal or spinal levels.

Many of the descending raphe-spinal neurons contain the neurotransmitter 5-HT, which appears to play an important role in the descending modulation of nociceptive transmission (Bowker et al. 1982). Intrathecal 5-HT raises the threshold for a variety of nociceptive reflexes in animals and inhibits the responses of nociceptive spinal neurons. These effects are potentiated by monoamine oxidase inhibitors or 5-HT agonists and are attenuated by 5-HT antagonists.

Although the descending system from the PAG and RM is the most extensively studied, several other nuclear groups and transmitter systems are likely involved in the central modulation of nociceptive transmission. For example, stimulation of the dorsolateral pons in the region of the locus coeruleus (LC) and the parabrachial nuclei produces behavioral analgesia in experimental animals and patients with clinical pain (Katayama et al. 1985).

The projection from this region of the pons is the source of a dense noradrenergic innervation to many zones of the spinal cord, including the dorsal horn. NE may therefore be another important transmitter in the descending control of nociception, since the behavioral analgesia produced by LC stimulation can be suppressed by adrenergic blockers applied at spinal levels. In findings consistent with the antinociceptive role postulated for the LC-dorsal horn projection, Mokha et al. (1985) have shown that electrical stimulation of the LC inhibits the nociceptive responses of dorsal horn neurons, although LC stimulation has little effect on non-nociceptive cells. This effect appears to be mediated by alpha-adrenergic receptors on the dorsal horn cells themselves, although presynaptic effects may also be important.

In addition to 5-HT and NE, a number of other neurotransmitters are contained in descending systems that terminate in the dorsal horn. The different roles for each descending pathway and transmitter system remain to be elucidated. It is likely, however, that these projections are responsible for the dynamic control of nociceptive transmission through both the trigeminal and spinal systems. Under normal conditions, for example, environmental stimuli may activate these pathways to modulate the response to painful stimuli. A wide variety of stressors, both noxious and non-noxious, can trigger behavioral analgesia. In fact, different animals can show either analgesic or hyperalgesic responses to the same stressor, and this result may correlate with indexes of the animal's emotional state.

Conclusion

The perception of pain is a fundamental experience relayed over a series of discrete pathways in the nervous system. These pathways engage specific transmitter systems that potentiate nociceptive transmission and may contribute to certain chronic pain states. The responses of pain transmission neurons are highly variable and may be modified by a variety of chemical, physical, and psychological manipulations.

In addition, the brain contains powerful endogenous mechanisms that gate the flow of noxious stimuli. Knowledge of these systems controlling pain transmission are, however, still rudimentary. Much work remains to be done in order to use the brain's own systems for pain modulation for clinical advantage.

References

Abols IA, Basbaum AI. Afferent connections of the rostral medulla of the cat: a neural substrate for midbrain-medullary interactions in the modulation of pain. J Comp Neurol 1981;201:285.

Basbaum AI, Wall PD. Chronic changes in the response of cells in cat dorsal horn following partial deafferentation. The appearance of responding cells in a previously nonresponding region. Brain Res 1976;116:181.

Bennett GJ. An animal model of neuropathic pain: a review. Muscle Nerve 1993;16:1040.

Bennett GJ, Xie Y-K. An Experimental Peripheral Neuropathy in Rat That Produces Abnormal Pain Sensation. In R Dubner, GF Gebhart, MR Bond (eds), Proceedings of the Fifth World Congress on Pain. Seattle: Elsevier BV, 1988a;129.

Bennett GJ, Xie Y-K. A peripheral mononeuropathy in rat that produces disorders of pain sensation like those seen in man. Pain 1988b;33:87.

Bowker RM, Westlund KN, Sullivan MC. Transmitters of the raphe-spinal complex: immunocytochemical studies. Peptides 1982;3:291.

Carstens E, Yokota T, Zimmerman M. Inhibition of spinal neuronal responses to noxious skin heating by stimulation of mesencephalic periaqueductal gray in the cat. J Neurophysiol 1979;42:558.

Cervero F. Visceral nociception: peripheral and central aspects of visceral nociceptive systems. Philos Trans R Soc Lond B Biol Sci 1985;308:107.

Cervero F, Iggo A. The substantia gelatinosa of the spinal cord. A critical review. Brain 1980;103:717.

Devor M, Wall PD. Plasticity in the spinal cord sensory map following peripheral nerve injury in rats. J Neurosci 1981;1:679.

Dong WK, Ryu H, Wagman IH. Nociceptive responses of neurons in medial thalamus and their relationship to spinothalamic pathways. J Neurophysiol 1978;41:1592.

Dubner R. Spinal Cord Neuronal Plasticity: Mechanisms of Persistent Pain Following Tissue Damage and Nerve Injury. In L Vecchiet, D Albe-Fessard, U Lindblom, MA Giamberardino (eds), New Trends in Referred Pain and Hyperalgesia. Amsterdam: Elsevier, 1993;109.

Gilman S, Newman SW. Manter and Gatz's Essentials of Clinical Neuro-anatomy and Neurophysiology (8th ed). Philadelphia: F.A. Davis, 1992;19.

Hargreaves KM, Roszkowski MT, Jackson DL, Swift JQ. Orofacial Pain: Peripheral Mechanisms. In JR Fricton, R Dubner (eds), Orofacial Pain and Temporomandibular Disorders. New York: Raven, 1995;33.

Henry JL. Effects of substance P on functionally identified units in cat spinal cord. Brain Res 1976;114:439.

Hokfelt T, Skirboll L, Lundberg JM, et al. Neuropeptides and Pain Pathways. In J Bonica, U Lindblom, A Iggo (eds), Advances in Pain Research and Therapy. New York: Raven, 1983;227.

Iggo A, Steedman WM, Fleetwood-Walker S. Spinal processing: anatomy and physiology of spinal nociceptive mechanisms. Philos Trans R Soc Lond B Biol Sci 1985;308:235.

Katayama Y, Tsubokawa T, Hirayama T, Yamamoto T. Pain relief following stimulation of the mesencephalic parabrachial region in humans: brain sites for nonopiate mediated pain control. Appl Neurophysiol 1985;48:195.

Lewis T. Pain. New York: Macmillan, 1942.

Loh L, Nathan PW. Painful peripheral states and sympathetic blocks. J Neurol Neurosurg Psychiatry 1978;41:664.

Lundeberg T. Pain physiology and principles of treatment. Scand J Rehabil Med Suppl 1995;32:13.

Maciewicz R, Bouckoms A, Martin JB. Drug therapy of neuropathic pain. Clin J Pain 1985;1:1.

Mark VH, Ervin FR, Hackett TP. Clinical aspects of stereotactic thalamotomy in the human. Part I. The treatment of chronic pain. Arch Neurol 1960;3:351.

Mehler WR, Feferman ME, Nauta WJH. Ascending axon degeneration following anterolateral cordotomy. An experimental study in the monkey. Brain 1960;83:715.

Mokha SS, McMillan JA, Iggo A. Descending control of spinal nociceptive transmission. Actions produced on spinal multireceptive neurons from the nuclei locus coeruleus (LC) and raphe magnus (RM). Exp Brain Res 1985;58:213.

Nathan PW. Pain and nociception in the clinical context. Philos Trans R Soc Lond B Biol Sci 1985;308:219.

Pearson J, Brandeis L, Cuello AC. Depletion of substance P containing axons in substantia gelatinosa of patients with diminished pain sensitivity. Nature 1983;295:61.

Perl ER. Myelinated afferent fibers innervating the primate skin and their response to noxious stimuli. J Physiol 1968;197:593.

Raj PP. Pain Mechanisms. In PP Raj (ed), Pain Medicine—A Comprehensive Review. St. Louis: Mosby 1996;12.

Reynolds DV. Surgery in the rat during electrical analgesia induced by focal brain stimulation. Science 1969;166:444.

Sweet WH, Poletti CE. Causalgia. In G Aronoff (ed), Evaluation and Treatment of Chronic Pain. Baltimore: Urban and Schwarzenberg, 1985.

Tasker RR. Deafferentation. In PD Wall, R Melzack (ed), Textbook of Pain. London: Churchill Livingstone, 1984;119.

Thompson JW. Neuropharmacology of the Pain Pathway. In PE Wells, V Frampton, D Bowsher (eds), Pain Management by Physical Therapy (2nd ed). Oxford: Butterworth–Heinemann, 1994;59.

Torebjork E. Nociceptor activation and pain. Philos Trans R Soc Lond B Biol Sci 1996;308:227.

Wall PD, Gutnick M. Properties of afferent nerve impulses originating from a neuroma. Nature 1974;248:740.

Wall PD, Devor M, Inbal R. Autotomy following peripheral nerve lesions: experimental anesthesia dolorosa. Pain 1979;7:103.

Wall PD, Devor M. The effect of peripheral nerve injury on dorsal root potentials and on transmission of afferent signals into the spinal cord. Brain Res 1981;209:95.

Willis WD. Nociceptive pathways: anatomy and physiology of ascending nociceptive pathways. Philos Trans R Soc Lond B Biol Sci 1985;308:253.

Woolf CJ, Wall PD. Chronic peripheral nerve section diminishes the primary A-fiber mediated inhibition of rat dorsal horn neurons. Brain Res 1982;242:77.

Yeung JC, Yaksh TL, Rudy TA. Concurrent mapping of brain sites for sensitivity to the direct application of morphine and focal electrical stimulation in the production of antinociception in the rat. 1977;4:23.

3   Medication Management

Raymond Maciewicz and Theresa Hoskins Michel

Somatic Pain

Pain can be a symptom of either somatic or neuropathic disease. Somatic pain results when a disease process activates nociceptive afferents in skin or viscera. Somatic pain is usually easily localized and proportionate to the amount of tissue injury and inflammation when it involves skin or subcutaneous tissues. On the other hand, pain of visceral origin is often poorly localized and may be referred to an area of skin supplied by the same sensory roots that innervate the diseased organ (Sessle et al. 1986, Foreman et al. 1977, Maciewicz et al. 1988).

Nonopioid Analgesics

Many acute or recurrent acute somatic pains can be effectively treated with oral, nonopioid analgesics such as aspirin, 650 mg, or acetaminophen (Tylenol), 650 mg, orally every 4 hours. Salicylates are the most widely used agents and can be divided into two groups: those that are acetylated, such as aspirin, and those that are not, such as choline magnesium salicylate (Trilisate). Both types of salicylates have pain-reducing, anti-inflammatory, and fever-reducing properties. The acetyl portion of the aspirin molecule inhibits platelet function and prolongs bleeding time. Nonacetylated salicylates do not interfere with platelet function.

Salicylates provide mild to moderate relief of pain by inhibiting prostaglandin synthesis, both peripherally and centrally. Uncoated aspirin induces gastrointestinal (GI) tract bleeding in about 70% of patients, although the amount is usually clinically insignificant. Prolonged use of salicylates in medically compromised patients may result in cumulative, severe GI symptoms, however.

Rarely, a patient may exhibit a sensitivity reaction to salicylates character-ized by bronchospasm. Tinnitus can occur in anyone using salicylates in large doses or after long-term use. It is reversible when salicylates are discontinued.

Eighteen nonsteroidal anti-inflammatory drugs that are not salicylates are also available in the United States. These agents have a mechanism of action similar to that of salicylates, and therefore their major side effects are similar.

Acetaminophen is a centrally acting analgesic. It has no anti-inflammatory action, but it is an effective antipyretic and analgesic. It works by blocking prostaglandin synthesis in the central nervous system and has less effect in the periphery.

Opioid Analgesics

Opioids are usually required for relief of severe pain. There is little rationale for the use of low-strength opioid analgesics such as propoxyphene, includ-ing those that also contain acetaminophen (e.g., Darvocet) (Collins and Kiefer 1981, Masten 1980), or mixed agonist/antagonist drugs such as penta-zocine (Talwin) (Goldstein 1985, Martin 1985). The analgesic effectiveness of these drugs is little better than aspirin, and the frequency of side effects is much greater. Mixed agonist/antagonist drugs can also precipitate with-drawal in patients habituated to stronger opioids. They should not be used routinely for pain management in any patient population.

It is reasonable to begin opioid therapy with an intermediate-strength opi-oid such as codeine, 30 mg, or oxycodone, 5 mg, every 4–6 hours. In oral doses, codeine is relatively safe, potent, and well tolerated. Both aspirin and acetaminophen potentiate the analgesic effect of codeine, so the two drugs can be used together. Oxycodone, 5 mg, is commonly available only in tablet form combined with aspirin or acetaminophen. If oral codeine, 60 mg (or oxycodone, 10 mg), fails to provide relief, however, it should be discon-tinued, as larger doses of codeine increase the frequency of side effects with-out clearly adding to its analgesic effectiveness. In these situations, codeine should be stopped and a higher potency opioid used, such as oral morphine, 30 mg every 4 hours, or oral hydromorphone (Dilaudid), 4 mg every 3–4 hours. There is substantial variation in the effective analgesic dose and the duration of action of opioids in individual patients. Dosages should therefore be adjusted according to the individual patient's needs.

It makes little sense to maintain a patient with long-term chronic pain on drugs that have a short half-life, such as oxycodone. Once a patient is regu-larly taking an opioid with benefit, the medication should be switched to a longer-acting opioid analgesic, such as sustained-release morphine (Dixon and Higginson 1991), transdermal fentanyl, or levorphanol. These agents will provide a more consistent blood level of the medication and therefore a more consistent analgesic action with fewer side effects. They are also more convenient for the patient to use.

The pharmacokinetics of opioids are greatly influenced by disease. Hepatic cirrhosis or renal failure can enhance the bioavailability and decrease the elimination of opioids. Decreased elimination is a particular problem with meperidine (Demerol). In debilitated patients receiving high doses of meperi-dine, the active metabolite normeperidine can accumulate, resulting in

TABLE 3.1 Therapeutic opioid trial for chronic noncancer pain

Proposed entry criteria
    Failure of reasonable pain management alternatives such as physical therapy, cognitive-behavioral techniques, and medical techniques
    Physical and psychosocial assessment, preferably by two specialists
    History of substance abuse and use of drug control services
    Final decision by a team of two or more medical practitioners
    Informed, written, witnessed consent by patient
Proposed practical guidelines
    Preference for mu-agonists that have a long duration of action such as slow-release morphine or methadone
    Scheduled, oral administration of drug
    Four-week trial period of planned therapy with frequent reviews to titrate dosage and assess clinical efficacy
    Demonstration of sustained improvement of pain control, function, or both

SOURCE: Reprinted with permission from SA Schug, RG Large. Opioids for chronic noncancer pain. Pain Clin Updates 1995;3:3.

tremor, confusion, and seizures. Morphine may be a superior drug to use when chronic, large doses of opioids are required in debilitated patients. The pharmacokinetics of morphine do not appear to be altered by cirrhosis.

A variety of drugs, including antihistamines, amphetamines, and antidepressants, may enhance the analgesic effects of opioids and can be useful in certain situations. Oral hydroxyzine, 25 mg four times daily, can potentiate opioid analgesia without adding to the sedative effects. Oral dextroamphetamine can make patients who are excessively sedated by opioids more alert while enhancing analgesia. Benzodiazepines, such as diazepam (Valium), and phenothiazines have numerous side effects and do not enhance analgesia. They should not be used as opioid adjuvants and could potentially exacerbate cognitive problems in certain patients.

The management of acute, painful exacerbations in a patient with chronic pain should be treated the same as any new, acute pain. Analgesics should be available to the patient when pain is present, with an understanding between the patient and physician that the drugs will be discontinued as the acute episode subsides. In a small group of patients, however, psychosocial factors and physical deconditioning may contribute to pain complaints and disability, making evaluation and management difficult. The interdisciplinary approach to management of such chronic pain patients is considered in Chapters 7 and 9–12.

Although opioids are clearly indicated for patients with ongoing pain due to a serious illness such as cancer, the use of opioid analgesics in patients with nonprogressive, chronic, painful conditions is controversial. Opioids are an option for such patients, particularly in the context of interdisciplinary management. Because opioid analgesics are associated with tolerance, dependence, and potential abuse, guidelines are available from various sources to help clinicians appropriately prescribe and monitor the effectiveness of these drugs in this patient group. One set of proposed guidelines is shown in Tables 3.1 and 3.2.

TABLE 3.2 Proposed guidelines for long-term management after successful therapeutic opioid trial for chronic noncancer pain

Prescriptions for a single medical practitioner (with deputy prescribers to cover absences)

Initially frequent, then at least monthly reviews and documentation of pain relief, functional status, appropriate medication use, and side effects

Review and discussion of concomitant education

Ongoing effort to improve social and physical function as a result of pain relief

Contract between patient and practitioner explicitly detailing termination of supply (with appropriate tapering of dose) and notification of drug control services in evidence of misuse such as diversion, loss or theft of medication, unexplained escalation of dosage, or request for opioids from other sources

Use of drug assays and/or supervised inpatient treatment in case of problems (especially unexplained exacerbation of pain or escalation of dosage)

Continuing review of overall situation with regard to nonopioid means of pain control

SOURCE: Reprinted with permission from SA Schug, RG Large. Opioids for chronic noncancer pain. Pain Clin Updates 1995;3:3.

Muscle Relaxants

Muscle relaxants are frequently prescribed to patients with acute and chronic pain states. The mode of action of these drugs and their therapeutic effectiveness in different pain disorders are inadequately studied and, in many cases, questionable.

Five centrally acting skeletal muscle relaxants are available: carisoprodol (Soma), chlorzoxazone (Paraflex), cyclobenzaprine (Flexeril), methocarbamol (Robaxin), and orphenadrine (Norflex SR). These drugs have many characteristics as those of tricyclic antidepressants due to their structural similarity. They have anticholinergic properties that produce a constellation of side effects, including dry mouth, blurred vision, and an increase in heart rate. Patients may complain of dizziness, drowsiness, weakness, and GI disturbances.

Neuropathic Pain

A number of patients consistently fail to achieve significant benefit from even large doses of opioids. Many of these patients suffer from neuropathic pain disorders. Pain usually occurs when a stimulus that is potentially tissue-damaging excites peripheral nociceptive afferents. When a noxious stimulus activates receptors in the skin, muscles, or joints, the pain that results is usually easily localized and described by the patient. However, pain can also result from injury to or chronic changes in peripheral or central somatosensory pathways, probably initially caused by an abnormal pattern of afferent activity that reaches the dorsal horn and more central structures. Changes in central sensory processing also occur after peripheral injury and are likely to be at least partially responsible for the nature and persistence of neuropathic pain symptoms that occur and persist without an obvious nociceptive stimulus. Many patients with difficult chronic pain problems have a neuropathic pain component.

Such patients can either present with a diffuse, painful neuropathy (e.g., alcoholic neuropathy), polyradiculopathy (e.g., diabetic mononeuritis multiplex), or a monoradiculopathy (e.g., postherpetic neuralgia [Strommen et al. 1988]). Central nervous system causes of pain, including myelopathy and thalamic syndrome, are also seen in clinical practice.

Neuropathic Sensory Symptoms

The sensory symptoms in neuropathic pain can be either focal or more generalized and are distinct from symptoms reported with somatic pain. Injury to nerve may result in a neuralgia, which is defined as pain in the distribution of a single nerve (Lindblom and Verrillo 1979, McFarland 1982, Dalessio 1991, Portenoy et al. 1986). Such pain is often accompanied by signs of nerve dysfunction. Frequently, the pain consists of a background, spontaneous burning or aching sensation that can be associated with paroxysmal jabs of sharp pain within the affected region. Nonpainful paresthesias may also be present. Despite an elevated sensory threshold, patients will often have an exaggerated response to a nociceptive stimulus (hyperalgesia) or perceive a non-nociceptive stimulus as painful (allodynia).

The clinical presentation of neuralgia is varied because of both the location of the affected nerve and the underlying pathogenesis of the lesion. In some forms of neuralgia, lancinating pain predominates with few other signs of nerve dysfunction. In contrast, causalgia after nerve injury is characterized by a continuous, severe, burning pain; allodynia; and often, evidence of sympathetic dysfunction.

Pain can also be a feature of more generalized disorders that affect sensory nerves. Disorders associated with degeneration of small-caliber axons, such as that seen in diabetic polyneuropathy, are more often painful conditions that selectively produce demyelination or loss of large-diameter fibers. In such cases, there can be multiple locations of the pain as well as a variety of types of pain. In diffuse sensory or sensorimotor neuropathies, the pain is usually symmetric and distal, affecting the feet and occasionally the hands (Jaspan et al. 1983, Riddle 1990, Cohen and Gross 1990). As with more focal neuralgias, the pain often consists of a spontaneous aching or burning sensation with superimposed paroxysmal jabs of pain. Allodynia and hyperalgesia are common features during acute, painful phases of the disease.

Pain may also be a debilitating symptom after damage to central somatosensory pathways (Gonzales et al. 1992). Lesions at the level of the spinal cord, brain stem, thalamus, or cortex can result in a syndrome of continuous, spontaneous pain that is referred to the periphery, often with superimposed sensory abnormalities, as discussed in Chapter 2.

Independent of the specific etiology or the pattern of involvement, however, neuropathic pain is often very different from other pains the patient has experienced and is frequently poorly described by the patient. Tasker (1984) reviewed the pain symptoms of 168 consecutive patients with pain after lesions of either the central or peripheral nervous system and found that the majority suffered from spontaneous burning or dysesthetic sensations. The words used by the patients to describe their symptoms were clearly different from those used by patients to describe normal nociceptive pains, suggesting that a common feature among patients with neuropathic pains may be a deafferentation state that can potentially induce chronic changes at many levels of the nervous system. These central and peripheral changes may contribute to the chronic nature of symptoms and partially explain the refractoriness of neuropathic states to opioid treatment.

Medical Management of Neuropathic Pain

The medical management of neuropathic pain is difficult, with often disappointing results. As discussed in Chapter 2, neuropathic pain can involve changes at many levels of the nervous system, so patients only rarely have substantial, lasting improvement with any single therapy. Furthermore, there are few well-designed studies of drug effects in neuropathic pain states. Most reports consist of anecdotal cases of uncontrolled series; when positive results are reported with a treatment, it is often unclear whether the clinical improvement is due to spontaneous remission, a primary analgesic effect of the drug, placebo effect, or treatment of concurrent depression. When there is apparent improvement, few studies distinguish which features of the patient's pain responded to a particular intervention, and very few studies have determined whether the clinical response lasted more than a few weeks or months. Nonetheless, several drugs are widely used clinically to treat patients with neuropathic pain, but they need further discussion and evaluation to determine their effectiveness.

Antisympathetic Agents

In some patients, neuralgias can present with spontaneous burning pain and evidence of sympathetic dysfunction in the affected limb. Mitchell, in his study of patients wounded in the Civil War, termed this painful state *causalgia* because of the continuous burning pain that characterized the disorder (Mitchell 1864). Causalgia appears to be a distinct form of sympathetic dystrophy, although its clinical presentations can be extremely varied. Patients usually develop dysesthesias distal to the nerve trauma, although the actual area affected may extend well beyond the distribution of a specific nerve. In some patients, the cutaneous hypersensitivity is severe, with pain evoked by light touch or "hairbending" (allodynia). Most patients also experience a continuous, spontaneous pain in the affected region. This pain is often exacerbated by any intense stimulus, such as bright light or loud noise. Emotional excitement may also increase the pain.

The sensory changes in causalgia are associated with disturbances in the sympathetic innervation of the affected area (Schwartzman and McLellan 1987, Rasmussen and Freedman 1946, Pak et al. 1970). Vasomotor changes are often seen, with the affected limb appearing pink and warm or cold and mottled. The skin is often thin and edematous, and bone resorption may occur (see also Chapter 7).

Disorders of sympathetic tone may be important in the development and maintenance of pain in the causalgic limb. Sympathectomy by either surgery or local anesthetic block frequently relieves the pain in causalgia, and in the opinion of some, pain relief by sympathetic block is an essential part of the diagnosis (Schwartzman and McLellan 1987, Pak et al. 1970, Loh and Nathan 1978).

Although there is no single, well-accepted explanation for the pain relief that follows sympathetic blockade, sympathetic efferents may potentially interact with cutaneous afferents to produce pain by several mechanisms: (1) There may be "cross-talk" between sympathetic efferents and unmyelinated sensory afferents; (2) there may be abnormal synaptic contacts between sensory afferents and fine-caliber cutaneous afferents within the skin; or (3) there may be an excessive sympathetic outflow that causes a change in vascular permeability and an elevation in extracellular algesic substances that produce pain. There is evidence for and against each of these potential mechanisms. The concept that there is an excessive or abnormal sympathetic contribution in these disorders has led to trials of regional and systemic antisympathetic agents.

Sympathetic Blockade.   A number of open studies have reported pain relief in patients with causalgia after sympathetic blockade with direct ganglionic blocks, an intravenous injection of guanethidine restricted to the painful limb below an arterial tourniquet, or systemic intravenous phentolamine. Clinically, patients may report an extended period of reduced pain that can last hours to months, well beyond the initial effect of the drug. There is evidence that the analgesic effect is related to the effectiveness of the chemical sympathectomy, as judged by objective tests. Unfortunately, despite the common use of sympathetic blocks, the reported studies of pain relief have been largely anecdotal case reports or open, uncontrolled patient series. Careful, controlled trials of antisympathetic treatments need to be performed to determine their true indications and effectiveness in patients with neuropathic pain states.

Oral Antisympathetic Agents.   Oral antisympathetic agents have been tried in a small number of open, uncontrolled series of patients with painful neuropathy. Loh and Nathan (1978) reported oral guanethidine to be effective in relieving pain in a small series of patients with a variety of neuropathic syndromes. Using oral phenoxybenzamine, an adrenergic blocker, Ghostine et al. (1984) reported relief in 40 consecutive patients with causalgia. Because oral or intravenous propranolol, a beta blocker, is reportedly ineffective in patients with painful neuralgia, these findings are consistent with experimental work on rat peripheral neuromas that suggests that damaged afferent fibers develop alpha- but not beta-adrenergic receptors.

Anticonvulsants

Although the findings in the reports cited above are consistent with the model of sympathetic mediation of pain in some patients with painful neuropathy, relatively few painful peripheral nerve disorders are associated with major evidence of sympathetic dysfunction, and even fewer respond to sympathetic blocks with local anesthetics. In patients with neuropathic pain with little or no sympathetic component, anticonvulsants and antidepressant drugs are frequently prescribed, although there is only limited evidence that such treatments are effective.

The anticonvulsant phenytoin (Dilantin) has a direct effect on both the peripheral nerve and the synaptic endings associated with a decrease in the inward sodium current across the axon membrane. Several studies provide evidence that phenytoin may have a role in the management of clinical neuropathic pain syndromes. The effectiveness of phenytoin has been studied most in the treatment of trigeminal neuralgia, for which phenytoin can provide sustained pain relief. With standard oral doses, the therapeutic effect usually begins within the first 3 days of treatment; the benefit includes both a reduction of the number of attacks of lancinating pain and a decrease in the severity of each attack. In anecdotal reports that include only a few patients, phenytoin is reported to have a beneficial effect on pain in other forms of specific neuralgia, including postherpetic neuralgia and glossopharyngeal neuralgia. Phenytoin has also been used for pain relief in more generalized neuropathies, including Fabry's disease and diabetic neuropathy.

Because phenytoin has direct effects on both axonal conduction and synaptic transmission, the principal site of action for pain relief in peripheral neuropathy could be at the level of the abnormal nerve or within the central nervous system. Since the lesion is peripheral, a peripheral site of action of drug effect would seem most likely. There is much evidence, however, that phenytoin also has a central effect in pain relief. Several open studies report that phenytoin and other anticonvulsants are effective in treating paroxysmal pain, including trigeminal neuralgia, in patients with multiple sclerosis, a central nervous system disorder. Anecdotal reports also describe beneficial responses in patients with central pain after stroke. Phenytoin seems particularly effective in treating sharp, lancinating pain; because the membrane effects of drug reduce the ability of axons to follow high rates of response, phenytoin may be of value in managing pain associated with high-frequency, synchronized discharges in peripheral or central axons.

Carbamazepine (Tegretol) is chemically related to the tricyclic antidepressants, especially imipramine. Its primary clinical usefulness, however, is as an anticonvulsant. Carbamazepine may have its principal effect on pain suppression at central synapses. Consistent with this view, carbamazepine depresses sensory transmission in the caudal trigeminal nucleus at low doses and may also have an effect at the thalamic level.

Like phenytoin, carbamazepine has been studied most extensively in the treatment of trigeminal neuralgia (Dalessio 1991). Carbamazepine is effective in 80% of trigeminal neuralgia patients within 24 hours, although the site of its action is only speculative. In treating trigeminal neuralgia, carbamazepine is clinically superior to phenytoin. Although results have been less well documented, carbamazepine is reported to be useful in a variety of other forms of neuropathic pain, including tabetic pain, postherpetic neuralgia, and diabetic neuropathy.

Pain due to primary central nervous system lesions may also occasionally respond to carbamazepine therapy. In two open-patient series, carbamazepine was reported to relieve the paroxysmal episodes of painful tonic spasm due to multiple sclerosis. It may also be useful in the management of pain in other forms of myelopathy.

Clonazepam (Klonopin) is a benzodiazepine frequently used in the management of neuropathic pain. Benzodiazepines facilitate both the presynaptic and postsynaptic inhibition, increase recurrent inhibition, and decrease the firing rate of normal and epileptic neurons in the brain. The pharmacologic effect appears to be due primarily to facilitation of the inhibitory neurotransmitter gamma-aminobutyric acid (GABA). This facilitation is mediated through benzodiazepine receptors, which are part of the GABA receptor complex.

There are several clinical reports that cite clonazepam as a treatment for chronic neuralgic pain. Most of these have studied the role of clonazepam in treating cranial neuralgias. In the majority of studies, clonazepam was found to be as effective as both carbamazepine and phenytoin, with few side effects.

Tricyclic antidepressant drugs are frequently used to treat pain after peripheral nerve injury. Tricyclic iminodibenzyl derivatives such as amitriptyline (Elavil) are the most commonly used drugs. Their major pharmacologic effect appears to be facilitation of monoamine transmission by inhibition of synaptic serotonin and norepinephrine reuptake. The site of action of tricyclic antidepressants in pain relief is not clear.

Nociceptive transmission through the dorsal horn is under powerful inhibition from descending brain stem pathways that arise in the region of the ventromedial medulla and the locus ceruleus of the pons (Mokha et al. 1986, Duggan 1985) (see Chapter 2). Serotonin and norepinephrine are important neurotransmitters in these descending systems. Extensive studies in animals provide evidence that these pathways may, in part, mediate the analgesia produced by systemic morphine as well as endogenous, conditioned analgesia (Basbaum and Fields 1978a, 1978b). Tricyclic antidepressant drugs may work by potentiating the effects of these descending analgesic pathways. Although tricyclic antidepressants have little analgesic potency by themselves, they strongly potentiate the analgesic effect of morphine. Botney and Fields (1983) demonstrated that spinal administration of amitriptyline potentiates the analgesic effects of systemic morphine, evidence that tricyclic antidepressants may work in part by influencing descending inhibitory systems at the level of the spinal cord.

Tricyclic antidepressants also have major effects on ascending monoaminergic systems that project into the forebrain. Changes in these pathways probably account for the antidepressant effect of these drugs. It seems likely that these ascending systems also are important in pain perception, although how antidepressant drugs influence sensory pathways at the level of the thalamus and cortex remains speculative. Also unresolved is the relationship between the antidepressant effect of tricyclic drugs and their beneficial effect on pain.

A number of studies report a beneficial effect of tricyclic antidepressants in patients with neuropathic pain. Unfortunately, most of these reports are anecdotal case studies using different tricyclics in varying dosages, often in combination with other medications. The number of patients who benefited from tricyclics varied greatly between studies, with anywhere from 27% to 100% of patients treated experiencing therapeutic benefit.

In open studies of clomipramine (Anafranil) in patients with neuralgias of varying etiology, several authors report a beneficial drug effect on clinical pain. Single-blind and double-blind studies confirmed these results. Watson et al. (1982) used a double-blind amitriptyline-placebo crossover protocol to convincingly demonstrate an analgesic effect in postherpetic neuralgia. Age and duration of symptoms did not correlate with outcome. Patients who were clinically depressed had better pain relief with amitriptyline; however, pain relief did not correlate with a change in clinical symptoms of depression. Tricyclic antidepressants also have been given to patients with painful diabetic neuropathy in a double-blind active placebo crossover study, with clear benefit independent of antidepressant effects (Max et al. 1987). The clinical studies to date provide evidence that adrenergic tricyclic drugs can reduce reported pain in patients with a variety of neuropathic pain states.

We know little about the basic mechanisms that produce and sustain pain after injury to the nervous system. Although recent studies demonstrate that peripheral lesions can induce changes in the dorsal horn, thalamus, and cortex, the factors that induce these changes and the relationship that such changes have to clinical pain are obscure (Zimmermann 1983a, 1983b, Pagni 1984, Sherman et al. 1984). Most patients with injury to the peripheral nerve or central somatosensory pathways do not develop clinically significant pain; it therefore remains unclear how patients with neuropathic pain differ in the responses to nervous system trauma. A better understanding of the basic mechanisms that underlie chronic neuropathic pain is essential to design more effective medical therapy.

The true effectiveness of any of these treatments depends on sustained functional improvement as judged by objective criteria and by the subjective assessment of the patient. Although a small number of well-controlled studies demonstrate that antidepressants and anticonvulsants do affect neuropathic pain, very few studies continued to follow up patients for longer than a few weeks, and it is unclear whether the therapeutic response was significant enough in most studies to make a functional improvement in the patient's condition. Addressing this issue, Sherman et al. (1984) polled more than 2,500 postamputation military veterans and found that 78% had persistent phantom limb pain. Although there are numerous reports of medical success in treatment of this problem, less than 1% of the patients in this sample reported any meaningful response to the treatments offered, including those discussed above.

Psychological Factors Affecting Response to Medications

Although there are a variety of studies of psychological profiles of chronic pain patients, there is little agreement about the frequency or nature of psychological diagnoses that contribute to the disability associated with chronic pain. Depressive symptoms are, however, common in patients with chronic pain, and a diagnosis of clinical depression can be made in approximately one-third of patients. There is also considerable symptomatic overlap between depression and anxiety. Between 60% and 70% of depressed patients are anxious, and 40–90% of anxious patients develop an episode of major depression (Dubrovsky 1993). The relationship between pain, anxiety, and depression in such patients is complex. The pain threshold is lowered in clinically depressed patients, and pain is a common complaint in patients who have primary depression. Patients with pain associated with chronic somatic disease also frequently develop depressive symptoms; however, the incidence of depression defined by strict clinical criteria is not clearly different in chronic pain patients when compared with medically ill patients without pain. Therefore, although patients with chronic pain often have symptoms of depression, it is not clear if these symptoms are a result of their pain problem or a contributory factor in their pain. For initial clinical management, the distinction may be unimportant. Antidepressant drugs can stabilize the sleep pattern and improve the dysphoric symptoms of patients with chronic pain. There is often a reduction in the intensity of reported pain that may be associated with a decrease in the requirement for analgesics. Antidepressants therefore have an important role in the management of chronic pain, although it is still uncertain whether these drugs act primarily to potentiate analgesics or to relieve depressive symptoms.

References

Basbaum AI, Fields HL. Endogenous pain control mechanisms: review and hypothesis. Ann Neurol 1978a;4:451.

Basbaum AI, Fields HL. Endogenous pain control systems: brainstem spinal pathways and endorphin circuitry. Rev Neurosci 1978b;7:309.

Botney M, Fields HL. Amitriptyline potentiates morphine analgesia by a direct action on the central nervous system. Ann Neurol 1983;13:160.

Cohen JA, Gross KF. Peripheral neuropathy: causes and management in the elderly. Geriatrics 1990;45:21.

Collins GB, Kiefer KS. Propoxyphene dependence: an update. Postgrad Med 1981;70:57.

Dalessio DJ. Diagnosis and treatment of cranial neuralgias. Med Clin North Am 1991;75:605.

Dixon P, Higginson I. AIDS and cancer pain treated with slow release morphine. Postgrad Med J 1991;67(suppl):S92.

Dubrovsky S. Approaches to developing new anxiolytics and antidepressants. J Clin Psychiatry 1993;54(suppl):5.

Duggan AW. Pharmacology of descending control systems. Philos Trans R Soc Lond B Biol Sci 1985;308:375.

Foreman RD, Schmidt RF, Willis WD. Convergence of muscle and cutaneous input onto primate spinothalamic tract neurons. Brain Res 1977; 124:555.

Ghostine SY, Comair YG, Turner DM. Phenoxybenzamine in the treatment of causalgia. Report of 40 cases. J Neurosurg 1984;60:1263.

Goldstein G. Pentazocine. Drug Alcohol Depend 1985;14:313.

Gonzales GR, Herskovitz S, Rosenblum M, et al. Central pain from cerebral abscess: thalamic syndrome in AIDS patients with toxoplasmosis. Neurology 1992;42:1107.

Jaspan J, Maselli R, Herold K, Bartkus C. Treatment of severely painful diabetic neuropathy with an aldose reductase inhibitor: relief of pain and improved somatic and autonomic nerve function. Lancet 1983; 2:758.

Lindblom U, Verrillo RT. Sensory functions in chronic neuralgia. J Neurol Neurosurg Psychiatry 1979;42:422.

Loh L, Nathan PW. Painful peripheral states and sympathetic blocks. J Neurol Neurosurg Psychiatry 1978;41:664.

Maciewicz R, Mason P, Strassman A, Potrebic S. Organization of trigeminal nociceptive pathways. Semin Neurol 1988;8:255.

Martin WR. Role of agonist/antagonist analgesics in medicine. Drug Alcohol Depend 1985;14:221.

Masten LW. Effect of repeated oral propoxyphene administration on toxicity and microsomal metabolism in the mouse. Drug Alcohol Depend 1980;5:87.

Max MB, Culnane M, Schafer SC. Amitriptyline relieves diabetic neuropathy pain in patients with normal or depressed mood. Neurology 1987;37:589.

McFarland HR. Chronic traumatic trigeminal neuralgia. South Med J 1982;75:814.

Mitchell SW, Morehouse GR, Keen WW. Gunshot Wounds and Other Injuries of Nerves. New York: Lippincott, 1864.

Mokha SS, McMillan JA, Iggo A. Pathways mediating descending control of spinal nociceptive transmission from the nuclei locus coeruleus (LC) and raphe magnus (NRM) in the cat. Exp Brain Res 1986;61:597.

Pagni C. Central Pain Due to Spinal Cord and Brainstem Damage. In PD Wall, R Melzack (eds), Textbook of Pain. London: Churchill Livingstone, 1984;481.

Pak TJ, Martin GM, Magness JL, Kavanaugh MD. Reflex sympathetic dystrophy. Minn Med 1970;53:507.

Portenoy RK, Duma C, Foley KM. Acute herpetic and postherpetic neuralgia: clinical review and current management. Ann Neurol 1986;20:651.

Rasmussen TB, Freedman H. Treatment of causalgia. An analysis of 100 cases. J Neurosurg 1946;3:165.

Riddle MC. Diabetic neuropathies in the elderly: management update. Geriatrics 1990;45:32.

Schwartzman RJ, McLellan TL. Reflex sympathetic dystrophy: a review. Arch Neurol 1987;44:555.

Sessle BJ, Hu JW, Amano N, Zhong G. Convergence of cutaneous, tooth pulp, visceral, neck, and muscle afferents onto nociceptive and nonnociceptive neurons in trigeminal subnucleus caudalis (medullary dorsal horn) and its implications for referred pain. Pain 1986;27:219.

Sherman R, Sherman CJ, Parker L. Chronic phantom and stump pain among American veterans: results of a survey. Pain 1984;18:83.

Strommen GL, Pucino F, Tight RR, Beck CL. Human infection with herpes zoster: etiology, pathophysiology, diagnosis, clinical course, and treatment. Pharmacotherapy 1988;8:52.

Tasker RR. Deafferentation. In PD Wall, R Melzack (eds), Textbook of Pain. London: Churchill Livingstone, 1984;119.

Watson CP, Evans RJ, Reed K, et al. Amitriptyline versus placebo in postherpetic neuralgia. Neurology 1982:32:671.

Zimmermann M. Central Nervous System Changes and Deafferentation: The Role of Reorganization and Gliosis. In JJ Bonica, U Lindblom, A Iggo (eds), Advances in Pain Research and Therapy (Vol 5). New York: Raven, 1983a;656.

Zimmermann M. Deafferentation Pain: Chairman's Introduction. In JJ Bonica, U Lindblom, A Iggo (eds), Advances in Pain Research and Therapy (Vol 5). New York: Raven, 1983b;661.

4   Evaluation of Chronic Pain Patients

Theresa Hoskins Michel

The term *evaluation* encompasses both assessment and measurement of a phenomenon. *Assessment* is a critical process that assists in the clinical management of a problem. *Measurement* is an objective quantification of an entity.

Assessment of Chronic Pain Patients

To assess chronic pain, as much as possible must be learned about the patient as a whole. Chronic pain is measured by breaking it down into component parts: intensity, quality, timing, and location. These parts are then quantified to have a basis for comparison with pain measurement at other times. The following purposes of evaluation can then be achieved:

1. Establish a baseline from which to plan and begin interventions.
2. Assist in the selection of appropriate interventions.
3. Make possible the evaluation of efficacy of interventions.

Chronic pain is a multidimensional condition and therefore involves a wide range of parameters that should be considered in its evaluation. Because pain is also a subjective experience unique to the individual, it presents a challenge to the person who evaluates it. Melzack and Casey (1968) suggest that pain is a sensory experience with motivational and affective properties. The following inclusive listing of assessment parameters was developed by McGuire and Sheidler (1993):

Physiologic Location, onset, associated factors, duration, type of pain, syndrome, anatomy, and physiology

Sensory Intensity, quality, and pattern

Affective Distress, anxiety, depression, mental state, perception of suffering, irritability, and agitation

Cognitive   Meaning of pain, thought processes, coping strategies, knowledge, attitudes, beliefs, previous treatments, and positive or negative influencing factors

Behavioral   Communication with others, interpersonal relationships, activities of daily living, behaviors (pain-related, preventive, or controlling), use of medications, sleep/rest patterns, and fatigue

Sociocultural   Ethnocultural background; family and social life; work and home responsibilities; environment; familial attitudes, beliefs, and behaviors; and personal attitudes and beliefs

It is clear from this list of pain dimensions that assessing the patient with chronic pain is not a simple and straightforward task. A number of problems are encountered when one is assessing pain in patients. The most significant problem is that it is sometimes difficult to see the pain from the patient's point of view. Patients are the foremost experts on their pain. McCaffery and Beebe (1989) have suggested their own definition of pain, as quoted in Chapter 1. They emphasize that "the person with the pain is the only authority about the existence and nature of the pain, since the sensation of pain can be felt only by the person who has it" (McCaffery and Beebe 1989).

Another problem encountered when assessing clinical pain is its variable nature and instability. Patients with identical etiologies do not experience pain in the same way. The individual perceptions of and responses to pain are diverse. Awareness of this makes it less likely for the clinician to fall into the trap of assuming how the pain must feel to a patient based on previous experience with similar patients or pain states. Furthermore, it is impossible to validate or invalidate any statements a patient makes about his or her pain. Particular measures of pain may mean different things to different people, and a patient's rating of his or her pain cannot be verified by comparison with another measure, a different pain state, or another person's opinion.

A number of different patient characteristics influence the assessment of pain, such as educational level; the nature of the problem; presence of affective disorders; biobehavioral influences, such as psychological, cognitive-perceptual, behavioral, and psychophysiologic factors (Feuerstein and Beattie 1995); age; motor coordination; visual acuity; and ethnic background (McGuire 1988). Environmental factors, including the presence or absence of family members and friends during the assessment and the establishment of a therapeutic relationship between assessor and patient, also influence the assessment of pain. The degree to which the patient experiences suffering as a result of his or her pain is also a significant factor. Suffering is paired with pain when the patient feels out of control of his or her life, the source of pain is unknown, the pain is especially serious, or the pain is chronic (Moon 1985).

Physical therapists are often very comfortable with assessment of physical impairments related to flexibility, strength, and endurance. The difficulty arises when these common assessment techniques are applied to the patient with chronic pain who demonstrates "illness behaviors." There is often a discrepancy between the physical findings and the patient's functional abilities;

TABLE 4.1 Comparison of symptoms and signs of physical disease and inappropriate illness behavior in chronic backache

	Physical disease	Inappropriate illness behavior
Symptoms		
Pain	Localized	Tailbone pain
		Whole-leg pain
Numbness	Dermatomal	Whole-leg numbness
Weakness	Myotomal	Whole-leg loss of function
Time pattern	Variable	No pain-free intervals
Response to treatment	Variable benefit	Intolerance of treatment
		Emergency admissions
Signs		
Tenderness	Localized	Superficial, widespread, nonanatomic
Simulated rotation	No pain	Pain
Simulated axial loading	No pain	Pain
Raising straight leg	No change on distraction	Improves with distraction
Sensory	Dermatomal	Regional
Motor	Myotomal	Regional
General reaction	Appropriate reaction to pain	Over-reaction to pain (e.g., crying out, facial expression, muscle tension, sweating, collapsing)

SOURCE: Reprinted with permission from G Waddell, M Bircher, D Finlayson, CJ Main. Symptoms and signs: physical disease or illness behaviour? BMJ 1984;289:739.

the chronic pain patient is much more disabled than one would have predicted based on physical impairments alone. Responding to the complexities of performing impairment measures in the population of chronic pain patients, Waddell et al. (1992) have commented on the inadequacies of a variety of clinical assessments of nonspecific low back pain patients and have developed their own approach. They have tried to develop a tool that provides a clinical assessment of impairment based solely on objective physical signs; examination techniques that are reliable; findings that are clearly separable from cognitive, psychological, or behavioral features of illness; findings specific to low back pain; and physical findings that are a cause of disability. In their efforts to develop such a tool, they also suggest that the most difficult task is separating physical disease from illness behavior. Among the numerous physical tests they used, many test results strongly correlated with behavioral signs. Based on this work with chronic low back pain patients, Waddell (1984) has published a table comparing symptoms and signs of physical disease with abnormal illness behaviors in chronic low back pain (Table 4.1).

The mismatch between physical findings and illness behavior has been described with various terms, including *abnormal illness behavior, symptom magnification,* and *disability exaggeration.* Many such cases may be generated by desire for financial gain, attention, or care or an excuse to avoid work. Assigning these motives implies malingering on the part of chronic pain patients; however, deliberate malingering is relatively rare among people with pain-related work disability (Ogden-Niemeyer 1989).

Despite efforts to evaluate the purely physical causes of pain, the final physical impairment scale developed by Waddell et al. was more closely related to the affective scale of the McGill Pain Questionnaire (MPQ) than to the sensory scale, and more to the various measures of illness behavior than to pain itself (Appendix 4.1). They believe the only measure that ensures recognition of the impact of physical impairments is the performance of adequate cognitive and behavioral assessments to determine their contribution to disability as well. This separation of physical signs and symptoms from behavioral disability is evident in patients who show real physical improvement yet continue to be crippled by chronic pain. They do still have potential for rehabilitation, since their primary disability is that of functional limitations.

Disability may be regarded as learned avoidance behavior, which means patients have learned to avoid certain movements or functional activities based on past experience of pain. By avoiding activities, the patient's repertoire of social, job, recreational, or role-related tasks is reduced. The result is most likely deconditioning—that is, loss of the physiologic support for performance of more tasks or higher energy–cost tasks. By avoiding certain movement patterns, the person develops secondary physical impairments of muscle-strain patterns and weakness, which can directly lead to new pain onset. Thus, new acute pain may be superimposed on the original chronic pain condition by secondary impairments. For this reason, overall body condition should be evaluated, with specific attention to patterns of muscle use and disuse.

The challenge to the physical therapist who assesses the patient with chronic pain is to identify all of the essential components of the total pain picture for the patient and develop a complete picture of the whole person within his or her environment, rather than a sense of a specific pain. To do so requires a thorough patient interview, a physical examination to identify impairments, a careful selection of pain measurement tools, and a disability evaluation. The information acquired must then be integrated with the information retrieved by other members of the health care team, especially information from psychosocial assessments. There are three major areas requiring evaluation in patients presenting with chronic pain: pain assessment and measurement, impairment definition, and disability assessment. Each of these three areas is addressed with different therapeutic goals, and therapy of each has different outcomes. Treatment is more likely to succeed if it is targeted toward goals in each of these three categories.

Patient Interview

The major goal of the interview is to develop a complete understanding of the properties of the patient's pain experience. Using a pain diary that the patient fills out in advance (Appendix 4.2) or a pain flow sheet (Appendix 4.3) helps in beginning this process.

Interview questions should address the nature of the physical problem and how the problem has affected the patient's life. The following sequence is suggested for determining the nature of the pain problem:

1.   *Identify the pain area.* Ask the patient where the present pain is experienced. A body diagram, such as the one found in the McGill-Melzack Pain Questionnaire (Appendix 4.4), is useful. Both the area where the initial pain was felt (e.g., at the site of original injury) and the area where the pain is now experienced should be identified. It is also useful to ask the patient to judge the intensity of the pain or pains by using a simple numeric scale (0–10) or Visual Analogue Scale (VAS) (Chapman et al. 1985). Ask what levels on the pain scale represent the present pain at its worst and best. The speed of onset of pain should be addressed. A graph of the pain intensity over time can also be helpful. Discuss what previous interventions have helped the pain, including home remedies and alternative therapies such as acupuncture.

2.   *Explore the mechanism of injury.* Ask the patient how and when the pain started and whether the pain is acute, persistent, or a result of repetitive injury. The pain could be related to a traumatic injury or previous surgery, be insidious in onset, or arise when specific motions are repeated.

3.   *Elicit the previous history of injuries.* Ask about time missed from work due to any injury.

4.   *Identify activities, positions, and actions that make the pain feel worse or better.* The pain diary should help determine what work or home activities contribute to the pain and whether sitting, standing, or movement relieve or aggravate the pain. Stressors in the life of the patient that result in altered postures, increases in anxiety and irritability, and changes in muscle use patterns should be identified. Muscle imbalances are often the result of positional changes, guarding postures, and muscle disuse patterns.

5.   *Determine the patient's functional limitations and disabilities.* Ask about the pain's effect on sleep patterns, ability to work or perform household tasks, and sex life. There are a number of questionnaires available to help assess disability, some of which are specific to entities such as low back pain (Oswestry Low Back Pain Disability Questionnaire) (Appendix 4.5), and others that are intended for use with all types of pain (Health Status Questionnaire or SF-36) (Appendix 4.6).

6.   *Discuss the patient's activity level and exercise habits.* Ask specifically about how long the patient is able to walk, stand, or sit and the amount of weight the patient can lift and carry. Ask the patient to describe a typical day, as outlined in the pain diary (see Appendix 4.2).

7.   *Identify the patient's interests in recreational activities and hobbies,* and whether pain interferes with the pursuit of these. Also ask about individuals whom the patient lives with and how they are responding to the patient's pain.

8.   *Identify the work situation of the patient,* how the pain has affected that work, and if the patient is receiving worker's compensation or is involved in litigation.

Medication use should also be discussed with the patient. Many patients take pain-control medications that influence their responses and ability to participate in physical therapy programs. A brief description of medications and their impact on physical therapy treatment programs is included in Chapter 3.

Tables 4.2, 4.3, and 4.4 are hypothetical cases that illustrate questions asked of three different types of chronic pain patients during the therapist's interview and their responses. The therapist's interpretation of their responses is also included.

The patient interview should accomplish three main goals. First, the therapist and the patient should each have a much better sense of each other and of their therapeutic relationship. Second, the therapist should be able to determine whether there are musculoskeletal concerns that are more acute or repetitive in nature and whether they can be dealt with effectively with hands-on approaches. The therapist should also rule out potential diagnoses that could mean serious disease and should be referred to a physician. Finally, the therapist may determine that the patient has chronic, persistent pain that is not amenable to physical interventions but interferes with the patient's functional capabilities, and that these functional limitations should be addressed in treatment.

Physical Examination

It is suggested that the patient interview and physical examination together offer nearly all of the necessary information required by a diagnostician to make the correct diagnosis (Kassirer and Kopelman 1991). In almost all cases, medical tests are much more costly and often more time consuming than the interview and physical examination and may yield less significant diagnostic information. The physical therapist has a large number of physical examination techniques available but needs to be selective in choosing which ones are appropriate to use with each patient. This selection process is determined by the patient's answers to the interview questions and the resulting hypotheses generated by the physical therapist. If the patient experiences reproducible back and hip pain with specific motions, the physical therapist would hypothesize that the problem is related to the musculoskeletal system and then test specific joint ranges, muscle lengths, and muscle strength. Thus, the physical examination of the patient with chronic pain may be very brief and simple or could become more involved, depending on the result of the interview process.

It may also be necessary to perform tests to determine postural alignment, breathing pattern, overload of cervical muscles involved in breathing, hyper- or hypomobility of joints, neural tension, muscle strength and endurance, tissue tenderness and soft-tissue tension, and vertebral position. These tests should help rule out certain diseases and rule in conditions treatable by the physical therapist. Basic observations of vital signs, mental status, gait, posture, and asymmetries should always be done.

The patient's ability to perform physically is often the most important part of the examination. It is better to actually observe patients performing transfers, ambulating, negotiating environmental barriers, and so on, rather than relying

TABLE 4.2 The patient interview: chronic pain in a patient without chronic pain syndrome

Question to patient	Examples of possible answers	Interpretation
When did your pain start?	In an accident 2 years ago—my car was struck from the rear.	This is a common injury.
Where is your pain?	In my neck, shoulders, back, and hips. I also feel numbness in both legs when I lie down.	This makes no anatomic sense. Be suspicious that this chronic pain has a major psychologic component.
On a scale of 0–10, how would you rate your pain?	0/10 up to 8/10. I have episodes of no pain, and some very bad days.	It is good that he reports episodes of no pain. He may not be a chronic pain patient.
How do you describe your pain?	Aching and pulling.	
How often do you get this pain?	I was fine until 2 weeks ago when it started again. It's been constant since then.	Is this recurrent pain or reinjury?
What makes your pain worse?	All physical activity, mostly with my arms.	This pattern could lead to avoidance of all activity.
What makes your pain better?	Heat, massage, and physical therapy.	These may be passive role therapies.
How often have you had physical therapy treatment?	I have had three separate physical therapists.	He is seeking complete relief.
What treatments?	Ice, ultrasound, massage, exercise. Every time I exercised I felt better.	This is a very good sign.
Are you exercising on your own?	No, I am afraid I will hurt myself. I have five kids to look after when I get home from work.	He does not follow through on a home program and takes a passive role for pain relief. He is looking for a complete cure. He uses family and work as an excuse to avoid his responsibility for caring for himself.
What is your work?	I am a salesman. I spend 40–50 hours per week driving in my car.	This is a very inactive job.
Is your sleep interrupted?	Yes, I have trouble falling asleep.	This is probably anxiety and is very common in chronic pain patients.
Your F-36 shows that your physical functioning is severely limited with severe pain and low vitality. Your mental health score is low enough to suspect depression. Are you depressed?	No, only because of the pain I have. Without pain my life would be perfect. I have wonderful children, my wife loves me, my business is fine.	Be suspicious of depression.
What are you most afraid that the pain will do to you?	That it will get worse and worse and I will end up in a wheelchair. I would not be able to provide for my family.	He is catastrophizing and exaggerating what could happen.

on patient recall of such activities. Signs of pain behaviors during activities, such as limping, guarding, rubbing, or grimacing, should be watched for. These signs may alert the diagnostician to the degree of behavioral factors involved in the patient's pain experience, as opposed to the physical or mechanical causes of pain. It is during the process of observation of functional activities that a pain behavioral assessment can be performed. Most chronic pain patients have

TABLE 4.3 The patient interview: chronic pain in a well-adjusted patient

Question to patient	Example of possible answers	Interpretation
When did your pain start?	Five years ago, but I'm not sure exactly when.	Chronic pain is lasting much longer than the expected healing period.
Where is your pain?	It is mostly in my legs.	
On a scale of 0 to 10, how would you rate your pain?	4/10 at best; 10/10 at worst. Sometimes it doesn't bother me at all; sometimes it interferes with the things I need to do.	She is coping well.
How do you describe your pain?	Pins and needles and shooting. It feels like ants crawling.	This sounds like peripheral neuropathy.
How often is your pain present?	Most of the time, but it fluctuates in intensity.	This is also a consistent description of peripheral neuropathy.
What makes your pain worse?	It is not consistent, but it worsens with all activity.	She functions in spite of pain.
What makes your pain better?	Medication and keeping busy.	She is coping well and using medications and distraction appropriately.
What do you do for your pain?	Heat, ice, self-massage.	She has good coping techniques.
What can you not do now that you would like to be able to do?	Stair climbing, going shopping for 3 hours at a time.	These are attainable goals.
How is your sleep?	Sometimes I have difficulty sleeping because of my pain.	This is probably a physical problem, not depression.
Do you work?	I house clean all day once a week, then I'm too tired the next day to do anything.	She needs to be provided with pacing information.
Did you ever have a job?	Yes, I was a schoolteacher, but now I'm retired.	This is consistent with age.
Was it early retirement?	Yes.	Did her pain influence her decision to retire? Ask!
Did you retire because of your pain?	No, I became caretaker for my son who died of AIDS.	Retirement was definitely not related to this pain.
How much does the pain interfere with your life?	I am more tired than usual. I cannot do as much as I would like. I can't keep up with my grandchildren.	This seems a realistic fatigue response. The impact on her life seems proportionate to the amount of pain she describes.
What can I help you with?	Help me walk better, climb stairs, and be less fatigued.	She may benefit from an ankle-foot orthosis.

AIDS = acquired immunodeficiency syndrome.

an activity intolerance problem rather than a medical problem. It is the activity intolerance that must be assessed in these cases.

Determining Impairments
Physical therapists have traditionally focused on impairments in their evaluation and treatment of patients. Muscle function problems involving strength and endurance, flexibility, joint range of motion, muscle tone, and structural

TABLE 4.4   The patient interview: chronic pain syndrome patient

Question to patient	Examples of possible answers	Interpretation
When did your pain start?	My pain started about 3 years ago when I had an accident at work.	This is chronic pain. Healing of tissues is finished.
Where is your pain?	In my back and down both legs.	This pattern of pain is plausible and warrants further questioning.
On a scale of 0–10, how would you rate your pain?	10 out of 10.	A maximal pain rating is suspicious for chronic pain syndrome.
What makes your pain worse?	Everything I do makes it worse.	He is catastrophizing. With deconditioning and secondary joint pathologies, his pain response to all activities seems likely.
What makes your pain better?	Medication and lying down make it better.	He has a passive lifestyle, is displaying avoidance behavior, and is dependent on medication.
How many hours do you lie down?	21 out of 24.	He is deconditioned and severely disabled.
How is your sleep?	I cannot sleep; I am too tense.	He is anxious and irritable. His waking up at night may be due to depression.
What can you now not do because of your pain that you used to do? General activity Bending Lifting Stooping Carrying Sitting Standing	I used to walk 20 minutes every day. Now I can't do anything. I never bend, lift, stoop, carry, sit, stand, or walk. My sitting tolerance is 10 minutes. I can walk 5 minutes. I can stand for 6 minutes.	He has a fear avoidance, fear of pain, and fear of reinjury. His sitting tolerance could be a misinterpretation of tolerance. His answers could be litigation driven and could be based on his low expectation for function.
What activities do you do outside of work?	I used to go bowling and socialize every weekend. Now I do not bowl, I never go out, and I watch TV.	This low activity tolerance could be depression or fear-avoidance based on low self-esteem and low self-efficacy.
Can you climb stairs?	No, I sleep on the sofa. I never have sex.	He demonstrates fear-avoidance.
Can you grocery shop? Can you perform housework?	I never used to need any help. Now I can't shop, cook, or clean. I get help from my mother or someone else.	His dependency on his family may be meeting his unmet dependency needs. There may be disturbed role functioning.
Do you live alone?	Yes.	
Who does chores for you?	Now my ex-wife or mother comes over to do everything.	The patient's family may contribute to his illness behavior.
Do you work?	No.	He does not perceive a need to work.
Do you like your job?	My job is too demanding. I hate my boss.	Apparent job dissatisfaction is a common problem contributing to disability.
How long were you working at this job?	6 months.	He does not have a stable work pattern.
Are you now receiving worker's compensation?	No, but I have a lawyer.	There are likely to be employer conflicts. This predicts a poor outcome in rehabilitation.
Are you thinking of going back to your job?	No, I am applying for disability benefits.	This answer demonstrates passive-dependence and probable secondary gains.
Are you planning to go back to work at any time?	I will go back to work when my pain is gone.	This is a pain-contingent behavior and is not realistic.

TABLE 4.4 *(continued)*

Question to patient	Examples of possible answers	Interpretation
It sounds like the pain that you have has had a great impact on your life.	[Patient bursts into tears.] Yes, I am worthless; I cry all the time. I can't live like this. I hate my life; if only something could be done for my pain.	Depression is very common in chronic pain patients. It is helped a lot by medications. Make use of psychiatrist's expertise for assistance. Check his MPI scores for dysfunctional profile and MMPI for depression scores.
Do you have a psychiatric diagnosis?	No.	Depression can run in families. If never diagnosed in the patient, find out about the family.
What would you do a year from now if you had no pain?	All my problems would be solved. I'd be just fine.	The patient has unrealistic expectations for treatment. Pain is the scapegoat for all of the patient's problems.

MPI = Multidimensional Pain Inventory; MMPI = Minnesota Multiphasic Personality Inventory.

deformities are most common. The goal of an objective musculoskeletal assessment is to determine which structures reproduce the patient's pain when stressed. To accomplish this, the patient is examined for active and passive range of motion, muscle strength, endurance, and motor control. Specific tests of muscle, ligament, and nerve structures can be performed. Mechanically derived pain is altered by movement or position and is most likely intermittent or variable. Chemically derived pain relates to inflammation, in which chemical irritants that are a part of the inflammatory process cause the pain. An unstable joint can result in chronic inflammation, which is worsened by movement into certain ranges. Thus, mechanical pain can provoke chemical pain or make it worse. Appropriate stabilization of the unstable joint can reduce inflammation and pain. Inflammatory pain is worsened by movement but gradually declines because inflammation is time limited and responsive to anti-inflammatory treatment.

Biomechanical assessments can also help the physical therapist determine patient physical impairments. Leg-length differences, pronated feet, ligamentous laxity, and bony hypertrophy are examples of impairments to assess in cases in which the history suggests that any of these factors may be involved in the patients symptomatology. Janda (1990) evaluated cases of chronic pain using electromyography (EMG) and developed a theoretical framework that describes the most frequently encountered muscle imbalances that contribute to pain. He describes a characteristic muscle pattern in which postural tonic muscles have a tendency to shorten, tighten, and become hyperactive. Phasic muscles, however, tend to weaken and become hypoactive. Both tonic and phasic muscle adaptations clearly lead to an even greater degree of impairment with muscle imbalances, postural deformities, potential for additional nociception, and damage. To evaluate impairments, palpation for muscle spasm and tightness, hypotonia, weakness, and trigger points may be substituted for EMG. Janda provides an example of the evaluation of a patient with cervical pain. With the patient standing, the positions of both scapulae and the interscapular space are observed. Tightness will pull one scapula closer to the thoracic spinous process, and weakness will flatten the space and make it appear hollow. Tightness in the upper trapezius presents as a more prominent muscle belly, with a straightening of the neck to shoulder line. A tight pectoralis major leads to rounded, protracted shoulders. In the forward head posture, the deep neck flexors are usually weak, whereas the sternocleidomastoids are tight and frequently acquire trigger points. Weakness is rarely discovered using manual muscle testing for these muscles. It is more instructive to observe movement patterns for coordination, timing, and the sequence of activation of muscles during simple weight-bearing activities. Weak postural muscles such as erector spinae will likely be activated inappropriately during certain movement patterns such as a sit-up. Instead of a reflex inhibition, these muscles are hyperactive during abdominal contractions, and sit-ups can actually worsen back pain in patients for this reason (Janda 1990). Alternative measures of muscle strength can include a maximum isometric lift test or a 10 RM (DeLorme) strength test. These are objective measures and relate more closely to functional limitations of patients. Range-of-motion measures with a standard goniometer and fingertip-to-floor distance tests are helpful in measuring flexibility (DiFabio et al. 1995). Evaluation of musculoskeletal problems includes observation of range of motion, muscle symmetry, body posture, movement symmetry; and arm- and leg-length discrepancies; manual muscle testing; identification of muscle trigger points by the "jump sign"; and examination for signs of scoliosis or other curvatures. Variations in strength between proximal and distal muscle groups should be checked. Stepping up and down steps or squatting and rising help in determining functional strength of hip extensors and knee extensors. Toe and heel rises help determine functional strength of lower leg muscles. Balance is necessarily a part of this evaluation. A neurologic examination may be necessary, including evaluation of neuro-ophthalmologic function, coordination, and motor performance. Disturbances of muscle tone, bulk, and symmetry and the presence of spasticity, rigidity, and tremor should also be evaluated. Sensory testing, including vision and hearing, light touch, pain, vibration, and deep tendon reflex testing, should be performed to assess neurologic integrity. In addition, impairments such as autonomic disturbances can be tested using evaluations of skin temperature, color, surface trophic changes, presence of edema, sweat or absence of sweat, hypersensitivity to touch, and allodynia (pain response to any light touch stimulation). Perceptual and cognitive deficits should be noted.

Impairments associated with neuropathic pain involve loss of sensory input and motor control. Sensory testing for light touch, vibration sense, temperature, and pain is useful. Cranial nerve testing is only slightly more complex and may be indicated for patients with headache or head trauma. Motor control testing clearly involves both muscle strength, endurance, and movement pattern assessment. Standard tests of coordination include the Romberg test, rapid alternating movements, and finger-to-nose tests. Neuropathic pain is often described as "shooting," "lancinating," "electric," or "lightning-like." Neuropathic pain can be accompanied by hypersensitivity to touch and allodynia.

Sympathetically maintained pain is a special form of neuropathic pain. In addition to allodynia and hyperalgesia, signs of autonomic dysfunction such as skin discoloration and temperature, edema, hair loss, and shiny skin surface are common. Some patients have a body part that is red, very hot, shiny, and swollen. Others have a white or mottled, cold, shiny, and hairless body part. Edema is variable. Over time, the patient loses muscle and atrophy becomes apparent. Deformities of feet and hands occur, with shortened tendons, hollow spaces where muscle bellies belong, and deformed joints. Osteopenia shows up on x-ray, and fractures may occur. Dysfunction is extreme, as patients protect their painful part and stop using it altogether. Disability and handicap commonly occur at later stages.

Secondary conditions occur as a result of a primary condition that disables a person (Pope and Tarlov 1991). The primary condition can be a pathology, an impairment, a functional limitation, or a different disability. Secondary impairments occur in the presence of a primary condition and can lead to additional disability. In chronic pain patients, common secondary conditions include depression, deconditioning, and loss of social role (inability to work). Secondary conditions can also include new sources of pain derived from muscle weakness that lead to altered movement patterns; shortened, weakened structures; and tight, overactive muscles. Secondary impairments are very common and will become worse if primary impairments are not identified and corrected. Neither primary nor secondary impairment necessarily leads to disability, however. There are examples of polio and rheumatoid arthritis patients who have major impairments in muscle weakness and painful joints but can function in spite of their pain by substitution of muscle groups. They may even be able to lead lives that include full-time employment, sports activities, and a relatively high quality of living. Patients with these conditions often develop more and more secondary conditions, however. In poliomyelitis, years of compensating for polio-wasted muscles causes the remaining muscle mass to be characterized by peripheral reinnervation by collateral sprouts from adjacent axons and muscle fiber hypertrophy (Grimby and Thoren Jonsson 1994). Eventually, these motor units succumb to the stresses of aging and their long-term loads, resulting in new impairments such as the development of joint instability, muscle weakness, joint and muscle pain, loss of function, and disability.

Usually, patients with chronic pain do not compensate well and avoid activities that result in pain. Indeed, fear of pain can frequently lead to fear of activity and a net decline in the number of functional activities a patient can perform. This leads to a very common secondary impairment of deconditioning. *Deconditioning* is defined as a loss of aerobic capacity or physical work capacity (Astrand and Rodahl 1986). To assess this impairment, it is possible to be very precise and obtain a measurement of the maximum oxygen consumption in patients using analysis of expired oxygen. Many chronic pain patients cannot perform even at their own low maximal level, however. To overcome this problem, there are a number of tests whose measurements correlate well with maximum oxygen consumption. One is a submaximal bicycle ergometer test. The workload-to–heart rate ratio obtained allows the therapist to predict maximum oxygen consumption using the Astrand nomogram (Astrand and Rodahl 1986). The 6-minute walk test is also a useful measure for prediction of maximum oxygen consumption. In this test the patient is encouraged to walk as far as possible in 6 minutes but may determine the speed and vary it as needed. The distance walked correlates with maximal oxygen consumption (Cooper 1968). Treadmill walking tests using specific protocols have been identified in the literature. Certain patients tolerate walking better than biking or tolerate a set speed on a treadmill better than being asked to set their own speed. Thus, the choice of test should be determined by the patient to be tested as much as by practicality issues or the therapist's preferences.

Pain Measurements

Many tools exist for the measurement of the sensory and emotional aspects of pain intensity. In the patient with chronic pain, however, it is best to keep such measurements short and simple so that pain is de-emphasized. An algorithm for helping the clinician select an appropriate pain measurement instrument is available (Figure 4.1). Often, patients are asked to rate their pain using a scale. The following Numeric Rating Scale also includes a verbal descriptor scale:

1 None
2 Mild
3 Moderate
4 Severe
5 Unbearable

Melzack's Present Pain Intensity Scale (PPI) on the MPQ is also useful:

0 No pain
1 Mild
2 Discomforting
3 Distressing
4 Horrible
5 Excruciating

Many clinicians simply ask for a number on a scale of 1–10, with 1 representing no pain and 10 the worst pain imaginable. This approach can also be used with a percentage scale or a scale of 1–100.

The VAS was first developed to measure subjective phenomena such as mood states (Maxwell 1978). It may be used as a pain intensity scale and consists of a horizontal or vertical line exactly 10 cm long with anchors at either end:

_____

No pain   Pain as bad as it
                                                 could possibly be

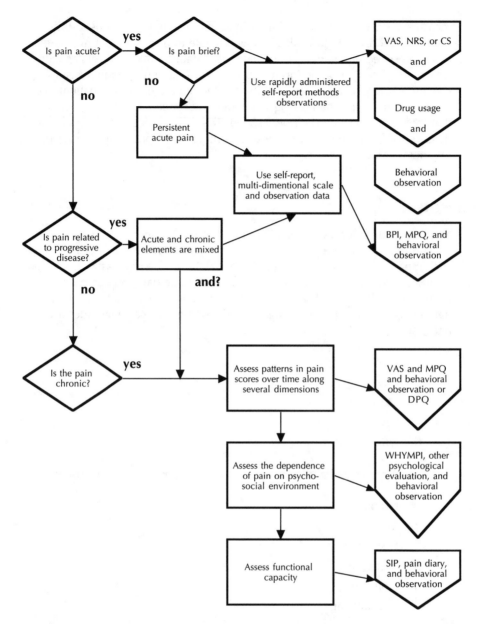

FIGURE 4.1 *Algorithm for selection of pain measurement instruments. (BPI = brief pain inventory; CS = category scale; DPQ = Dartmouth Pain Questionnaire; MPQ = McGill Pain Questionnaire; NRS = Numeric Rating Scale; SIP = Sickness Impact Profile; VAS = Visual Analogue Scale; WHYMPI = West Haven-Yale Multidimensional Pain Inventory.) (Modified with permission from J Bonica. The Management of Pain [2nd ed]. Philadelphia: Lea & Febiger, 1990;592.)*

The patient is asked to place a mark through the line at the point that best describes how much pain is experienced at a certain point. The measurement is taken as the distance in millimeters from the zero end to the mark made by the patient. The mark is the patient's pain rating and can be read as a number or a percent.

Measures that include the affective or emotional dimension of the pain experience generally include both the sensory dimension (pain intensity) and a subjective or reactive component. The Johnson Two-Component Scale is such a scale:

Pain sensation scale

0 ———————————————————————————— 10

No sensations   Medium   Maximum sensations

Pain distress scale

0 ———————————————————————————— 10

None   Slight   Moderate   Significant   Extreme

The MPQ is a multidimensional approach to measurement of pain (see Appendix 4.4). The MPQ includes a body diagram on which the patient draws the location and sensory aspects of pain using symbols or colors to differentiate aspects of pain. It also includes Melzack's PPI (illustrated above) and a section dedicated to differentiating the qualities of pain. This part consists of 20 different word lists used to measure the sensory, affective, evaluative, and other dimensions of pain. Patients are instructed to select only one word from any list and only those that apply to their pain experience. The final parts of the MPQ address the pattern of pain and factors that relieve and aggravate the pain. The patient's choice of words on the PPI are related to the pattern. This complex questionnaire has been used with many different pain populations and has been shown to have excellent reliability and predictive validity because it discriminates among groups of patients and different pain syndromes. It permits assessment of physiologic characteristics in the realms of sensory, affective, and cognitive experiences of pain and addresses the complexities of chronic pain (Turk et al. 1985).

Disability Assessment

Assessment of disability becomes the most important aspect of the evaluation once the patient's status as a chronic pain patient has been established. According to the data on disability from the 1983–1985 National Health Interview Surveys, the two leading causes of disability in the United States are orthopedic impairments and arthritis (National Institute on Disability and Rehabilitation Research 1988). Both conditions often lead to chronic pain. The relationship between chronic pain and disability depends on activity intolerance and failure to return to work (Hazard et al. 1994).

Because chronic pain becomes the major focus of the patient, pain becomes the single explanation for many problems the patient may be having and allows the patient to avoid dealing with these problems. Disability assessment is the most important part of the assessment of the patient with chronic pain.

The simplest approach to disability assessment is to determine the functional activities that cannot be performed and those that can be performed in spite of increasing or continuing pain. The therapist can create a list of relevant functional activities or choose a scale such as those developed for low back and neck pain. A pain scale or verbal analogue scale associated with each activity on the list can then yield specific data about functional limitations due to pain. Work-related disability assessment should list job specific tasks. See Chapter 11 for information on task analysis in disability assessment.

There are a number of health-related quality of life instruments that are applicable to many different types of patients. These questionnaires ask patients about functional abilities (see the Roland-Morris Disability Questionnaire in Appendix 4.7). The Health Status Questionnaire (SF-36) of the Medical Outcome Study (Ware and Sherbourne 1992) is also widely used (see Appendix 4.6). This questionnaire addresses physical functioning, role limitations due to physical and emotional problems, social functioning, general mental health, pain, energy, fatigue, and general health perceptions. It takes a patient approximately 10 minutes to fill out. A second, simpler option is the COOP chart method, which addresses physical, mental, and social aspects of pain; overall health change; social resources; and quality of life (COOP stands for Dartmouth Primary Care Cooperative Information Project) (Nelson et al. 1987). There are nine items the patient can fill out alone or with a clinician rating. The chart takes less than 10 minutes to complete (Nelson et al. 1987). A third option is the Duke University Health Profile (Parkerson et al. 1981). This scale permits assessment of symptom status and physical, emotional, and social function. It uses 64 self-report items and takes 20 minutes to complete. The Sickness Impact Profile (SIP) (Bergner et al. 1981) addresses physical and psychosocial aspects of the condition. This form has 136 items and takes 30 minutes to complete. The scale a-dapted for chronic pain patients specifically from the SIP is called the SIP Roland-Morris scale (Jensen et al. 1992). This disease-specific measure requires less time and correlates well with the MPQ and the Beck Depression Inventory.

The McMaster Health Index Questionnaire (MHIQ) covers physical, social, and emotional aspects of the patient's condition. Items addressing mobility, self-care, communication, global physical function, general well-being, work/social role, performance, social support, participation, global self-function, self-esteem, personal relationships, critical life events, and global emotional function are all included. Completion of the 59 questions takes 20 minutes (Chambers et al. 1982). The Nottingham Health Profile (McEwen 1988) is a 45-item self-report measure covering pain, physical mobility, sleep, emotional reactions, energy, social isolation, employment, household work, relationships, personal life, sex, hobbies, and vacations. It requires 10 minutes to complete. The Quality of Well-Being Scale is a 50-item scale covering functional performance in self-care, mobility, institutionalization, and social activities. Symptoms and problems are also addressed. This self-report measure takes 12 minutes (Fanshel and Bush 1970). The Functional Status Questionnaire is a 10-minute, 34-item self-report scale that addresses basic and intermediate activities of daily living, emotional function, anxiety, depression, quality of social interaction, social performance, occupational function, social activities, sexual function, global disability, global health satisfaction, and social contacts (Jette et al. 1986).

A number of disease-specific health status indexes are also available. For low back pain, four disability questionnaires, which are reprinted in their entirety (see Appendixes 4.1, 4.5, 4.6, and 4.8), are widely used.

More specific measures for chronic pain and disability exist as well. The Multidimensional Pain Inventory is an example (Kerns et al. 1985). A brief screening version of this inventory is included in Appendix 4.9.

Because psychosocial factors are extremely important in the problems of chronic pain patients, there are a number of psychological tests and social indexes available. In most cases, these tests are best administered by behavioral sciences professionals. The results can then be taken into account by the physical therapist. Coping attributes, major life adversity, and social support affect the presentation of chronic pain states. Clearly, identification of such factors will be most useful in planning physical therapy intervention strategies. One group of evaluators has clustered the following clinical subgroups of chronic pain patients based on their responses to measures of pain, disability, and depression: (1) chronic pain syndrome patients, who have high levels of pain, disability, and depression; (2) positive adaptation-to-pain patients, who have high levels of pain but low levels of disability and depression; and (3) good pain-control patients, with low levels of pain, disability, and depression (Klapow et al. 1993). Poor clinical presentations across all three dimensions of pain, disability, and depression are associated with high life adversity, passive/avoidance coping, and low satisfaction with social supports (Klapow et al. 1995). The Life Events and Difficulties Schedule (Brown and Harris 1978), and the Psychiatric Epidemiology Research Interview (Grant et al. 1989) are recommended to measure life adversity.

For measuring coping, the revised Ways of Coping Checklist (Vitaliano et al. 1985) has been used. The social support variable can be measured using the Sarason Social Support Questionnaire (Sarason et al. 1983).

Additional dimensions of pain and function that should be taken into account include the patient's beliefs regarding pain and treatment, perceptions of the work environment, fear of pain, and the patient's beliefs regarding his or her own ability to improve function and use pain-coping strategies (Feuerstein and Beattie 1995).

The Minnesota Multiphasic Personality Inventory is widely used to assess all disability groups and yields a great deal of information about the psychological status of patients (Hathaway and McKinley 1967). The shorter SCL-90 is a self-report scale developed in 1976 that yields equally valuable information (Derogatis et al. 1976).

Conclusion

Physical therapists have been taught to evaluate impairments and probably feel most comfortable in this realm. In many patients with chronic pain, however, there is little relationship between diagnostic findings and the degree of disability identified. It is for this reason that the schema of pathology leading to impairments, disability, and handicap are important to apply in this group of patients. The complexity of the performance restrictions found during functional testing must be emphasized and remembered during evaluation of chronic pain patients. The therapist's ability to integrate findings on many different levels of evaluation becomes important.

References

Astrand P-O, Rodahl K. Textbook of Work Physiology (3rd ed). New York: McGraw-Hill, 1986;296, 365.

Bergner MB, Bobbitt RA, Carter WB, Gilson BS. The SIP: development and final revision of a health status measure. Med Care 1981;19:787.

Brown GW, Harris T. Social Origins of Depression: Study of Psychiatric Disorders in Women. London: Tavistock, 1978.

Chambers LW, MacDonald LA, Tugwell P, et al. The McMaster health index questionnaire as a measure of quality of life for patients with rheumatoid disease. J Rheumatol 1982;9:780.

Chapman DDL, Casey KL, Dubner R, et al. Pain measurement: an overview. Pain 1985;22:1.

Cooper KH. A means of assessing maximal oxygen intake. JAMA 1968; 203:201.

Derogatis IR, Rickels K, Rock AF. The SCL-90 and the MMPI, a step in the validation of a new self-report scale. Br J Psychol 1976;128:280.

DiFabio RP, Mackey G, Holte JB. Disability and functional status in patients with low back pain receiving workers' compensation: a descriptive study with implications for the efficacy of physical therapy. Phys Ther 1995;75:180.

Fanshel S, Bush JW. A health-status index and its application to health-services outcomes. Operations Res 1970;18:1021.

Feuerstein M, Beattie P. Biobehavioral factors affecting pain and disability in low back pain: mechanisms and assessment. Phys Ther 1995;75:267.

Grant I, McDonald WI, Patterson TL, Trimble MR. Life Events and Multiple Sclerosis. In GW Brown, T Harris (eds), Life Events and Illness. New York: Guilford, 1989;295.

Grimby G, Thoren Jonsson A-L. Disability in poliomyelitis sequelae. Phys Ther 1994;74:415.

Hathaway SR, McKinley JC. The Minnesota Multiphasic Personality Inventory Manual. New York: The Psychological Corporation, 1967.

Hazard RG, Haugh LD, Green PA, Jones PL. Chronic low back pain: the relationship between patient satisfaction and pain, impairment, and disability outcomes. Spine 1994;19:881.

Janda V. Muscles and Cervicogenic Pain Syndromes: Physical Therapy of the Cervical and Thoracic Spine. In R Grant (ed), Clinics in Physical Therapy (Vol 19). New York: Churchill Livingstone, 1990.

Jensen MP, Strom SE, Turner JA, Romano JM. Validity of the Sickness Impact

Profile Roland scale as a measure of dysfunction in chronic pain patients. Pain 1992;50:157.

Jette AM, Davies AR, Cleary PD, et al. The Functional Status questionnaire: reliability and validity when used in primary care. J Gen Intern Med 1986;1:143.

Kassirer JP, Kopelman RI. Learning Clinical Reasoning. Baltimore: Williams & Wilkins, 1991;15.

Kerns RD, Turk DC, Rudy TE. The West Haven-Yale Multidimensional Pain Inventory (WHYMPI). Pain 1985;23:345.

Klapow JC, Slater MA, Patterson TL, et al. An empirical evaluation of multidimensional clinical outcome in chronic low back pain patients. Pain 1993;55:107.

Klapow JC, Slater MA, Patterson TL, et al. Psychosocial factors discriminate multidimensional clinical groups of chronic low back pain patients. Pain 1995;62:349.

Maxwell C. Sensitivity and accuracy of the visual analogue: a psychophysical classroom experiment. Br J Clin Pharmacol 1978;6:15.

McCaffery M, Beebe A. Pain: A Clinical Manual for Nursing Practice. St. Louis: Mosby, 1989.

McEwen J. The Nottingham Health Profile. In S Walker, R Rosser (eds), Quality of Life: Assessment and Application. Lancaster, England: 1988;95.

McGuire DB. Measuring Pain. In M Frank-Stromborg (ed), Instruments for Assessing Clinical Problems. East Norwalk, CT: Appleton & Lange, 1988;336.

McGuire DB, Sheidler VR. Pain. In SL Groenwald, MH Frogge, M Goodman, CH Yarbro (eds), Cancer Nursing Principles and Practice. Boston: Jones & Bartlett, 1993;516.

Melzack R, Casey KL. Sensory, Motivational, and Central Control Determinants of Pain: A New Conceptual Model. In D Kenshalo (ed), The Skin Senses. Springfield, IL: Thomas, 1968;42.

Moon MH. Psychological Approaches to the Treatment of Chronic Pain. In TH Michel (ed), Pain. International Perspectives in Physical Therapy (Vol I). Edinburgh: Churchill Livingstone, 1985;49.

National Institute on Disability and Rehabilitation Research. Data on Disability from the National Health Interview Surveys: 1983–1985. Washington, DC: National Institute on Disability and Rehabilitation Research, 1988;5.

Nelson E, Wasson J, Kirk J, et al. Assessment of function in routine clinical practice; description of the COOP chart method and preliminary findings. J Chronic Disability 1987;40:55S.

Ogden-Niemeyer L. The Issue of Abnormal Illness Behavior in Work Hardening. In L Ogden-Niemeyer, K Jacobs (eds), Work Hardening: State of the Art. Thorofare, NJ: Slack, 1989;67.

Parkerson GR, Gehlbach SH, Wagner EH, et al. The Duke-UNC Health Profile: an adult health status instrument for primary care. Med Care 1981;19:806.

Pope A, Tarlov A. Disability in America: Toward a National Agenda for Prevention. Washington, DC: National Academy, 1991.

Sarason IG, Levine HM, Basham R, et al. Assessing social support: the social support questionnaire. J Pers Soc Psychol 1983;44:127.

Turk DC, Rudy TE, Salovey P. The McGill Pain Questionnaire reconsidered: confirming the factor structure and examining appropriate uses. Pain 1985;21:385.

Vitaliano PP, Russo J, Carr JE, et al. The Ways of Coping Checklist: revision and psychometric properties. Multivar Behav Res 1985;20:3.

Waddell G, Bircher M, Finlayson D, Main CJ. Symptoms and signs: physical disease or illness behaviour? BMJ 1984;289:739.

Waddell G, Somerville D, Henderson I, Newton M. Objective clinical evaluation of physical impairment in chronic low back pain. Spine 1992;17:617.

Ware J, Sherbourne C. The MOS 36-item Short Form Health Survey (SF-36). Med Care 1992;30:473.

Waddell and Main Back Questionnaire

WADDELL AND MAIN BACK QUESTIONNAIRE

NAME _____   PHONE _____

DATE _____   TIME _____   SUBJECT CODE _____

ADMINISTRATION # _____   ORDER _____

	YES	NO
1. Do you require help or avoid heavy lifting (i.e., 30–40 lb, a heavy suitcase, or a 3- to 4-year-old child)?	_____	_____
2. Have you limited your sitting to less than 30 minutes?		
3. Have you limited traveling in a bus or car to less than 30 minutes?	_____	_____
4. Have you limited standing in one place to less than 30 minutes?	_____	_____
5. Do you limit walking to less than 30 minutes?	_____	_____
6. Is your sleep disturbed regularly (i.e., more than 2–3 times per week)?	_____	_____
7. Do you regularly miss or curtail social activities (excluding sports)?	_____	_____
8. Has your sexual activity diminished in frequency?	_____	_____
9. Do you regularly require help with footwear (i.e., tights, socks, or tying laces)?	_____	_____

Restriction has to be since the onset of and because of low back pain. The common or usual effect is assessed, discounting occasional limitations or special efforts.

SOURCE: Reprinted from Physical Therapy. Delitto A. Are measures of function and disability important in low back care? 1994;74:460, with the permission of the American Physical Therapy Association.

Pain Diary Page for One Day

DAILY DIARY

Name _____ Date _____

Time	Pain rating scale	Medication type & amount taken	Other pain relief measures tried or anything that influences your pain	Major activity being done: lying sitting standing/walking
12 MIDNIGHT				
1 AM				
2				
3				
4				
5				
6				
7				
8				
9				
10				
11				
noon 12				
1				
2				
3				
4				
5				
6				
7				
8				
9				
10				
11				

Comments: _____

_____

_____

SOURCE: Reprinted with permission from M McCaffery, A Beebe. Pain: A Clinical Manual for Nursing Practice. St. Louis: Mosby, 1989;27.

FLOW SHEET—PAIN

Patient _____   Date _____

*Pain rating scale used _____

Purpose: To evaluate the safety and effectiveness of the analgesic(s).

Analgesic(s) prescribed: _____

Time	Pain rating	Analgesic	R	P	BP	Level of arousal	Other†	Plan & comments

*Pain rating: A number of different scales may be used. Indicate which scale is used and use the same one each time. For example, 0-10 (0 = no pain, 10 = worst pain).

† Possibilities for other columns: bowel function, activities, nausea and vomiting, other pain relief measures. Identify the side effects of greatest concern to patient, family, physician, nurses.

R = respirations; P = pulse; BP = blood pressure (mm Hg).

SOURCE: Reprinted with permission from M McCaffery, A Beebe. Pain: A Clinical Manual for Nursing Practice. St. Louis: Mosby, 1989;27.

McGill-Melzack Pain Assessment Questionnaire

Cover sheet:

Patient's name: _____ Age: _____

Hospital No.: _____

Clinical category (e.g., cardiac, neurologic, etc.): _____

Diagnosis: _____

_____

_____

Analgesic (if already administered):

  1. Type: _____

  2. Dosage: _____

  3. Time given in relation to this test: _____

Patient's intelligence: Circle number that represents best estimate:

  1 (low)   2   3   4   5 (high)

This questionnaire has been designed to tell us more about your pain. Four major questions we ask are:

  1. Where is your pain?
  2. What does it feel like?
  3. How does it change with time?
  4. How strong is it?

It is important that you tell us how your pain feels now. Please follow the instructions at the beginning of each part.

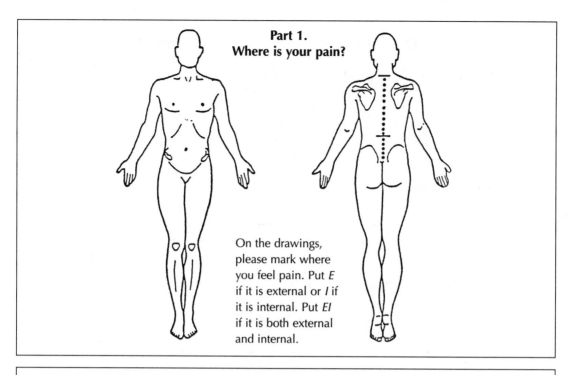

**Part 1.
Where is your pain?**

On the drawings, please mark where you feel pain. Put *E* if it is external or *I* if it is internal. Put *EI* if it is both external and internal.

Part 2. What does your pain feel like?

Some of the words below should describe your present pain. Circle only those words that best describe it. Use only a *single word* in each appropriate category—the one that applies best. Leave out any category that is not suitable.

1	2	3	4	5
Flickering	Jumping	Pricking	Sharp	Pinching
Quivering	Flashing	Boring	Cutting	Pressing
Pulsing	Shooting	Drilling	Lacerating	Gnawing
Throbbing		Stabbing		Cramping
Beating		Lancinating		Crushing

6	7	8	9	10
Tugging	Hot	Tingling	Dull	Tender
Pulling	Burning	Itchy	Sore	Taut
Wrenching	Scalding	Smarting	Hurting	Rasping
	Searing	Stinging	Aching	Splitting
			Heavy	

11	12	13	14	15
Tiring	Sickening	Fearful	Punishing	Wretched
Exhausting	Suffocating	Frightful	Grueling	Blinding
		Terrifying	Cruel	
			Vicious	
			Killing	

16	17	18	19	20
Annoying	Spreading	Tight	Cool	Nagging
Troublesome	Radiating	Numb	Cold	Nauseating
Miserable	Penetrating	Drawing	Freezing	Agonizing
Intense	Piercing	Squeezing		Dreadful
Unbearable		Tearing		Torturing

Part 3. How does your pain change with time?

1. Which word or words would you use to describe the pattern of your pain?

1	2	3
Continuous	Rhythmic	Brief
Steady	Periodic	Momentary
Constant	Intermittent	Transient

2. What kind of things relieve your pain?

_____
_____
_____
_____

3. What kind of things increase your pain?

_____
_____
_____
_____

Part 4. How strong is your pain?

People agree that the following five words represent pain of increasing intensity.
They are:

1	2	3	4	5
Mild	Discomforting	Distressing	Horrible	Excruciating

To answer each question below, write the number of the most appropriate word in the space beside the question.

1. Which word describes your pain right now? _____
2. Which word describes it at its worst? _____
3. Which word describes it when it is the least? _____
4. Which word describes the worst toothache you ever had? _____
5. Which word describes the worst headache you ever had? _____
6. Which word describes the worst stomachache you ever had? _____

SOURCE: Reprinted from R Melzack. The McGill Pain Questionnaire: major properties and scoring methods. Pain 1975;1:275–277 with kind permission of Elsevier Science — NL, Sara Burgerhartstraat 25, 1055 KV Amsterdam, The Netherlands.

Appendix
4.5

Oswestry Low Back Pain Disability Questionnaire

(The Robert Jones and Agnes Hunt Orthopaedic Hospital, Oswestry, Shropshire, Department for Spinal Disorders)

NAME _____   PHONE _____

DATE _____   TIME _____   SUBJECT CODE _____

ADMINISTRATION # _____   ORDER _____

Please read:

This questionnaire has been designed to give the doctor information as to how your back pain has affected your ability to manage in everyday life. Please answer every section, and mark in each section only the one box which applies to you. We realize you may consider that two of the statements in any one section relate to you, but please just mark the box which most closely describes your problem.

Section 1 - Pain Intensity

☐ I can tolerate the pain I have without having to use pain killers.
☐ The pain is bad but I manage without taking pain killers.
☐ Pain killers give complete relief from pain.
☐ Pain killers give moderate relief from pain.
☐ Pain killers give very little relief from pain.
☐ Pain killers have no effect on the pain and I do not use them.

Section 2 - Personal Care (washing, dressing, etc.)

☐ I can look after myself normally without causing extra pain.
☐ I can look after myself normally but it causes extra pain.
☐ It is painful to look after myself and I am slow and careful.
☐ I need some help but manage most of my personal care.
☐ I need help every day in most aspects of self care.
☐ I do not get dressed, wash with difficulty and stay in bed.

Section 3 - Lifting

☐ I can lift heavy weights without extra pain.
☐ I can lift heavy weights but it gives extra pain.
☐ Pain prevents me from lifting heavy weights off the floor, but I can manage if they are conveniently positioned, e.g. on a table.
☐ I can lift only very light weights.
☐ I cannot lift or carry anything at all.

Section 4 - Walking

☐ Pain does not prevent me walking any distance.
☐ Pain prevents me walking more than 1 mile.
☐ Pain prevents me from walking more than ½ mile.
☐ Pain prevents me from walking more than ¼ mile.
☐ I can only walk using a cane or crutches.
☐ I am in bed most of the time and have to crawl to the toilet.

Section 5 - Sitting

☐ I can sit in any chair as long as I like.
☐ I can only sit in my favorite chair as long as I like.
☐ Pain prevents me sitting more than 1 hour.
☐ Pain prevents me from sitting more than ½ hour.
☐ Pain prevents me from sitting more than 10 minutes.
☐ Pain prevents me from sitting at all.

Section 6 - Standing

☐ I can stand as long as I want without extra pain.
☐ I can stand as long as I want but it gives me extra pain.
☐ Pain prevents me from standing for more than 1 hour.
☐ Pain prevents me from standing for more than 30 minutes.
☐ Pain prevents me from standing for more than 10 minutes.
☐ Pain prevents me from standing at all.

Section 7 - Sleeping

☐ Pain does not prevent me from sleeping well.
☐ I can sleep well only by using tablets.
☐ Even when I take pills, I have less than six hours sleep.
☐ Even when I take pills, I have less than four hours sleep.
☐ Even when I take pills, I have less than two hours sleep.
☐ Pain prevents me from sleeping at all.

Section 8 - Sex Life

☐ My sex life is normal and causes no extra pain.
☐ My sex life is normal but causes some extra pain.
☐ My sex life is nearly normal but is very painful.
☐ My sex life is severely restricted by pain.
☐ My sex life is nearly absent because of pain.
☐ Pain prevents any sex life at all.

Section 9 - Social Life

☐ My social life is normal and gives me no extra pain.
☐ My social life is normal but increases the degree of pain.
☐ Pain has no significant effect on my social life apart from limiting my more energetic interests, e.g., dancing, etc.
☐ Pain has restricted my social life and I do not go out as often.
☐ Pain has restricted my social life to my home.
☐ I have no social life because of pain.

Section 10 - Traveling

☐ I can travel anywhere without extra pain.
☐ I can travel anywhere but it gives me extra pain.
☐ Pain is bad but I manage journeys over two hours.
☐ Pain restricts me to journeys of less than one hour.
☐ Pain restricts me to short necessary journeys under 30 minutes.
☐ Pain prevents me from traveling except to the doctor or hospital.

SOURCE: Reprinted with permission from JCT Fairbanks, J Couper, JB Davies, et al. The Oswestry Low Back Pain Disability Questionnaire. Physiotherapy 1980;66:271.

SF-36 Health Survey

INSTRUCTIONS: This survey asks for your views about your health. This information will help keep track of how you feel and how well you are able to do your usual activities.

Answer every question by marking the answer as indicated. If you are unsure about how to answer a question, please give the best answer you can.

1. In general, would you say your health is: (Circle one)

Excellent 1
Very good 2
Good 3
Fair 4
Poor 5

2. *Compared to one week ago,* how would you rate your health in general now? (Circle one)

Much better now than one week ago 1
Somewhat better now than one week ago 2
About the same as one week ago 3
Somewhat worse now than one week ago 4
Much worse now than one week ago 5

3. The following items are about activities you might do during a typical day. Does *your health now limit you* in these activities? If so, how much?

(Circle one number on each line)

ACTIVITIES	Yes, Limited A Lot	Yes, Limited A Little	No, Not Limited At All
a. *Vigorous activities*, such as running, lifting heavy objects, participating in strenuous sports	1	2	3
b. *Moderate activities,* such as moving a table, pushing a vacuum cleaner, bowling, or playing golf	1	2	3
c. Lifting or carrying groceries	1	2	3
d. Climbing *several* flights of stairs	1	2	3
e. Climbing *one* flight of stairs	1	2	3
f. Bending, kneeling, or stooping	1	2	3
g. Walking *more than one mile*	1	2	3
h. Walking *several blocks*	1	2	3
i. Walking *one block*	1	2	3
j. Bathing or dressing yourself	1	2	3

4. During the *past week,* have you had any of the following problems with your work or other regular daily activities *as a result of your physical health*?

(Circle one number on each line)

	Yes	No
a. Cut down on the *amount of time* you spent on work or other activities	1	2
b. *Accomplished less* than you would like	1	2
c. Were limited in the *kind* of work or other activities	1	2
d. Had *difficulty* performing the work or other activities (for example, it took extra effort)	1	2

5. During the *past week*, have you had any of the following problems with your work or other regular daily activities *as a result of any emotional problems* (such as feeling depressed or anxious)?

(Circle one number on each line)

	Yes	No
a. Cut down on the *amount of time* you spent on work or other activities	1	2
b. *Accomplished less* than you would like	1	2
c. Didn't do work or other activities *as carefully* as usual	1	2

6. During the *past week*, to what extent has your physical health or emotional problems interfered with your normal social activities with family, friends, neighbors, or groups?　　　　　　　　　　　　　(Circle one)

Not at all 1
Slightly 2
Moderately 3
Quite a bit 4
Extremely 5

7. How much *bodily* pain have you had during the *past week?*　　　(Circle one)

None 1
Very mild 2
Mild 3
Moderate 4
Severe 5
Very severe 6

8. During the *past week*, how much did *pain* interfere with your normal work (including both work outside the home and housework)?　　　(Circle one)

Not at all 1
A little bit 2
Moderately 3
Quite a bit 4
Extremely 5

9. These questions are about how you feel and how things have been with you *during the past week*. For each question, please give the one answer that comes closest to the way you have been feeling. How much of the time during the *past week*:

(Circle one number on each line)

	All of the Time	Most of the Time	A Good Bit of the Time	Some of the Time	A Little of the Time	None of the Time
a. Did you feel full of pep?	1	2	3	4	5	6
b. Have you been a very nervous person?	1	2	3	4	5	6
c. Have you felt so down in the dumps that nothing could cheer you up?	1	2	3	4	5	6
d. Have you felt calm and peaceful?	1	2	3	4	5	6
e. Did you have a lot of energy?	1	2	3	4	5	6
f. Have you felt downhearted and blue?	1	2	3	4	5	6
g. Did you feel worn out?	1	2	3	4	5	6
h. Have you been a happy person?	1	2	3	4	5	6
i. Did you feel tired?	1	2	3	4	5	6

10. During the *past week*, how much of the time has your *physical health or emotional problems* interfered with your social activities (like visiting with friends, relatives, etc). (Circle one)

All of the time 1
Most of the time 2
Some of the time 3
A little of the time 4
None of the time 5

11. How true or false is *each* of the following statements for you?

(Circle one number on each line)

	Definitely True	Mostly True	Don't Know	Mostly False	Definitely False
a. I seem to get sick a little easier than other people	1	2	3	4	5
b. I am as healthy as anybody I know	1	2	3	4	5
c. I expect my health to get worse	1	2	3	4	5
d. My health is excellent	1	2	3	4	5

Appendix
4.7

Roland-Morris Disability Questionnaire

Roland/Morris Disability Questionnaire

NAME _____ PHONE _____

DATE _____ TIME _____ SUBJECT CODE _____

ADMINISTRATION # _____ ORDER _____

When your back hurts, you may find it difficult to do some of the things you normally do.

This list contains some sentences that people have used to describe themselves when they have back pain. When you read them, you may find that some stand out because they describe you *today*. As you read the list, think of yourself *today*. When you read a sentence that describes you *today*, put a check beside the number of the sentence. If the sentence does not describe you, then leave the space blank and go on to the next one. Remember, only check the sentence if you are sure that it describes you *today*.

_____ 1. I stay at home most of the time because of my back.

_____ 2. I change position frequently to try and get my back comfortable.

_____ 3. I walk more slowly than usual because of my back.

_____ 4. Because of my back, I am not doing any of the jobs that I usually do around the house.

_____ 5. Because of my back, I use a handrail to get upstairs.

_____ 6. Because of my back, I lie down to rest more often.

_____ 7. Because of my back, I have to hold onto something to get out of an easy chair.

_____ 8. Because of my back, I try to get other people to do things for me.

_____ 9. I get dressed more slowly than usual because of my back.

_____ 10. I only stand up for short periods of time because of my back.

_____ 11. Because of my back, I try not to bend or kneel down.

_____ 12. I find it difficult to get out of a chair because of my back.

_____ 13. My back is painful almost all the time.

_____ 14. I find it difficult to turn over in bed because of my back.

_____ 15. My appetite is not very good because of my back pain.

_____ 16. I have trouble putting on my socks (or stockings) because of the pain in my back.

_____ 17. I only walk short distances because of my back pain.

_____ 18. I sleep less well because of my back.

_____ 19. Because of my back pain, I get dressed with help from someone else.

_____ 20. I sit down for most of the day because of my back.

_____ 21. I avoid heavy jobs around the house because of my back.

_____ 22. Because of my back pain, I am more irritable and bad tempered with people than usual.

_____ 23. Because of my back, I go upstairs more slowly than usual.

_____ 24. I stay in bed most of the time because of my back.

SOURCE: Adapted with permission from M Roland, R Morris. A study of the natural history of back pain. Part I: The development of a reliable and sensitive measure of disability in low-back pain. Spine 1983;8:141.

Dallas Pain Questionnaire

DALLAS PAIN QUESTIONNAIRE

Patient # _____

Name: _____ Today's Date: _____

Date of Birth: _____ Examiner _____

Please read carefully: This questionnaire has been designed to give your doctor information as to how your pain has affected your life. Be sure that these are your answers. Do not ask someone else to fill out the questionnaire for you. Please mark an "X" in the appropriate box that expresses your thoughts from 0 to 100% in each section.

Section I: Pain and Intensity

To what degree do you rely on pain medications or pain relieving substances for you to be comfortable?

None   Some   All the time

0% [ ][ ][ ][ ][ ][ ] 100%

Section II: Personal Care

How much does pain interfere with your personal care (getting out of bed, teeth brushing, etc)?

None (no pain)   Some   I cannot get out of bed

0% [ ][ ][ ][ ][ ][ ] 100%

Section III: Lifting

How much limitation do you notice in lifting?

None (I can lift as I did)   Some   None

0% [ ][ ][ ][ ][ ][ ] 100%

Section IV: Walking

Compared with how far you could walk before your injury or back trouble, how much does pain restrict your walking now?

I can walk the same Almost the same Very little I cannot walk

0% [ ][ ][ ][ ][ ][ ] 100%

Section V: Sitting

Back pain limits my sitting in a chair to?

None, pain same as before   Some   I cannot sit at all

0% [ ][ ][ ][ ][ ][ ] 100%

Section VI: Standing

How much does your pain interfere with your tolerance to stand for long periods?

None, same as before   Some   I cannot stand

0% [ ][ ][ ][ ][ ][ ] 100%

Section VII: Sleeping

How much does pain interfere with your sleeping?

None, same as before   Some   I cannot sleep at all

0% [ ][ ][ ][ ][ ][ ] 100%

Section VIII: Social Life

How much does pain interfere with your social life (dancing, games, going out, eating with friends, etc)?

None, same as before   Some   No activities total loss

0% [ ][ ][ ][ ][ ][ ] 100%

Section IX: Traveling

How much does pain interfere with traveling in a car?

None, same as before   Some   I cannot travel

0% [ ][ ][ ][ ][ ][ ] 100%

Section X: Vocational

How much does pain interfere with your job?

None, no interference   Some   I cannot work

0% [ ][ ][ ][ ][ ][ ] 100%

Section XI: Anxiety/Mood

How much control do you feel that you have over demands made on you?

(No change) Total   Some   None

100% [ ][ ][ ][ ][ ][ ] 0%

Section XII: Emotional Control

How much control do you feel that you have over your emotions?

Total   Some   None

100% [ ][ ][ ][ ][ ][ ] 0%

Section XIII: Depression

How depressed have you been since the onset of pain?

Not depressed significantly   Overwhelmed by depression

0% [ ][ ][ ][ ][ ][ ] 100%

Section XIV: Interpersonal Relationships

How much do you think your pain had changed your relationships with others?

Not changed   Drastically changed

0% [ ][ ][ ][ ][ ][ ] 100%

Section XV: Social Support

How much support do you need from others to help you during this onset of pain (taking over chores, fixing meals, etc)?

None needed   All the time

0% [ ][ ][ ][ ][ ][ ] 100%

Section XVI: Punishing Responses

How much do you think others express irritation, frustration, or anger toward you because of your pain?

None   Some   All the time

0% [ ][ ][ ][ ][ ][ ] 100%

SOURCE: Modified with permission from GF Lawlis, R Cuencas, D Selby, et al. The development of the Dallas Pain Questionnaire: an assessment of the impact of spinal pain on behavior. Spine 1989;14:512.

Screening Questions for Dysfunctional Chronic Pain from the Multidimensional Pain Inventory

1. Rate your level of pain at the present moment.

No pain   Very intense pain

0   1   2   3   4   5   6

2. How much has your pain changed the amount of satisfaction or enjoyment you get from taking part in social and recreational activities?

No change   Extreme change

0   1   2   3   4   5   6

3. During the past week how tense or anxious have you been?

Not at all   Extremely

0   1   2   3   4   5   6

4. How much has pain changed your ability to take part in recreational and other social activities?

No change   Extreme change

0   1   2   3   4   5   6

5. During the past week how well do you feel you've been able to deal with your problems?

Not at all   Extremely well

0   1   2   3   4   5   6

6. On the average, how severe has your pain been during the past week?

Not at all   Extremely severe

0   1   2   3   4   5   6

7. During the past week, how successful were you in coping with stressful situations in your life?

Not at all successful   Extremely successful

0   1   2   3   4   5   6

8. During the past week, how irritable have you been?

Not at all irritable   Extremely irritable

0   1   2   3   4   5   6

Scoring for the above scale is suggested based on the following rules:

Pain severity (PS) = Questions 1 and 6
Interference (I) = Questions 2 and 4
Life control (LC) = Questions 5 and 7
Affective distress (AD) = Questions 3 and 8
A score greater than 9 indicates a dysfunctional response for PS, greater than 10 is dysfunctional for I, greater than 6 is dysfunctional for LC, and greater than 8 is dysfunctional for AD.

SOURCE: Modified from RD Kerns, DC Turk, TE Rudy. The West Haven-Yale Multidimensional Pain Inventory (WHYMPI). Pain 1985;23:345.

5	# Pathophysiology of Activity Intolerance

Theresa Hoskins Michel and Harriët Wittink

Activity intolerance is a major source of disability in the chronic pain patient population. The principles of deconditioning, the 12 landmark studies that describe physical fitness in this population, and the basic theory and practical considerations in exercise reconditioning are discussed in this chapter.

The measurement of aerobic fitness or aerobic power is maximal oxygen consumption ($\dot{V}O_2$max), which is affected by cardiac output (Q) and arteriovenous oxygen difference (a–$\dot{V}O_2$). The Fick equation describes the determinants of $\dot{V}O_2$max:

$$\dot{V}O_2\text{max} = Q(a–\dot{V}O_2)$$

Thus, aerobic power is determined by the performance of the cardiac muscle and efficiency of the muscular system in extracting oxygen from blood for use in generating energy. For each liter of oxygen consumed, approximately 5 kcal of energy is produced. Therefore, the higher the oxygen uptake, the higher the aerobic energy output (Astrand and Rodahl 1986). Aerobic fitness directly affects the physical activities an individual is able to perform. Most activities are described in terms of their energy cost (Astrand and Rodahl 1986).

Deconditioning

The term *deconditioning* refers to a condition that makes a number of pathologies more likely and places affected individuals at increased risk. In 1986, data from the Public Health Service (U.S. Department of Health and Human Services 1986) showed that scarcely more than one in 10 people reported performing physical activity for at least 30 minutes daily. Approximately one in five people reported activity for at least 30 minutes five or more times a week. Nearly one in four people ages 18 or older reported no leisure-time physical activity, and among people ages 65 and over, more than two of every five reported essentially sedentary lifestyles.

One of the highest risks of deconditioning is coronary artery disease (CAD). Physically inactive people have almost twice the risk of developing CAD than those who engage in regular physical activity. Habitual activity can also help in the management of non–insulin-dependent diabetes mellitus and osteoporosis. It has been associated with lower rates of stroke and may reduce the risk of colon cancer (Astrand and Rodahl 1986).

All physical activity involves muscular contractions powered by energy. The currency of energy expenditure is adenosine triphosphate (ATP). The phosphorolysis of ATP to adenosine diphosphate (ADP) and inorganic phosphate releases the energy. The amount of ATP stored in muscle at any time is small and must be resynthesized continuously if exercise continues for more than a few seconds. The synthesis of ATP requires a substrate for energy. Carbohydrate and fat act as substrates under usual conditions and in the presence of ADP, adenosine monophosphate (AMP), creatine phosphate (CP), and inorganic phosphate. Synthesis takes place by different aerobic or anaerobic enzyme pathways. Only carbohydrates (glycogen) use the anaerobic pathway for the generation of energy, whereas glycogen, fat, and protein can be used aerobically. These aerobic and anaerobic synthesis processes are summarized as follows:

Anaerobic

$$ADP + CP \rightarrow ATP + C$$
$$\text{Glycolysis} \rightarrow \text{Pyruvate} + ATP + \text{lactate}$$
One molecule of glycogen yields 4 ATP.

Aerobic

$$\text{Free fatty acids} + O_2 \rightarrow ATP + CO_2 + H_2O$$
$$\text{Glycolysis} + O_2 \rightarrow ATP + CO_2 + H_2O$$
$$\text{Amino acids} + O_2 \rightarrow ATP + CO_2 + H_2O$$
One molecule of free fatty acid (palmitate) yields 138 ATP or 5.8 ATP/O_2.
One molecule of glycogen yields 38 ATP or 8.5 ATP/O_2.

These outlines demonstrate that the aerobic energy yield from glycolysis is much lower than that for free fatty acids. However, glycogen is in limited supply, whereas fatty acids are the largest supplier of stored energy. A man weighing 160 pounds has 80–85% of calories (approximately 140,000) stored as fat. Less than 2,000 calories are stored as carbohydrates (Fisher and Jensen 1990). The ability to use fat depends on oxygen transport capacity because fat can be metabolized only in the muscle cell in the presence of oxygen.

At the initiation of any activity after rest or a lower energy state, there is insufficient oxygen at the muscle cell level to permit aerobic pathways to operate. The only mechanisms to support the energy requirement in this condition of relative oxygen deprivation (oxygen deficit period) are anaerobic. When CP, AMP, and ADP are exhausted in a few seconds, only anaerobic glycolysis is available. Once the delay of oxygen transport has caught up and the demand for energy can be supplied by an oxygen-dependent pathway, it is possible to generate ATP aerobically. This delay in oxygen transport is related to the time it takes for respiratory and heart rates to meet the demands of the activity. This period of oxygen deficit is generally about 3–5 minutes. After this period, a steady state of oxygen delivery can be achieved as long as the demand for energy does not change. The *steady state condition* is defined as the period when energy demand is met exactly by energy delivery and can be measured in terms of a steady heart and respiratory rate response. There is no accumulation of lactate in the body. Steady state can be maintained at 40% of $\dot{V}O_2$max without undue fatigue. Higher levels can be maintained by well-trained individuals. If the activity is stopped or slowed down, a period of oxygen debt ensues during which a recovery heart rate and respiratory rate can be recorded. If activity is shifted upward so that there is an even higher level of energy demand, a new oxygen deficit period begins, and a new steady state may be achieved after a few minutes of adjustment unless the new level is too high (higher than 60% of maximum effort).

Whenever there is an upward shift in demand, there is a delay in delivery of oxygen based on the ability of the cardiopulmonary system to respond. This delay means there is insufficient oxygen in the muscle cell to deliver ATP aerobically and anaerobic metabolism must supply the ATP. As oxygen becomes available aerobic metabolism is used more. During steady state, all energy can be supplied aerobically. Even at early phases of steady state exercise free fatty acids are not in use. Because these are large, complicated, multicarbon chain molecules, the process of breakdown takes longer. The fragments of three carbon fatty acids are gradually made available after 15 or more minutes of steady state exercise. Only after about 30 minutes of steady-state exercise is it expected that fat metabolism is preferred over carbohydrate metabolism for sustaining ATP production.

There is an intensity of exercise that, while submaximal, is too demanding to be sustained by aerobic metabolism. The delivery of ATP through aerobic pathways becomes inadequate at 60–70% of maximal effort, perhaps because the aerobic pathways are complicated, fairly slow, and dependent on one molecule of oxygen at the end of the respiratory chain. As the demand at this high level continues or increases, ATP continues to be delivered via aerobic metabolism. The demand is supplemented by anaerobic glycolysis, which uses up carbohydrate rather quickly and generates more ATP at the rate of 4 ATP more per molecule of glycogen. This production is added to the 38 ATP molecules still available from each glycogen molecule in the aerobic pathway.

Adding more ATP by using both pathways causes lactate to accumulate in muscle cells and in the blood stream. This relative acidosis is detected by homeostatic sensors that maintain constant pH. As the pH drops, the kidneys are signaled to retain bicarbonate to buffer the acid in the blood. This process results in the production of additional CO_2, which is added to the metabolic byproduct of CO_2 in muscle cells. The quick accumulation of CO_2 results in the stimulation of the ventilatory system to rid the body of the excess CO_2. A significant increase in respiratory rate occurs that marks the respiratory threshold. Although the level of exercise intensity can continue to increase, no long-term steady state can occur above this threshold. Fat metabolism will be too slow, and glycogen metabolism will be used above this threshold.

These changes can be marked by the respiratory quotient (RQ), which is usually measured by collecting a sample of expired air during exercise. The percentage of CO_2 is divided by the percentage of O_2 in the expired air sample. When fat or a mixture of fat and carbohydrate is being burned for energy, the RQ is less than 1.0 because CO_2 production is not in excess of oxygen use in aerobic metabolism. Once the anaerobic pathway is used again and lactate begins to accumulate, however, much higher concentrations of CO_2 are present in expired air due to the burning of carbohydrates in aerobic and anaerobic pathways. RQ values become 1.0 and above, signaling anaerobic metabolism and a truly maximal effort. Use of carbohydrates exclusively for energy means that glycogen depletion will eventually occur. Glycogen depletion occurs in all prolonged activity; however, the higher the intensity of activity, the faster depletion occurs.

Deconditioning results in a lowering of the respiratory threshold from the normal 60–70% of maximal effort to a lower percentage. This is a relative change, even as the absolute maximal capacity is being reduced to a lower value. Thus, deconditioned individuals experience dyspnea and fatigue earlier in their aerobic exercise and have a difficult time maintaining a steady state of exercise without undue fatigue. If their deconditioned state has altered their respiratory threshold to 40% of their maximal oxygen consumption and they attempt to exert themselves at a level higher than 40%, they will rely on anaerobic metabolism for energy supply. This pathway requires use of the limited supply of glycogen and results in the formation of lactate.

$\dot{V}O_2$max is the aerobic capacity of the individual. This value is influenced by all of the energy delivery systems of the body and is measured by collecting expired air during a progressive exercise test. At a person's maximal level, the content of oxygen in the expired air is at a plateau representing a lower oxygen content than that which was breathed in. This occurs because the body required the use of some of the oxygen that was taken in. Essentially, the difference in oxygen content between inspired and expired air represents the oxygen uptake of the body and, at maximum, is at a plateau value in spite of increases in workload. Table 5.1 lists normative values of $\dot{V}O_2$max. It is difficult to get deconditioned patients who also have pain to continue exercise at these high levels of workload in order to demonstrate the plateau in the value of oxygen. Therefore, RQ and respiratory threshold measurements are often used, and the maximal oxygen uptake is estimated by extrapolation from these submaximal levels.

Deconditioned individuals also have an inefficient oxygen delivery system that relies on the ventilatory pump, the pulmonary gas exchange system, and the cardiac pump. With inactivity, skeletal muscles, including those involved in inspiration (the diaphragm, intercostals, and accessory muscles of breathing) atrophy, lose mitochondrial enzymes, and may lose capillary blood supply to nutritive beds. As these changes occur, motor nerve conduction velocity is reduced. Thus, the ability of the ventilatory pump to respond to the stimulus for deeper and more frequent ventilations is weakened. The car-

TABLE 5.1 Cardiorespiratory fitness classification measured in maximal oxygen uptake (ml/kg/min)

Age (years)	Low	Fair	Average	Good	High
Women					
20–29	<24	24–30	31–17	38–48	49+
30–39	<20	20–27	28–33	34–44	45+
40–49	<17	17–23	24–30	31–41	42+
50–59	<15	15–20	21–27	28–37	38+
60–69	<13	13–17	18–23	24–34	35+
Men					
20–29	<25	25–33	34–42	43–52	53+
30–39	<23	23–30	31–38	39–48	49+
40–49	<20	20–26	27–35	36–44	45+
50–59	<18	18–24	25–33	34–42	43+
60–69	<16	16–22	23–30	31–40	41+

SOURCE: Reproduced with permission. © "Exercise Testing and Training of Apparently Healthy Individuals: A Handbook for Physicians," 1972 Copyright American Heart Association.

diac muscle does not atrophy but does change in its performance efficiency. With detraining, heart rates are markedly elevated at rest and show excessive response at all submaximal levels of exercise. This is due in part to sympathetic stimulation, enhanced drive, and loss of stroke volume. The stroke volume is the volume of blood delivered by the heart with each stroke. Cardiac output is the stroke volume per unit of time. With a loss of volume capacity, the pump becomes smaller and must beat faster to meet the cardiac output demand. This cardiac output demand is determined by the activities being performed and their ATP (and therefore oxygen) requirements. Most activities performed in a standard way will have a predictable energy requirement. This requirement will change when muscles become inefficient due to spasticity or weakness. It will also become higher when the patient is heavier than the standard body weight. Deconditioned, nonobese patients who do not have peripheral muscle loss, spasticity, or rigidity still have an additional burden in meeting the energy demand of an activity because they are using an inefficient oxygen transport system. Deconditioned patients who also have inefficient muscle-use patterns have additional energy requirements that increase the burden to the oxygen transport system even more.

All of these factors mean that the deconditioned individual has limited oxygen available in the working tissue and less ability to utilize it in muscle. Therefore, carbohydrates are used for fuel, leading to formation of lactate in muscle. This accumulation decreases muscle contractility, causes muscle fatigue, and puts the individual at considerable risk for injury.

Muscle fiber types include type I and type II fibers. Type I (also called slow-twitch or red) fibers are predominantly oxidative fibers and have a low glycolytic capacity. They have a rich capillary supply and high myoglobin content that facilitates the delivery of oxygen to muscle cells. These fibers contain numerous large mitochondria. The high oxidative capacity and low threshold for tetanization make the type I fibers well suited for prolonged tonic contractions such as those required by postural muscles. Because of their high oxidative capacity, oxygen delivery role, and heavy reliance on fat oxidation, these fibers are also fatigue resistant. Type II (fast-twitch or white) fibers have a high glycolytic capacity but few mitochondria and a low oxidative capacity, making them well suited for anaerobic processes.

One peripheral adaptation to inactivity in muscle tissue is loss of mitochondrial enzyme activity. This can even occur in individuals who trained intensely for 10 or more years and started with enzyme activity twice as high as untrained individuals. These individuals lose enzyme activity progressively during the first 56 days of detraining but then stabilize at levels 50% more than those obtained from sedentary control subjects (Coyle et al. 1984, 1985). Single muscle fiber analysis reveals that the persistent elevation of mitochondrial enzyme levels above control values is more marked in type II fibers than in type I fibers (Holloszy and Coyle 1984). This information is consistent with the findings on atrophy of muscles with disuse or immobilization. Type I fibers have been reported to atrophy to a greater extent than type II fibers (St. Pierre and Gardiner 1987). This observation is supported by bedrest studies in which a proportionately higher percentage loss of torque in the antigravity muscles was found (Gogia et al. 1988). The loss of torque may also be attributed to the reduction in reflex potentiation, suggesting an impaired ability to activate motor units during voluntary contractions (Dudley et al. 1989). Altered activity patterns have been found to result in pronounced physiologic and morphologic adaptations of the neuromuscular junction. These adaptations are dependent on the model and duration of increased or decreased use and are, in part, specific to the type of muscle fiber. Studies suggest that muscle inactivity results in a reduction in neuromuscular transmission with a concomitant increase in transmission in the neuromuscular junction area. Muscle force is also reduced during this time (Deschenes et al. 1994). Therefore, loss of muscle strength and endurance with inactivity is a function of the following factors: (1) loss of muscle mass, (2) decreased ability to utilize energy substrates efficiently, (3) decreased neuromuscular transmission, and (4) decreased efficiency in muscle fiber recruitment.

Muscle Pathophysiology and Deconditioning

Myofascial pain syndromes are a group of muscle disorders characterized by the presence of hypersensitive points called trigger points (TPs). TPs may be the result of muscle weakness, muscle imbalance, trauma, stress, and visceral pathology. These points occur within one or more muscles, the investing connective tissue, or both. They are associated with a syndrome of pain, muscle spasm, tenderness, stiffness, limitation of motion, weakness, and occasionally, autonomic dysfunction (Sola and Bonica 1990). A TP is so named because its stimulation produces effects at another place, called the area of reference. TPs can develop in any muscle in the body and can be active or latent. An active TP is associated with spontaneous pain at rest or with motion that stretches or overloads the muscle. A latent TP does not cause spontaneous pain but can be diagnosed by applying discrete pressure on the TP that is likely to refer pain locally and to the area of reference. It is

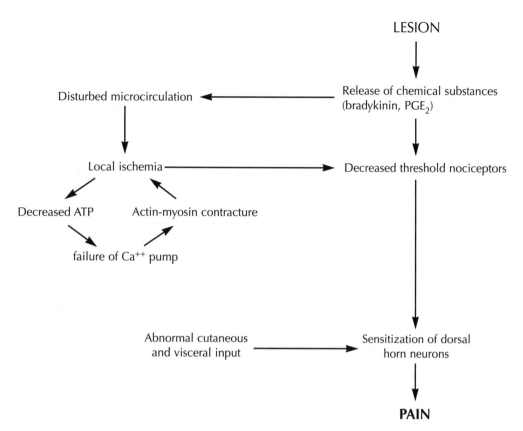

FIGURE 5.1   *Model of myofascial pain generation. (ATP = adenosine triphosphate; PGE = prostaglandin E.)*

still unclear exactly what TPs are, how they become hypersensitive, and how they produce pain. A hypothesis is outlined in Figure 5.1.

Joint Pathophysiology and Deconditioning

The biochemical and mechanical changes arising with stress deprivation of the joint structures and their dynamic movers (the musculotendinous unit) are important to physical therapy treatment. Inactivity and bedrest cause substantial weakness and loss of tissue from all elements of the musculoskeletal system. These changes include a loss of bone, muscle, and connective tissues; a reduction in joint range of motion, muscle strength, and endurance; and a marked decline in physical fitness (Twomey 1992). Muscle responds to disuse with atrophy and loss of contractile strength and mitochondrial enzymes. Tendons and ligaments lose tensile and insertion strength, tissue elasticity, and stretch resistance.

Marked changes in fiber appearance and orientation in the joint capsule have been observed with immobilization and disuse of joints (Akeson et al. 1987). These tissues become brittle and connective tissues become weaker and less stress resistant. According to Wolff's law, connective tissue responds to mechanical loading the same way bone does. The more demand that is placed on connective tissue, the stronger it will become. Tendons and ligaments respond to exercise with thickening and increased tensile strength (Tipton et al. 1975). Articular cartilage demands regular mechanical loading to remain healthy. Exercise ensures the passage of synovial fluid over articular surfaces. The alternate compression and relaxation of articular cartilage that occur during movement enable the synovial fluid to be taken back into the articular cartilage as the area of pressure changes over the joint surfaces (Twomey 1992, Frank et al. 1984, Salter and Field 1960, Salter 1989). The intervertebral disc is heavily dependent on movement in the same way. Lumbar sagittal movement brings about the largest fluid exchange between the discs and the interstitial fluid surrounding the spine (Adams and Hutton 1985, 1986). Low-metabolism structures such as tendons, ligaments, intervertebral discs, and articular cartilage require hundreds of controlled repetitions to increase their metabolism and remodeling response (Olson and Svendsen 1992). In the absence of movement, weight bearing, and repetitions, there is no remodeling influence, no demand for strengthening of connective tissue, and no nutritive bathing by synovial fluid. Structures lose strength and nutrition, are subject to rapid tearing with minor stresses, become unhealthy, and are at high risk for damage.

In addition to these mechanical factors, there are neurophysiologic changes with inactivity. The fibrous capsules and ligaments act as joint stabilizers to guide tracking of the articulating surfaces. These fibrous structures contain proprioceptive endings that signal higher centers to compensate using muscle response when strains are applied to the joint. The passive stabilization by ligaments is reinforced by the dynamic stabilization of muscle, and they are interlocked via the central nervous system (Figure 5.2).

Articular tissues are innervated by nociceptive afferents as well as by large-diameter, fast-conducting primary afferents. The latter are associated with low-threshold receptors that respond to non-noxious mechanical stimuli or movements. Many of the group III and IV primary afferents, and perhaps some group II afferents, are involved in responses to noxious stimulation of articular and other musculoskeletal tissues. These afferents, which can be activated by chemical and mechanical stimuli, terminate in the peripheral tissues as free nerve endings and encode a nociceptive stimulus. Recent studies have shown that some of these afferents may respond instead to low-threshold, non-noxious mechanical distortion of articular tissues (Schaible and Grubb 1993).

The term *sensitization* refers to a situation in which the activation threshold of the afferents is lowered by the application of substances such as bradykinin or prostaglandins (see Chapter 2). An enhancement of articular afferent activity has also been shown in animals with experimentally induced arthritis: Articular afferents become responsive to gentle innocuous movements or develop an increased resting discharge. The period of the increased excitability of the nociceptive afferents corresponds closely with the onset and duration of pain behavior and hyperalgesia in these animals. In addition to the enhanced responsiveness of nociceptive afferents, the experimental arthritis appears to be associated with mechanosensitivity in

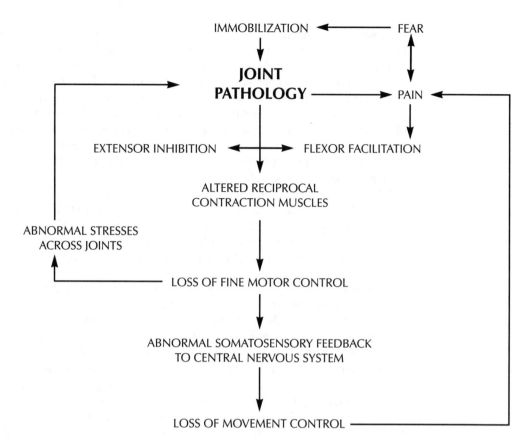

FIGURE 5.2   *A hypothesis of the relationship of joint pathology to loss of movement control.*

afferents previously unresponsive to joint movement or local stimulation and with an enhanced response of some low-threshold, non-nociceptive afferents. These various features of the responses of articular afferents point to peripheral mechanisms that may contribute to our ability to code the intensity of articular pain, to the hyperalgesia and allodynia that can occur in a traumatized or inflamed joint, and to the spontaneous and movement-related pain that is commonly seen in a damaged or inflamed joint (Sessle and Hu 1991).

Reconditioning

Aerobic exercise increases the maximal extraction of oxygen by the contracting muscles (increased difference in a–$\dot{V}o_2$). Endurance training increases the capillary density, decreases the diffusion distance from blood to muscles, and increases both the size and number of skeletal muscle mitochondria. This increased mitochondrial content is accompanied by training-induced increases in the enzyme levels involved in the oxidation of free fatty acids. Responses to endurance exercise after training include increased fatty acid oxidation, reduced carbohydrate oxidation and lactate production, and an improved endurance capacity ($\dot{V}o_2$max). Therefore, total body carbohydrate stores are conserved during exercise of the same absolute intensity.

Simply, endurance training promotes system efficiency by increased supply of oxygen (through increased number of capillaries, increased diameter of capillaries, and decreased diffusion distance) and increased oxygen use (through increases in size and number of mitochondria and an increase in the number of enzymes in the mitochondria).

With endurance training the aerobic capacities of all muscle fiber types increase. The greatest increases are observed in type I fibers after continuous training and in type II fibers after interval training. The oxidative capacities of type I and II fibers become more similar after a period of endurance training. There is no evidence that type I fibers can be converted into type II or vice versa.

Anaerobic exercise generally refers to heavy-resistance, static forms of muscular contraction. The active muscle must generate very high tensions to balance a high load. When intramuscular tension exceeds the functional strength of the walls of arteries inside the muscle, there is a collapse of arterial walls, especially in the capillaries, where walls are thin and tissue nutrition takes place. When collapse occurs, there is no delivery of oxygen, and exercise can be sustained only anaerobically. Therefore, anaerobic exercise is characterized by strengthening contractions of muscle or high-load, static contractions. This is in contrast to aerobic exercise, which involves moderate-intensity, dynamic contractions of muscles and cardiopulmonary delivery of oxygen and fuel substrates.

Effects of Exercise on Mood

A large body of literature exists suggesting that both aerobic and anaerobic exercise can decrease depression and anxiety and buffer stress. Because pain has repeatedly been found to be associated with psychological illness, these effects should be considered in the treatment of chronic pain patients. The incidence of depression in chronic pain populations (more than 80%) has been shown to be substantially higher than in normal or acute pain populations (Gamsa and Vikis-Freibergs 1991). Overall, the empiric evidence for a link between exercise and depression is mixed. Depressed people are unlikely to engage in physical activity. It may be that physical activity is actually indirectly associated with depression through its association with other related characteristics, such as self-efficacy, health belief system, and physical health status. The most obvious association of depression and physical activity is physical health status, as those suffering from physical impairment are more likely to be depressed and less likely to engage in physical activity (Camacho et al. 1991).

North et al. (1990) conducted a meta-analysis of 80 recent studies on the effects of exercise on depression. This analysis included all reported forms of depression and aerobic, strength, and endurance exercise. It concluded that both immediate and long-term exercise significantly decreased depression and that the antidepressant effects continued in follow-up measures. Subjects from most of the populations studied demonstrated decreased depression with exercise. Subjects requiring medical or psychological care for their depression demonstrated the largest increases. The data suggest that exercise was as effective as an antidepressant as psychotherapy and that anaerobic exercise was as effective as aerobic exercise. Exercise was not as effective an antidepressant as exercise and psychotherapy together, suggesting that an additive effect of treatments may exist. Subjects undergoing medical rehabilitation for other conditions such as hypertension or diabetes demonstrated a larger decrease in depression than did other groups not receiving rehabilitation but needing psychotherapy. The greatest decreases of depression were seen in programs of 17 weeks or longer. A significant correlation was found between total number of exercise sessions and the amount of decrease in depression. The data suggest that the longer the exercise program and the greater the total number of exercise sessions, the greater the decrease in depression. The number of times exercise was performed per week and the length of exercise session were found to have no influence.

Crews and Landers (1987) performed a meta-analysis of 34 studies in an attempt to examine moderator variables and statistically assess whether the literature supports the hypothesis that aerobically fit subjects actually experience a reduced stress response. The results of their analysis show that regardless of the type of physiologic and psychological measure used, aerobically fit subjects had a reduced psychosocial stress response. All of the studies in their review used acute, short-term stressors, meaning that these results may not necessarily apply to real-life situations in which individuals may experience more long-term, chronic levels of high stress.

Petruzzello et al. (1991) conducted a meta-analysis of the anxiety-reducing effects of exercise. Data were collected from studies reporting the effects of exercise on self-reported state (acute) or trait (chronic) anxiety and psychophysiologic correlates of anxiety (e.g., electromyography, electroencephalography, alpha waves, blood pressure, and galvanic skin response). One hundred and four studies were reviewed, and 408 effect sizes were calculated based on a population of 3,048 subjects. Aerobic exercise was associated with lower anxiety in those subjects reporting state anxiety. Exercise did not achieve better effects than medication, relaxation, or quiet rest, however. Exercise lasting 0–20 minutes yielded significantly lower effect sizes than exercise lasting 21–30 minutes. Regular exercise was associated with a reduction of self-reported trait anxiety of more than 0.3 standard deviation units below comparison groups. The length of the exercise training program had much stronger effects when the program exceeded 9 weeks. The strongest effects were seen for programs lasting more than 16 weeks. The overall mean effect size for psychophysiologic correlates of anxiety was 0.56, indicating that exercise was associated with a change in anxiety of more than 0.5 standard deviation units below comparison groups.

Martinsen (1990) concluded in a review that depressed people have normal pulmonary function but are physically sedentary and have reduced physical work capacity compared with the general population. This indicates that their reduced physical fitness level is caused by physical inactivity. He found that the results of all studies indicated the same conclusion: Aerobic exercise is more effective than no treatment and not significantly different from other forms of treatment, including psychotherapy. Exercise is associated with an antidepressive effect in patients with mild to moderate forms of non-bipolar depressive disorders. An increase in aerobic fitness does not seem to be essential for the antidepressive effect because similar effects are obtained with nonaerobic forms of exercise.

LaFontaine et al. (1992) found that researchers unanimously concluded that aerobic exercise and anxiety are related in an inverse and consistent manner. Yet, they have consistently refrained from suggesting that this relationship involves causality. They also found that studies consistently reported that aerobic exercise is effective in the treatment of mild to moderate forms of depression and anxiety. It was consistently reported that the benefits were greatest in those who were more depressed and more anxious and that an increase in cardiovascular health was not necessary for mood enhancement.

Byrne and Byrne (1993) reviewed 50 studies published between 1976 and 1989 in refereed journals and concluded that 90% of the studies support both the antidepressive properties of exercise and the effect of exercise in combating anxiety. Their data suggest that improvements in aerobic capacity are not responsible for mood improvement and that a nonaerobic activity such as weight training has equally positive effects on the alleviation of depression.

Stein and Motta (1992) evaluated the effects of aerobic and nonaerobic exercise on depression and self-concept. They used a pretest and post-test control group design with 89 undergraduate students who engaged in either the aerobic exercise of swimming, the nonaerobic exercise of weight training, or a control introductory psychology class. Cardiovascular fitness was estimated by the 12-minute Cooper swim test. Their analysis indicated that both aerobic and nonaerobic training was equally effective in significantly reducing self-reported depression when compared with the control group. The nonaerobic condition was superior to the aerobic condition for enhancing self-concept.

Lennox et al. (1990) studied the effect of exercise on normal mood by evaluating the effect of 13 weeks of aerobic exercise on the mood of 47 nondepressed men and women. Fitness was assessed by estimating $\dot{V}O_2$max from a modified treadmill test before and after the training program. Though the subjects demonstrated significant improvements in physical fitness, they did not show a significant change in mood.

Thirlaway and Benton (1992) investigated the hypothesis that participation in physical activity, rather than improved cardiovascular fitness, is the factor associated with better mental health and mood. Their sample was comprised of 246 normal men and women. Cardiovascular fitness ($\dot{V}O_2$max) was estimated by a submaximal bicycle ergometer test. Physical activity level was estimated by a self-report questionnaire, and a Profile of Mood States was used to assess mood. They found that higher levels of physical activity are associated with a tendency to report a positive mood. This relationship was independent of sex and age factors unless the individuals were unfit. Inactive but fit subjects were reported to have a poorer mood than those who were inactive and unfit. They concluded that the effect of physical activity on mental health and mood is not mediated by the level of fitness. Therefore, prescribing physical activity needs to emphasize performing physical activity rather than improving fitness.

Brown (1991) designed a study to determine whether the stress-buffering role of physical fitness could be found using relatively objective measurements of fitness and health status and whether the buffering effect of fitness was independent of measures of psychological distress. Subjects were 37 male and 73 female undergraduates. Fitness was estimated using a submaximal bicycle ergometer test; self-reports of physical exercise were assessed with the Physical Activity questionnaire; and life stress was measured with the Life Experiences Survey. Doctor visits for physical illnesses served as the main dependent variable in this research. Brown showed that stress was linked to increased medical visits only among subjects who scored low in fitness. Stress had virtually no negative impact on illness behavior in physically fit subjects. Self-reported exercise and physical fitness appeared to buffer the negative effects of life stress. He concluded that people who are physically fit are less vulnerable to the adverse effects of stress than those who are less fit.

Norris et al. (1990) investigated the effect of fitness on psychological and physiologic indices of well-being. One hundred police officers were assigned nonrandomly to an aerobic or nonaerobic training group, and an additional 50 subjects were recruited to serve as a control group. Heart rate and blood pressure were recorded before and after the program. Fitness was assessed by a timed 1.5-mile run. The Job Stress Questionnaire, Life Situation Survey, and General Health Questionnaire were used to assess psychological stress. The aerobic group experienced the greatest reductions in resting heart rate and blood pressure and the greatest improvement in the 1.5-mile run. The nonaerobic group experienced reduction in resting heart rate and blood pressure. Their performance in the timed run did not improve. The aerobic training group registered substantially improved scores in self-reported stress, health, and well-being on all three tests, whereas the nonaerobic group improved scores on the Life Situation Survey and General Health Questionnaire but not on the Job Stress Questionnaire. The control group improved on none of the measures and scored higher on the Life Situation Survey at the second test time.

In summary, general agreement exists on a relationship between exercise and improvement of mood, although researchers tend to avoid statements of causality.

The association between improved mood and exercise is extraordinarily important for the treatment of chronic pain and chronic pain syndrome patients. These patients often have complaints of depression and anxiety as comorbid expressions of their pain. Although treating anxiety and depression may not fit into the historic role of the physical therapist, the effects of exercise on these mood states should not be underestimated in their importance.

Effects of Exercise on Pain

A number of studies have shown that exercise plays a role in increasing pain tolerance (Haier et al. 1981, Janal et al. 1984, De Meirleir et al. 1985, Gurevich et al. 1994). Both single sessions of exercise (Atkinson 1977,

Ekbom and Lindahl 1970) and a regular aerobic exercise regimen (Fitterling et al. 1988, Lockett and Campbell 1992) have been shown to reduce the intensity, frequency, and duration of migraine headache. Patients with rheumatoid arthritis or osteoarthritis who participate in an aerobic exercise regimen show significant improvements in pain tolerance and overall joint pain (Ike et al. 1989). Dental pain thresholds have been elevated by aerobic exercise (Petrovaara et al. 1984, Droste et al. 1991, Gurevich 1994).

Physical Fitness in the Chronic Pain Population

Mayer coined the term *deconditioning syndrome* to describe the physical changes observed in chronic low back pain patients (Mayer 1968). Cady et al. (1979) wrote the earliest paper that evaluated strength and fitness variables in workers with back injury. It examined five variables as they related to subsequent back injury occurrence in 1,652 firefighters during 1971–1974. The five variables were (1) endurance work (measured in watts at the end of 20 minutes of steady state exercise with a heart rate response of 160 beats per minute [physical work capacity (PWC)160]), (2) total isometric strength of selected muscle groups, (3) total spine flexibility, (4) diastolic blood pressure during exercise at a heart rate of 160 beats per minute, and (5) heart rate 2 minutes after standardized bicycle exercise. Three groups of firefighters were identified based on their fitness levels. The high-fitness group had a PWC160 of 181 W; the middle-fitness group had a PWC160 of 147 W; and the low-fitness group's PWC160 was 115 W. Subsequent frequency of injuries and cost per injury claim were analyzed in relation to fitness classifications. The frequency of injuries was 10 times higher for the least fit group than for the most fit group ($n = 266$ in least fit group, $n = 259$ in most fit group). The cost per claim for the 19 injured men from the least fit group was 13% more than for the 36 injured men from the middle-fitness group. There were too few claims made by the most fit group for an accurate estimation of cost per claim. These data show that good physical fitness is associated with fewer injuries at work and lower costs of worker's compensation claims.

A second publication in 1985 followed the earlier paper in which the results of a fitness program and a self-insurance system for worker's compensation were reported (Cady et al. 1985). After a 3-year period, average PWC160 had increased by 16%, with the oldest group (>50 years of age) showing the most improvement. Higher levels of PWC160, strength, and flexibility were found to be inversely related to worker's compensation cost. Individuals with greater flexibility, higher strength values, or higher watts at PWC160 were characterized by a much lower frequency of back pain and lower total injury costs. A correlation coefficient of r = 0.50 was found between the level of PWC160 and general activity level as obtained by interview.

In 1980, a study of seven men and eight women enrolled in a multifaceted inpatient pain program was reported in which the effects of a gradually progressive activity program on gait and physiologic capacity were evaluated (Thomas et al. 1980). The average treatment period was 6 weeks. During this period, patients exercised twice daily and worked toward individualized target walking distances and bicycling levels. Three walking tests were used for evaluation, one each at free, fast, and slow speeds on a 60-m level concrete track. The energy cost of walking was examined with measurements of oxygen consumption per minute, oxygen consumption per meter walked, and the oxygen-pulse value calculated from oxygen consumption per minute divided by heart rate. This study reported that chronic low back pain patients, at their self-selected speed, consumed 11% more oxygen than values expected for a normal population walking at the same velocity. After the treatment program, the mean velocity of walking at a self-selected speed went up by 19 m per minute, which brought the energy cost of walking to within 5% of a normal population. Thus, there was a decline in energy cost per meter with training that was equivalent to an 18% increase in walking efficiency. The predicted maximal aerobic capacity after the treatment program was 21.4–48.5 ml per kg per minute for men, and 25.6–45.1 ml per kg per minute for women. There was a 14% improvement in men and a 38% improvement in women. It is clear that chronic pain can cause a measurable reduction in aerobic capacity and that it may be reversed in a relatively short time with a suitable activity program. It is also important to note that these data point out the inefficient movement patterns adopted by chronic pain patients that result in inefficient walking. Patterns such as muscle guarding, limping, tightness, or weakness may account for this result. An activity program appears to benefit patients with this problem as well.

Schmidt (1985) investigated whether differences could be established between physical performance in chronic low back pain patients and a control group and whether differences between groups could be explained by increased pain. Thirty-nine subjects were in each group. The mean age for both groups was 41 years. Patients reported a mean pain duration of 104 months. All subjects performed a treadmill test at 5 km per hour on a 5% incline for 1 minute. The incline then increased by 1% at 1-minute intervals. The total time on the treadmill, RQ, and heart rate at the end of exercise were used to determine group differences. Pain was measured on a Visual Analogue Scale (VAS) before and after the test. There was a significant difference in performance between groups. The chronic low back pain patients spent much less time on the treadmill (a mean of 10 minutes, 40 seconds vs. 14 minutes, 42 seconds), had a lower peak heart rate at the end (a mean of 159 vs. 170), and a lower RQ (a mean of 0.98 vs. 1.04). Pain before the test in the chronic low back pain group was rated at an average of 45 and increased to an average of 53 at the end of the test. Schmidt concluded that the poorer physical performance of the chronic low back pain group could not necessarily be attributed to an increase of pain during the test since their VAS scores increased only slightly. He stated that chronic low back pain patients are poorer at discriminating between their chronic pain and muscular pain arising from an intensive exercise involving infrequently used muscles. The mean difference of 8 mm on the VAS was slight but may be clinically meaningful to chronic low back pain patients.

McQuade (1988) described the association between physical fitness, pain, depression, physical dysfunction, and psychological dysfunction in a sample of 96 chronic low back pain patients. All measures were taken at the same time. Pain was measured using the McGill Pain Questionnaire and the VAS to determine an average pain value during the previous week. The average hourly level of pain over the week was measured using an activity diary. Physical and psychosocial disability were measured with the Sickness Impact Profile. Depression was assessed with the Center for Epidemiologic Studies Depression Scale. Physical work capacity was measured by calculating a workload-to-heart rate ratio and then standardizing this to a heart rate of 150 on a bicycle ergometer (PWC150). Oxygen consumption was estimated from the heart rate/oxygen consumption relationship at submaximal workloads.

For 50 males and 49 females, the mean estimated maximum oxygen consumption was 20.5 ml per kg per minute. This value is comparable to an expected value for an elderly unfit 70-year-old subject with no pain. There was a modest association between aerobic capacity and self-reported activity levels. Those with fewer physical limitations had a higher activity level and a higher aerobic capacity. There was no relationship between pain and physical fitness and a negative relationship between fitness and psychosocial dysfunction.

The benefits of a 3-week functional restoration program over a 1-year observation period in 59 people disabled with chronic low back pain was reported in 1989 (Hazard et al. 1989) Thirty-eight males and 19 females with a mean age of 37 who were disabled for an average of 19 months without evidence of surgically correctable disease participated in the program. The program ran for 53 hours per week and included physical therapy (stretching, strengthening, and reconditioning), occupational therapy (work hardening), psychological treatment, and behavioral counseling. Pain was assessed using a VAS, and functional status was measured by the Oswestry Questionnaire. Aerobic capacity was assessed by a cycling endurance test in which work demands were increased by 100 kilopond meters (kpm) per minute at 2-minute intervals until patient intolerance or a target heart rate of 85% of predicted maximal heart rate (220 – age) was reached.

Working patients differed significantly in age from nonworking patients. This could be a confounding factor in the reported differences. Working men had an initial cycling endurance of 90 kpm per minute and an improved postprogram endurance of 196 kpm per minute. Working women began at 36 kpm per minute and ended at 80 kpm per minute. Nonworking men began with 53 kpm per minute and ended at 106 kpm per minute. Nonworking women had an initial endurance of 49 kpm per minute and a postprogram endurance of 90 kpm per minute. After 1 year postprogram, working men had values of 129 kpm per minute, working women 55 kpm per minute, nonworking men 78 kpm per minute, and nonworking women 80 kpm per minute. All groups lost cycling endurance during the year after the program but did not regress to pretreatment levels. This suggests that the exercise program was not adhered to vigorously by these subjects. Hazard et al. also suggested that graduates of the program were not distinguishable from unemployed counterparts when they did return to work, except by their cycling endurance and Oswestry scores, but that these two values could not explain why some patients returned to work and others did not. They all showed similar scores on trunk isokinetic flexion and extension, lifting capacity, pain, and depression regardless of whether they were working.

After a second year of postprogram follow-up, Hazard et al. (1991) reported that subjects who did return to work 1 year after treatment had greater cycling capacity, as well as lower Minnesota Multiphasic Personality Inventory schizophrenia scores, higher Wechsler Adult Intelligence Scale-Revised scores, and lower levels of cigarette smoking. Initial and discharge cycling endurance were the best physical score predictors of employment status 1 year after treatment, but cycling endurance did not correlate with program completion. Initial pain intensity scores were higher for program graduates than for program dropouts.

In the largest study of this kind to date, 3,020 employees at the Boeing plant in the Seattle area were enrolled in an investigation of the role of cardiovascular risk factors and fitness in industrial back pain complaints (Battie et al. 1989). The subjects ranged in age from 21 to 67 years, with a mean age of 36.2 years. Men comprised 78% of the study participants. A cardiovascular risk questionnaire was administered that screened for high blood pressure and history of heart disease. Subjects with these risks ($n = 399$) were eliminated. All of the remaining subjects were tested submaximally on a treadmill to determine predicted maximal aerobic capacity. Test endpoints were 80% of predicted maximal heart rate or physical discomfort. Maximal oxygen consumption estimates were obtained on 2,434 subjects who were then followed for more than 3 years in order to track subsequent back problems.

Both men and women, 28.5% and 28.3% respectively, reported a history of back problems for which they had sought some medical help. Only in men was there a relationship between back pain and a high risk for cardiovascular disease. The maximal oxygen consumption values did not differ significantly between subjects with or without back problems when controlling for sex and age. This finding conflicts with the earlier study of Cady et al. (1979), who suggest that fitness may not affect the risk of having low back pain but may affect the response to the problem and recovery. A closer examination of the first 26 subjects to develop chronic, disabling back pain in the Boeing study group revealed a significantly lower fitness level compared with unaffected age- and sex-matched subjects. This finding suggests that people who are less fit do not recover as well from back injury or chronic pain as patients with higher levels of fitness do.

In 1991, a report was published comparing aerobic training in three different intervention groups (inpatient, outpatient, and control groups) (Hurri et al. 1991). The 245 participants were all blue-collar workers ages 35–54 years who were randomly assigned to the three groups. Treatment consisted of physical exercise, relaxation exercise, and massage. Testing was performed with a bicycle ergometer, beginning with a 25-W load and increased by 25 W every fourth minute until the subject reported maximum effort. Pain was rated on an index that was the sum of pain VAS ratings for morning, after a workday, and evening. Subjects also rated their disability during the preceding month in 15 different situations. Results showed no differences in aerobic capacity between these three groups either before or after treatment, and therefore analyses were carried out on the whole sample as one group. $\dot{V}O_2$max values were within the range of normal reference values but somewhat low for age. These values also did not correlate significantly with the pain or short-term or long-term changes in the pain or disability index. This study seems to suggest that blue-collar workers are only slightly deconditioned compared with other chronic pain patients and that exercise, relaxation, and massage are not able to make a difference in aerobic capacity, pain, or disability measures over the period of treatment.

A study investigating the effects of an exercise program enrolled 111 industrial employees who were on sick leave due to back pain (Kellett et al. 1991). An exercise program was instituted during working hours, with an additional exercise session at least once per week outside working hours, for 1½ years. Before initiation of the exercise program, a baseline period of 1½ years was used to establish the number of days of sick leave due to back pain and the number of episodes of back pain occurring. Then the group was divided into an exercise group (n = 59) and a control group (n = 53), with comparable mean ages.

The exercise program included a warm-up, gentle stretching exercise, alternate strengthening and aerobic conditioning exercises, and 10-minute lectures about traditional theories regarding back pain. Each exercise session lasted 30 minutes and was followed by 10 minutes of relaxation. Attendance averaged 77% at each session. For the pre- and post-test of physical fitness, the participants rode a bicycle ergometer at an intensity that provoked a steady state heart rate of at least 120 beats per minute. Both the exercise and control group subjects performed this test. The mean preprogram estimated aerobic capacity for the exercise group was 43.28 ml per kg per minute and 44.36 ml per kg per minute for the control group. These preprogram differences were not significant. The exercise group experienced a 36% dropout rate, whereas the control group had a 9% dropout rate.

At the end of the program, the exercise group had a 51.2% decrease in sick days due to back pain, whereas the control group had a 65% increase. There was no significant difference between the groups in the number of back pain episodes reported. Aerobic capacity was not significantly different postprogram in the exercise group; however, it had dropped significantly in the control group. Thus, the reduction in sick days in the exercise group could not be attributed to an increase in fitness. Enrollment in the exercise program did have a significant impact on subjective improvement of back pain, however.

In 1992 a study reported on the differences in mobility, strength, and fitness between an operant conditioning approach and a traditional approach to treating subacute low back pain (Lindstrom et al. 1992). Physical fitness was estimated using a bicycle ergometer on which the baseline load of 50 W was increased stepwise by 50 W every 6 minutes until a steady-state heart rate of 130 beats per minute was achieved. The VAS was used to rate pain, which was not different between the two groups before treatment. The estimated maximal oxygen consumption for the operant conditioning group before and after treatment was 20.7 ml per kg per minute and 28.2 ml per kg per minute, respectively. The mean number of appointments with the physical therapist was 10.7. After 1 year, the operant conditioning group had an estimated maximal oxygen consumption of 33 ml per kg per minute compared with the control group mean (18.6 ml per kg per minute). Patients in the operant conditioning group returned to work 5 weeks earlier than the patients in the control group. After 2 years, the average duration of sick time taken due to low back pain was 12.1 weeks in the operant conditioning group and 19.6 weeks in the traditional care group. Thus, this study supports the idea that more physically fit patients recover from back injury better and return to work sooner.

Aerobic power in 46 chronic pain patients was assessed before and after a residential multidisciplinary treatment program (Davis et al. 1992). Twenty-seven males and 19 females were tested for physical fitness on a bicycle ergometer using increments of 20 W per minute for women and 30 W per minute for men. The average age of these subjects was 38.4 years, and the predominant complaint was low back pain. The mean duration of pain was 41.2 months (range of 7–216 months), and the mean number of surgical procedures per patient was 1.1. The mean pretreatment aerobic capacity for the group was 16.2 ml per kg per minute. The mean group RQ on the bicycle ergometer test was 1.05. After treatment, the mean group aerobic capacity was 19.1 ml per kg per minute with a RQ of 1.11. Thus, the patients were able to achieve a higher exercise effort on their post-treatment exercise test and moved from the sedentary category to the sedentary/light or light activity level of functioning. This change was due to a physical conditioning effect, an ability to desensitize to the symptoms accompanying physical exertion, or both.

A study evaluating the effects of aerobic exercise after lumbar micro-discectomy was reported in 1994 (Brennan et al. 1994). Thirteen men and six women from one neurosurgical practice (mean age 35.8 years) participated in the aerobic exercise program, whereas 11 men and six women from a second neurosurgical practice (mean age 32.6 years) did not. Initial testing was done 4 weeks after surgery. Patients were asked to rate their pain on a VAS and to complete the Activity Pattern Indicator Questionnaire. Treadmill testing using the Balke protocol was done, and oxygen consumption was measured. The treatment program lasted for 12 weeks, during which exercise was performed five times per week at 70–80% of maximal heart rate. The nontraining group performed stretching and strengthening exercise. Maximal oxygen consumption values for the training group were 30.3 ml per kg per minute pretreatment and 38.1 ml per kg per minute post-treatment. For the nontraining group these values were 29.6 ml per kg per minute pretreatment and 32.3 ml per kg per minute post-treatment. These differences between groups were statistically significant. No differences were found between groups for VAS and Activity Pattern Indicator scores, even after the training period. It is clear that after surgery both groups are in a very low fitness category (fifth percentile). After the treatment period, the training group improved to a fair level of fitness (thirty-fifth percentile) and the nontraining group remained in a low fitness rating (tenth percentile).

These studies all found that chronic pain patients fall into the very low fitness or sedentary category, with the highest values found in working blue-collar subjects, and the lowest found at 16.2 ml per kg per minute by Davis et al. (1992). The subjects' capacity to improve with aerobic conditioning is clearly demonstrated. Improvement in aerobic capacity has an impact on their ability to return to work sooner and results in an apparently quicker recovery from back injury. These data provide a convincing argument that chronic pain patients can and should engage in aerobic training during their rehabilitation.

Practical Considerations for Exercise and the Chronic Pain Patient

In considering these findings, it is important to explore what type of exercise increases the threshold of pain, what types of pain exercise affects, and what the mechanism of this increased pain tolerance after exercise is.

Type of Exercise: Aerobic or Anaerobic

Although some work has been done to investigate the effect of exercise on pain threshold, it appears that exercise has been understood to mean aerobic training. Very little research exists on whether strength or aerobic exercise has greater pain threshold-raising benefits. Only one investigation could be found (Anshel and Russell 1994) on the effect of aerobic and strength conditioning on pain tolerance. They found that exercise incorporating aerobic fitness results in greater pain tolerance than strength training alone. Markedly increased pain tolerance for those undergoing aerobic training occurred between weeks 6 and 12 of the study. According to the authors, because an aerobic training effect usually occurs after 6 weeks, it appears that marked improvement in cardiovascular functioning is a relevant component in linking the role of aerobic work to pain tolerance.

Intensity of Exercise Required for Pain Control

The analgesic effects of exercise are generally attributed to the production of beta-endorphins during physical exercise (De Meirleir et al. 1985, Janal et al. 1984). The hypothesis that endorphins are necessary to mediate exercise-induced analgesia is called into question by recent evidence that a significant elevation in circulating beta-endorphins occurs only in exercise intensities of 75–80% $\dot{V}O_2$max or above (Donovan and Andrew 1987). Analgesic effects of exercise have been found at submaximal work loads of around 63% of $\dot{V}O_2$max, however (Gurevich et al. 1994). Droste et al. (1991) found that pain threshold elevations were most pronounced during maximal exertion, when the subjects reported the greatest fatigue. Elevations in pain threshold were correlated with rating of perceived exertion. This exercise-induced elevation in pain threshold did not appear to be directly related to plasma endorphin levels.

Reconditioning Exercises

The primary goal of reconditioning exercise in chronic pain patients is to improve functional performance. A general weakening of all tissues takes place with disuse. Exercise treatment should be directed at increasing the strength of the tissues so the body can respond to the functional demands placed on it. This can be done effectively with high repetition, low-load exercise and motions. Low loads prevent damage to the tissues, and high repetitions have been shown to be most effective in increasing metabolism in low-metabolism structures. This kind of exercise can be achieved with small dumbbells or other weights, pulleys, or Nautilus equipment. Placing stress on the low-metabolism structures can be done indirectly by muscle contractions. For instance, increasing the fluid exchange between the disc and the interstitial fluid surrounding the spine can be achieved by having the patient maximally flex and extend the lumbar spine repetitively. The patient can also be asked to perform a latissimus pull-down exercise with high repetitions. The contraction and relaxation of the muscle will have a pumping effect on the intervertebral disc, increasing its metabolic activity. Low-load, high-repetition exercise will increase muscle endurance. This is especially beneficial for postural muscles.

As the patient becomes stronger, the load can be increased and the number of repetitions decreased to increase the patient's muscle strength. The body will respond to the demands placed on it, but the challenge must not be punishing or damaging. The physical therapist must ensure that the exercise program matches the physical capacity of the patient's body.

The body responds to the demands placed on it by using a variety of homeostatic mechanisms. In the person with chronic pain, activity intolerance secondary to pain leads to physiologic and pathologic changes in almost all organ systems but specifically in those organ systems that are related to activity performance. Reconditioning the patient with chronic pain can restore health to many organ systems and specific tissues. This approach deals directly with pain as a symptom, changes the health status of the individual and has a profound effect on the perception of health status (and therefore on physical performance) in individuals in pain.

The aerobic challenge should follow the general guidelines for physical fitness development. The prescription includes (1) mode of exercise (any dynamic, freely moving, freely breathing form, preferably one that is enjoyable to the patient), (2) intensity of exercise (moderate, below the respiratory threshold of fatigue and dyspnea), (3) duration of exercise (at least 30 minutes, but can be in intervals), (4) frequency of exercise (four or five times per week unless the duration is less than 30 minutes, then at least once per day).

The quota system of exercise prescription is described in detail in Chapter 6. This system allows patients to achieve short-term goals that build up their tolerance so that they achieve the above exercise prescription. In some ways, they must be conditioned to exercise in a cardiovascular and pulmonary fitness program before they can be fully reconditioned for muscular strength and endurance. In the end, the program will recondition all systems supporting movement and functional improvement.

Mechanism of Exercise-Induced Analgesia

It appears that pain inhibition through exercise can be mediated through the opiate and the nonopiate systems. Rhythmic exercise stimulates the A-delta or group III afferents arising from muscle. Histologically, A-delta or group III afferents are a prominent group of fine myelinated fibers located in skeletal muscle nerves. More recent investigations indicate that these afferents respond to muscle stretch and contraction with low-frequency discharge (Thoren et al. 1990). For this reason, Kniffki et al. (1981) called the endings of these afferents *ergoreceptors*. Group III afferents do not respond to small movements of the limb and therefore are unlikely to be of major importance in motor control (Thoren et al. 1990).

Both a single session and repeated brief sessions of aerobic exercise have been shown to induce marked postexercise decreases in blood pressure that often last for several hours (Thoren et al. 1990). This decrease has been linked with inhibition of sympathetic nerve activity (Thoren et al. 1990)

Thoren et al. (1990) and Lundeberg (1995) hypothesize that rhythmic exercise activates the ergoreceptors. Impulses are then transmitted to the spinal cord and reach the periaqueductal gray nucleus (PAG), the hypothalamus, and the thalamus through ascending pathways (see Chapter 2). The thalamus, which is involved in pain perception, has opiate receptors of several types and contains enkephalinergic nerve cells. The PAG and nucleus raphe magnus (NRM) are part of the descending pain modulatory system and are involved in the central nervous system regulation of blood pressure. Both the midbrain PAG and the brain stem NRM are rich in opiate receptors. In the NRM, the descending inhibitory serotonergic neurons to the spinal cord are stimulated. The terminals of the descending fibers synapse on enkephalin-containing neurons, which inhibit spinal neurons that mediate pain sensation. Preganglionic sympathetic nerve fibers may possibly be influenced through this pathway also. In addition to the descending serotonergic pathway, there is another descending pathway that most likely originates in the reticular formation.

The hypothalamus is involved in autonomic control, including blood pressure and pain modulation, and contains the nucleus arcuatus, which is the major beta-endorphinergic nerve cell site in the central nervous system. The nucleus arcuatus has endorphinergic projections to the thalamus, the PAG, and the brain stem. The released beta-endorphin probably acts as a neurotransmitter or neuromodulator. The mechanism for analgesia induced by acupuncture and low frequency is probably similar to this (Lundeberg 1995).

There is some recent evidence that pain modulation mechanisms may have sex differences (Touchette 1993). Males may have more powerful opiate-dependent pathways than females. Males and females may have distinct nonopiate pathways (Mogil et al. 1993).

The hypothesis that pain control systems become more active with longlasting muscle exercise is supported by the finding that immobilized and inactive patients suffer more from pain than active ones do. It is important to keep the patient mentally and physically stimulated. Muscle training programs should be included in the rehabilitation of pain patients (Lundeberg 1995).

The results from the studies described above may not be directly transferable to patients with chronic pain states. Pain elicited in a laboratory setting in normal volunteers may or may not be comparable to clinical pain states. It is our experience that the majority of patients feel good when they are exercising. Although it may be interesting to find the mechanism of this feeling, the mechanism does not matter as long as the result of exercise is the desired one. Whether patients experience less pain after aerobic exercise because of distraction, a greater sense of control, improved body image, improved mood, activation of the pain-inhibiting descending systems, or reduced activity of the sympathetic system is unclear. Exercise appears to be an excellent tool to use in the treatment of chronic pain patients.

References

Adams MA, Hutton WC. The effect of posture on the lumbar spine. J Bone Joint Surg Br 1985;67:625.

Adams MA, Hutton WC. The effects of posture on diffusion into the lumbar intervertebral discs. J Anat 1986;147:121.

Akeson WH, Amiel D, Abel MF, et al. Effects of immobilization on joints. Clin Orthop 1987;219:28.

Anshel M, Russell K. Effect of aerobic and strength training on pain tolerance, pain appraisal and mood of unfit males as a function of pain location. J Sports Sci 1994;12:535.

Astrand P, Rodahl K. Textbook of Work Physiology, Physiological Base of Exercise (3rd ed). New York: McGraw-Hill, 1986.

Atkinson R. Physical fitness and headache. Headache 1977;17:189.

Battie MC, Bigos SJ, Fischer LO, et al. A prospective study of the role of cardiovascular risk factors and fitness in industrial back pain complaints. Spine 1989;14:141.

Brennan GP, Shultz BB, Hood RS, et al. The effects of aerobic exercise after lumbar microdiscectomy. Spine 1994;19:735.

Brown J. Staying fit and staying well: physical fitness as a moderator of life stress. J Pers Soc Psychol 1991;60:555.

Byrne A, Byrne DG. The effect of exercise on depression, anxiety and other mood states: a review. J Psychosom Res 1993;17:565.

Cady L, Bischoff D, O'Connell E, et al. Strength and fitness and subsequent back injuries in firefighters. J Occup Med 1979;21:269.

Cady L, Thomas P, Karwasky R. Program for increasing health and physical fitness of firefighters. J Occup Med 1985;27:110.

Camacho TC, Roberts RE, Lazarus NB, et al. Physical activity and depression: evidence from the Alameda County study. Am J Epidemiol 1991;134:220.

Coyle EF, Martin WH, Sinacore DR, et al. Time course of loss of adaptations after stopping prolonged intense endurance training. J Appl Physiol 1984;57:1857.

Coyle EF, Martin WH, Blomfield SA, et al. Effects of detraining on responses to submaximal exercise. J Appl Physiol 1985;59:853.

Crews DJ, Landers DM. A meta-analytic review of aerobic fitness and reactivity to psychosocial stressors. Med Sci Sports Exerc 1987;19.

Davis V, Fillingim R, Doleys D, Davis M. Assessment of aerobic power in chronic pain patients before and after a multi-disciplinary treatment program. Arch Phys Med Rehabil 1992;73.

De Meirleir K, Arentz T, Smitz J, et al. Effects of opiate antagonism on physiological and hormonal responses to acute dynamic exercise. Med Sci Sports Exerc 1985;17:235.

Deschenes MR, Covault J, Kraemer W, Maresh CM. The neuromuscular junction. Muscle fiber type differences, plasticity and adaptability to increased and decreased activity. Sports Med 1994;17:358.

Donovan R, Andrew G. Plasma beta endorphin immunoreaction during graded cycle ergometry. Med Sci Sports Exerc 1987;19:229.

Droste C, Greenlee M, Schreck M, Roskamm H. Experimental pain thresholds and plasma beta endorphin levels during exercise. Med Sci Sports Exer 1991;23:334.

Dudley GA, Gollnick PD, Convertino VA, et al. Changes of muscle function and size with bedrest. Physiologist 1989;32(Suppl):1.

Ekbom K, Lindahl J. Effect of induced rise of blood pressure on pain in cluster headache. Acta Neurol Scand 1970;46:585.

Fisher AG, Jensen CR. Scientific Base of Athletic Conditioning. Philadelphia: Lea & Febiger, 1990.

Fitterling JM, Martin JE, Gramling S, et al. Behavioral management of exercise training in vascular headache patients: an investigation of exercise adherence and headache activity. J Appl Behav Anal 1988;21:9.

Frank C, Akesow WH, Woo SL-Y, et al. Physiology and therapeutic value of passive joint motion. Clin Orthop 1984;185:113.

Gamsa A, Vikis-Freibergs V. Psychological events are both risk factors in and consequences of chronic pain. Pain 1991;44:208.

Gogia PP, Schneider VS, LeBlanc AD, et al. Bedrest effect on extremity muscle torque in healthy men. Arch Phys Med Rehabil 1988;69.

Gurevich M, Kohn P, Davis C. Exercise induced analgesia and the role of reactivity in pain sensitivity. J Sports Med 1994;12:549.

Haier R, Quaid K, Mills J. Naloxone alters pain perception after jogging. Psychiatry Res 1981;5:231.

Hazard RG, Fenwick JW, Kausch SM, et al. Functional restoration with prospective study of patients with chronic low back pain. Spine 1989;14:157.

Hazard RG, Bendix A, Fenwick JW. Disability exaggerations as a predictor of functional and restoration outcomes for patients with chronic low back pain. Spine 1991;16:1062.

Holloszy JO, Coyle EF. Adaptations of skeletal muscle to endurance exercise and their metabolic consequences. J Appl Physiol 1984;56.

Hurri H, Mellin G, Korhonen O, et al. Aerobic capacity among chronic low back-pain patients. J Spinal Disord 1991;4:34.

Ike RW, Lampman RM, Castor CW. Arthritis and aerobic exercise: a review. Physician Sportsmed 1989;17:128.

Janal M, Colt E, Clark W, Glusman M. Pain sensitivity, mood and plasma endocrine levels in man after long distance running: effects of naloxone. Pain 1984;19:13.

Kellett K, Kellett D, Nordholm L. Effects of an exercise program on sick leave due to back pain. Phys Ther 1991;71:283.

Kniffki K, Mense S, Schmidt R. Muscle receptors with fine afferent fibers which may evoke circulatory reflexes. Circ Res 1981;48(suppl I):125.

LaFontaine TP, DiLorenzo TM, Frensch PA, et al. Aerobic exercise and mood. A brief review, 1985–1990. Sports Med 1992;13:160.

Lennox SS, Bedell JR, Stone AA. The effect of exercise on normal mood. J Psychosom Res 1990;34:629.

Lindstrom I, Ohlund C, Eek C, et al. The effect of graded activity on patients with subacute low back pain: a randomized prospective clinical study with an operant conditioning behavioral approach. Phys Ther 1992;72:279.

Lockett DM, Campbell JF. The effects of aerobic training on migraine. Headache 1992;32:50.

Lundeberg T. Pain physiology and principles of treatment. Scand J Rehabil Med 1995;32(Suppl):13.

Martinsen EW. Benefits of exercise for the treatment of depression. Sports Med 1990;9:380.

Mayer J. Overweight: Causes, Costs, and Control. Englewood Cliffs, NJ: Prentice-Hall, 1968;69.

McQuade K, Turner J, Buchner DM. Physical fitness and chronic low back pain. An analysis of the relationship among fitness, functional limitations and depression. Clin Orthop 1988;233.

Mogil J, Sternberg W, Kest B, et al. Sex differences in the antagonism of swim stress-induced analgesia effects of gonadectomy and estrogen replacement. Pain 1993;53.

Norris R, Carroll D, Cochrane R. The effects of aerobic and anaerobic training on fitness, blood pressure and psychological stress and well being. J Psychosom Res 1990;34:368.

North TC, McCullagh P, Tran ZV. Effect of exercise on depression. Exerc Sport Sci Rev 1990;18:379.

Olson J, Svendsen B. Medical exercise therapy: an adjunct to orthopaedic manual therapy. Orthop Phys Ther Prac 1992;4:7.

Petrovaara A, Huopaniemi T, Virtanen A, Johansson G. The influence of exercise on the dental pain thresholds and the release of stress hormones. Physiol Behav 1984;33:923.

Petruzzello SJ, Landers DM, Hatfield BD, et al. A meta-analysis on the anxiety reducing effects of acute and chronic exercise. Outcomes and mechanisms. Sports Med 1991;11:143.

Salter RB. The biologic concept of continuous passive motion of synovial joints. J Bone Joint Surg Am 1989;242:12.

Salter RB, Field P. The effects of continuous compression on living articular cartilage. J Bone Joint Surg Am 1960;42:31.

Schaible HG, Grubb BD. Afferent and spinal mechanisms of joint pain: review article. Pain 1993;55:5.

Schmidt A. Cognitive factors in the performance level of chronic low back pain patients. J Psychosom Res 1985;29:183.

Sessle BJ, Hu JW. Mechanisms of pain arising from articular tissues. Can J Physiol Pharmacol 1991;69:617.

Sola AE, Bonica JJ. Myofascial Pain Syndromes. In JJ Bonica (ed), The Management of Pain (2nd ed). Philadelphia: Lea & Febiger, 1990;352.

Stein PN, Motta RW. Effects of aerobic and non-aerobic exercise on depression and self concept. Percept Mot Skills 1992;74:79.

St. Pierre D, Gardiner PF. The effect of immobilization and exercise on muscle function, a review. Physiother Can 1987;39:24.

Thirlaway K, Benton D. Participation in physical activity and cardiovascular fitness have different effects on mental health and mood. J Psychosom Res 1992;36:657.

Thomas LK, Hislop H, Waters R. Physiological work performance in chronic low back disability—effects of a progressive activity program. Phys Ther 1980;60.

Thoren P, Floras J, Hoffman P, Seals D. Endorphins and exercise: physiological mechanisms and clinical implications. Med Sci Sports Exerc 1990;22:417.

Tipton CM, Matthes RD, Maynard JA, Cary RA. The influence of physical activity on ligaments and tendons. Med Sci Sports Exerc 1975;7:165.

Touchette N. Estrogen signals a new route to pain relief. J NIH Res 1993;5:53.

Twomey L. A rationale for the treatment of back pain and joint pain by manual therapy. Phys Ther 1992;72.

US Department of Health and Human Services: United States Health and Prevention Profile, Washington, DC, 1986.

6   Physical Therapy Treatment

Harriët Wittink, Theresa Hoskins Michel, Lisa Janice Cohen, and Scott M. Fishman

All treatment plans should be based on an understanding of the physical and psychopathophysiologic changes associated with pain and should include treatment that limits the dysfunctional impact of chronic pain by changing the patient's behaviors and appraisal of pain (Dworkin et al. 1992).

Physical therapy treatment of pain patients includes the following goals:

1. Reduction of the impact of pain
2. Improvement in the patient's knowledge of independent pain management
3. Resolution of treatable impairments and an improved aerobic capacity
4. Improvement of functional capacity or attainment of measurable functional goals within a certain time frame

Common Physical Therapy Treatment Approaches for Pain Patients

Commonly used physical therapy treatment approaches for pain patients include operant conditioning, functional restoration, or modified functional restoration.

Operant Conditioning

The operant conditioning approach was first developed by Fordyce and colleagues at the University of Washington's department of rehabilitation. This program involved a 4- to 8-week inpatient period designed to gradually increase the patient's activity level and to decrease or end medication, crutch, cane, and brace use. The program is based on the assumption that, although pain may initially result from some underlying organic pathologic condition, environmental reinforcement can modify and further maintain various aspects of pain behavior.

The term *operant conditioning* refers to the modification of pain behavior and the shaping of pain-incompatible behavior (e.g., lying down, avoiding physical and social activities) not to the attempt to "cure" pain (Fordyce et al. 1968). This method addresses excess disability and expressions of suffering (Fordyce et al. 1985) and substitutes rewards for healthy behavior (such as productive activity directed toward achievement of goals) for traditional expressions of sympathy and concern. The goal of this approach is to ignore pain behavior so it is not reinforced, whereas the desired behavior is reinforced with compliments and attention (Greenhoot and Sternbach 1977).

Physical therapy treatment in the program uses exercises that take into account the nature and site of the pain problem and general physical status considerations (Fordyce et al. 1981). According to Fordyce et al. (1981),

> The exercises also perform the function of identifying the starting point or baseline of each patient in regard to exercise tolerance. The operant treatment program emphasizes increasing exercise and activity level. Early exercises are termed baseline sessions. For each baseline session and for each exercise, the instructions are given in a working-to-tolerance mode. Specifically, the patient is instructed by the therapist as follows: "Do as many as you can until pain, weakness, or fatigue cause you to stop."

Quotas are then set for each exercise. Each quota should be less than the average baseline number of repetitions. This ensures that the patient can meet the first quota so that he or she receives positive feedback for achieving a goal. Quotas are then increased at a predetermined rate regardless of how the patient feels. This separates fear of pain from activity and allows the patient to relearn healthy behaviors.

Case Example

The patient is a 42-year-old nursing aide who has had low back pain radiating into her right leg for 2 years after a work-related injury. She had a discectomy approximately 1½ years ago that did not alleviate her pain. She has been told by her health care providers to get bed rest and limit activity. She has had two trials of physical therapy, including ultrasound, heat, joint mobilization, and neural stretching. None of these treatments decreased her pain. She is not working, and her children, ages 9 and 12 years old, take care of most of the housework and grocery shopping. The most amount of activity she does is walking from her bed to the living room and kitchen. Recently, she saw a new physical therapist who was unable to reproduce her pain by physical examination. Objective findings included decreased lumbar range of motion (ROM) in flexion and decreased hip flexion bilaterally. Lower extremity strength, reflexes, and sensation were normal. Straight-leg raising (SLR) was negative for radicular pain bilaterally. Her physical therapist assigned a daily walking program and set of exercises. The next day, she woke up with increased pain in her back and leg—she was afraid she had reherniated her disc. She went to the emergency room and was told to stop the exercises, thus reinforcing the idea that activity causes harm to her back. Her physical therapist told her to stop the exercises and began treatment with hot packs and massage. Her pain behavior is now doubly reinforced. Her increased pain is most likely the result of movement of her stiff joints and deconditioned muscles and is misinterpreted as a new pain by both herself and her physical therapist. Treatment would have been more effective if the physical therapist had told her she would be sore the next day after exercise and that she might have increased pain in her back and leg. She should have been told to manage the soreness with local heat or ice and to continue exercising despite her increased pain. This patient had avoided physical activities because she was afraid she would harm her back. Instead of being reassured by her health care providers that soreness is a natural result of moving stiff body parts and that this will decrease as she exercises more, the response of her providers to her complaint of increased pain confirms her fear.

Functional Restoration

The term *functional restoration* was coined by Thomas Mayer. This approach integrates a functional rehabilitation emphasis with a multimodal pain management program that uses a comprehensive cognitive-behavioral treatment orientation to help patients better cope with and manage their pain, temporarily increased while undergoing the "sports medicine" approach to back care (Mayer et al. 1986). The philosophy of the functional restoration approach is that almost all patients suffering from chronic low back pain can be returned to a productive lifestyle (i.e., work). The primary goal for each patient is restoring high levels of function rather than eliminating pain and to reduce reliance on health care providers (Mayer and Gatchel 1988).

The central assumption in this treatment approach is that the major physical deficit in chronic low back patients is the "deconditioning syndrome," caused by prolonged disuse of spinal joints and muscles. Physical therapy treatment consists of aggressive individualized physical reconditioning based on the objective quantification (i.e., isokinetic testing) of physical functioning.

In this program, no hands-on techniques are used, and modalities such as heat, ice, and transcutaneous electrical nerve stimulation (TENS) are discouraged. Patients are weaned from their braces, canes, and crutches, as well as from their pain medications. The goal is return to work, and more emphasis is placed on work simulation.

The program consists of four phases. In the preprogram phase, the patient is instructed in a generic stretching program at home to normalize ROM. The second phase involves the most contact with and supervision of the patient. During an intensive 3-week program, there are 150 contact hours, with 50% spent in training and 50% in counseling. The physical therapy part of the comprehensive program focuses on the patient's strength, endurance, and aerobic capacity.

Mayer and Gatchel (1988) emphasized that physical therapists should rely increasingly on objective, functional-capacity assessment technology for mobility, strength, and endurance tests. Exercises progress based on these tests, with the goal of attainment of normative values for strength and endurance. Therefore, patient's progress is based on the outcome of their testing regardless of their pain.

The follow-up phase is of variable frequency and duration. Patients are responsible for maintaining a home exercise program, using an exercise facility, or both. The fourth phase tracks long-term outcomes.

Modified Functional Restoration

In the changing health care environment, the focus of physical therapy treatment has shifted from dealing with impairments to emphasizing the achievement of functional outcomes. Treatment of impairments must be linked to improved physical functioning. Also, the patient is no longer seen as a passive recipient of health care. Instead, an active partnership between the patient and the physical therapist is formed to achieve treatment goals. Patients are expected to take an active role and to learn to manage their problems independently. Education and instruction in home programs are extremely important. These changes are not new to treatment approaches for chronic pain patients.

Since the development of the initial treatment philosophies for chronic pain patients described above, progress has been made in understanding of tissue behavior, motor planning and execution, exercise specificity, and pain mechanisms. Guarding and limping may not be just pain behaviors, but rather a reflection of abnormal sensory feedback resulting in abnormal motor output. Extinguishing pain behaviors without changing a patient's cognition (see Chapter 9) may not lead to an optimal outcome. The relationship of high-technology equipment to both assessment and treatment of functional ability remains unclear. The use of pain modalities such as TENS, ice, and heat can be used to increase functional levels without increasing pain behaviors. Physical therapists now have a wide range of techniques to help patients regain optimal functional ability. Earlier treatment philosophies must be updated, and the original functional restoration model for spinal dysfunction patients must be expanded for all chronic pain patients. Thus, although the treatment focus still is on functional restoration, this program deviates from the program initially conceptualized by Mayer and Gatchel (1988). Ideally, chronic pain and chronic pain syndrome patients are treated by a team of health care professionals who address the multifaceted nature of their pain.

Physical therapy treatment for chronic pain and chronic pain syndrome patients can include ice, heat, TENS, traction, massage, and exercise. The decision about whether treatment should include hands-on techniques is based on assessment tools described in Chapter 4 and on the evaluation of the patient.

Although it is appropriate to treat patients with acute pain with hands-on techniques, this approach may not be appropriate for chronic pain patients. Chronic pain patients can be helped only with hands-on techniques if their pain is reproducible. In fact, the use of hands-on techniques can be disastrous for chronic pain syndrome patients. If pain and functional limitations are no longer related, treating the pain will not change the functional level.

Furthermore, if a patient has had pain for a long time, it is unlikely that it can be "fixed." Chronic pain patients have often seen a variety of health care providers who all promise to cure the pain and who have tried and failed. During this process, patients become passive and increasingly dependent on, yet disillusioned with, the medical system. Physical therapy treatment of chronic pain should not focus on passive treatment techniques that deny patients control over their own physical health. The focus of physical therapy treatment should be on helping patients regain control over their lives by active participation in their pain therapy program and independent management of their pain. To achieve this, an active partnership should be established between the patient and the physical therapist. The physical therapist becomes a guide, helping the patient achieve the desired goals of independent pain management; improved functioning; and control through education, behavioral modification, and appropriate physical therapy treatment in an environment sufficiently secure to reduce fear and promote self-confidence. The role of the physical therapist is that of motivator, challenger, and educator. The patient participates by following through with the home program and taking responsibility for pain management and achievement of functional goals. The following aspects of treatment are central to the management of chronic pain patients:

1. Education
2. Instruction in self-management of pain
3. Functional goal setting
4. Behavior modification techniques
5. Exercise
6. Modalities

Education
Patients are often surprisingly poorly informed about the nature of their pain, about the anatomy of their affected body part, and about the difference between acute and chronic pain. Education about the anatomy of the affected body part(s) and the pathophysiology of pain will help increase the patient's understanding of the nature of the problem, reduce anxiety, and increase his or her compliance with and participation in physical therapy treatment. Because referral to behavioral medicine is almost always necessary, good patient comprehension of the multidimensional nature of pain, involving both physical and emotional components, will help facilitate the patient's acceptance of the need for this referral. It should also dispel the patient's notion that he or she is being referred to a psychologist because the pain is "all in his or her head." Patients often complain that they feel they have not been given a diagnosis for their pain. They believe that if they had a diagnosis, their pain could be cured. The physical therapist should explain that diagnosing a specific type of pain (e.g., atypical facial pain, fibromyalgia, myofascial pain syndrome, complex regional pain syndrome) does not mean there is a specific cure for it. Patients need to know that there is no "magic bullet" capable of curing them from their pain and that health care providers do not have all the answers. Occasionally, patients suggest that for some reason treatment to cure their pain is being withheld.

Education about the range of treatments available for the patient's condition and pointing out that the patient has tried and failed these treatments should help dispel this notion.

Sometimes, patients are waiting for their health care providers to tell them what they already know: that their pain may never go away completely. The physical therapist should explain that this is why the focus of treatment is on improved functional ability and independent management of pain rather than on pain relief.

Education about the effects of deconditioning helps patients understand what is happening to their bodies as they start to exercise. Chronic pain patients should understand that their muscles have lost strength and endurance because of inactivity and that they are likely to experience soreness and fatigue with exercise for at least the first few weeks after starting an exercise program. Many patients are afraid to exercise because they think they will do more damage to their bodies, which will lead to more pain and possibly serious complications such as paralysis. The difference between hurt and harm should be explained. Patients must understand that increased pain with increased activity (hurt) does not equal a new injury (harm), but rather that muscle soreness and the aching of joints that have not been used for a long time are part of initiating an exercise program.

Education about pacing is also important. Many patients who have been inactive become disgusted with themselves and decide to undertake significant activity. This may mean cleaning the entire house in 1 day or shopping for 6 hours. Even though they are in a great deal of pain, they continue until they have completed their task. They are then in bed for the next week. Pacing is quota setting by the patient, in which the patient undertakes an activity but stops when the pain begins to increase and then takes time out to do some relaxation or physical exercises. Tracking how much activity time it takes before the pain noticeably increases helps the patient set quotas for the next time this activity is undertaken. (Sternbach 1987). The duration of the activity can then slowly be increased, and many patients find that, with this approach, their tolerance to activity increases without an increase of pain.

Perhaps most important is education about pain treatment itself and the expectations of the patient and the health care providers involved. Commonality between the goals of the program and the patient's goals increases patient compliance and participation, which is associated with a better treatment outcome. Shutty et al. (1990) showed that common treatment goals were strongly related to increased treatment satisfaction and, to a lesser extent, decreased ratings of disability 1 month after treatment.

Self-Management Techniques

One of the more striking differences between acute illness and chronic illness is the extent to which the patient takes an active role in management. For example, treatment of acute renal failure requires that the patient allow the medical treatment team to perform procedures, administer medications, and care for the patient's well-being. In contrast, insulin-dependent diabetes mellitus (IDDM) requires the patient to learn to measure blood sugars, administer insulin, and make major changes in lifestyle, especially in diet and activity level. It would not be appropriate for an otherwise competent and physically able person with IDDM to be a passive recipient of health care services to manage daily insulin needs. This expectation is applicable to the management of chronic pain as well. Self-management is a cornerstone of pain management. This is even more critical as shrinking health care resources continue to limit payment for physical therapy services. The therapist must be able to have a greater impact on the patient's function in a shorter period of time than ever before. This can be accomplished only by having the patient become an active participant in the process of rehabilitation.

Self-management techniques include the use of pain-control modalities (e.g., heat, ice, and self-massage) and a structured home exercise program. These tools may seem simplistic and obvious; however, the process of instructing and investing the patient in their use is difficult and complex. Part of the difficulty lies in the history of treatment failures with which patients often present. At best, past physical therapy will have had no impact on the patient's pain. It is common for a patient to state in the initial interview that physical therapy worsens his or her pain. A number of factors may be responsible for past treatment failures, including persistent failure of physical therapists to recognize and treat the differences between acute and chronic pain states, past treatment that did not address the emotional and cognitive aspects of chronic pain, and an inability of the patient to recognize anything less than total pain relief as success. It is the responsibility of the physical therapist treating chronic pain to work with a patient to change his or her perception of physical therapy. The tools of physical therapy must be reframed in a positive and functional light. This can be accomplished by helping the patient invest himself or herself in the treatment process. The simpler and more accessible the tools given to the patient, the more likely he or she will be compliant in the use of those tools.

The benefits of exercise have already been discussed in Chapter 5. Those benefits, however, can be realized only by consistent performance. Exercise in the context of the physical therapy clinic is of limited benefit without independent performance at home. Success in an exercise program can make the difference between function and failure for a patient with chronic pain. It is the responsibility of the physical therapist to ensure that the home program is structured, appropriate, and meaningful.

Many patients with chronic pain fail to exercise appropriately because they have lost the ability to self-assess and self-regulate activity. Patients have a tendency to do less when they feel more pain and fatigue and more on days when they feel reasonably well. Although this is understandable, it is detrimental to progress. It allows for continued linking of pain with function and results in a discontinuous course of many exercises performed on good days and none on a bad day, without any clear progression toward a goal. Furthermore, there is the danger the patient will overexercise when he or she feels well, to make up for not exercising previously. Overuse or postexercise soreness often results from this pattern. Patients have difficulty choosing between the conflicting philosophies of "let pain be your guide" and "no pain, no gain." With appropriate structure, patients can learn to adequately listen to their bodies and make intelligent choices about exercise intensity.

That structure should include therapist-directed quotas set at a submaximal level to ensure early success with an appropriate rate of increase built in.

Exercise must be compatible with a person's lifestyle, or compliance will be poor. The type of exercise should have meaning in a patient's life, and the ritual of performing it should fit into his or her daily schedule. The therapist should work with the patient to find the types of activities the patient has enjoyed in the past or has interest in pursuing currently. It may be necessary for the therapist to help the patient modify the activity or his or her expectations about performance for the patient to feel successful.

Case Example

The patient is a 37-year-old former construction worker who had a work-related lifting injury 5 years ago. He has had chronic low back and lower extremity pain, with several unsuccessful trials of physical therapy in the past. He is fearful of beginning an exercise program. He is also frustrated at his low level of physical conditioning and constantly talks about how much he was previously able to bench press when he was actively weightlifting. Working with the patient, the therapist chooses an exercise regimen consisting of a stationary bicycle program (he wants to bike with his children) and exercises to encourage self-mobilization of the pelvis/low back area (he has difficulty with any activity that involves lumbar motion). The patient is instructed in the use of the bicycle, including proper height adjustment and use of low-resistance settings. He is asked to ride the bicycle for as long as he can until pain or fatigue limits him. He is instructed in pelvic tilt, lower trunk rotation, knee-to-chest, and bridging exercises. He is told to perform as many repetitions as he can until pain or fatigue limits him. He is asked to do this once a day for 3 days and to keep a chart of the results. On the next physical therapy visit, the therapist reviews the following numbers:

	Day 1	Day 2	Day 3
Bicycle	3 min	10 min	2 min
Pelvic tilt	5 repetitions	12 repetitions	0 repetitions
Trunk rotation	5 repetitions	8 repetitions	2 repetitions
Knee-to-chest	5 repetitions	10 repetitions	2 repetitions
Bridging	5 repetitions	7 repetitions	0 repetitions

The patient shows a pattern of poor self-regulation, with an overdo/underdo cyclic response. The therapist averages the three trial results and chooses to begin the patient at 60% of the average of each exercise because the trial results are so widely divergent. The following baselines are chosen for this patient's home program:

Bicycle	3 min
Pelvic tilt	4 repetitions
Trunk rotations	3 repetitions
Knee-to-chest	4 repetitions
Bridging	3 repetitions

He is also given a structured rate of increase of one repetition or 1 minute every third day until he reaches 20 minutes on the bicycle and 12 repetitions of each exercise. At that time, the program will be revised to increase its level of difficulty. He is told to adhere to the schedule regardless of his pain level. He is told that he may modify the way he does the exercises by going slower, using less force or range of motion, or taking more frequent rest breaks; however, he must perform the program daily.

Case Example

The patient is a 72-year-old female with osteoporosis and arthritis. She understands that she must exercise to help slow her bone loss, as well as to help manage her pain, but she has always been a sedentary person. Her husband plays golf 3 days a week and walks daily at 5:30 A.M. He has been trying to convince her to walk with him, but she has difficulty with stiffness in the mornings. She is also afraid of hurting herself by trying to keep up with her husband. She lives in a condominium complex with a senior center. There is an indoor track that is reserved for walking three afternoons per week. The therapist helps the patient plot out a structured walking program on this track. Because people of differing abilities walk there, she does not feel compelled to meet her husband's standard of appropriate exercise. She can also take advantage of the time of day when it is easiest for her to move. Walking was the activity of choice for this patient because, although she had never formally exercised, she had always lived in a city and walked a great deal.

Functional Goal Setting

Function drives the treatment process. When functioning is increased, the subjective components of pain and disability are said to have decreased. Focusing on function allows the entire treatment team and patient to avoid issues that may disrupt a successful rehabilitation approach (Gatchel 1994).

The assessment should clarify patient's current level of functioning. Chronic pain patients most often report intolerance to sitting, standing, and walking and difficulty lifting and carrying. These problems limit ability to perform housework, shop, work, and play. Treatment begins with patients setting their own goals. This can be amazingly difficult for many patients. Greenhoot and Sternbach (1977) note that

> An extraordinary number of patients have literally never considered the possibility that they may have to adjust to their pain. It is as if time spent with the pain has been suspended, as if it "doesn't count" in one's life, and that when relieved these patients expect to start again in life where they were suspended, despite the fact that many years have usually elapsed since they were pain free.

Because many patients have viewed their pain this way, goals must be practical and attainable within a reasonable time frame (6–8 weeks). Some patients have no sense that they might be able to do anything at all because they are overwhelmed by their pain and need help in determining functional goals. Because their lives seem to have stopped when they started to have pain, it is not uncommon to have patients be unrealistic about their goals because they base them on the things they could do before the prolonged inactivity due to their pain set in. Occupational therapists are very skilled in functional goal setting, and joint assessment and treatment is recommended.

A patient who is unable to set functional goals even with help from the physical therapist is not likely to achieve a good outcome. It is possible that the patient has no functional goals. He or she may still seek complete pain relief or be involved in litigation that necessitates the amassing of medical bills.

Case Example

A 32-year-old male complaining of headache had insidious onset of headache 1½ years ago. Since then, he has seen 64 different specialists in three states. The results of computed tomography scan of the head, magnetic resonance imaging of the cervical spine, and blood work were all negative. When he was told his headache was muscular in origin, he disagreed. "I know something is wrong with me and I am not going to stop until I find someone who can find out what this is and fix it," he said.

When a patient has clearly unrealistic goals, further exploration of why the patient is seeking treatment is necessary. Some patients are happily disabled, meaning that, although they function at low levels, they are not distressed and have no real desire to change their current situation. They may have applied for social security disability insurance, and improving their function is not their goal because that may mean return to work, which they seek to avoid. These patients may just want some temporary symptomatic relief from their pain. It is up to the physical therapist to decide whether such expectations can be met.

Setting functional goals helps direct treatment and makes it more meaningful for the patient. The ideal program for a patient with chronic pain is related to the functional goals the patient has identified at the start of treatment. Specificity in training is an important factor. A stationary bicycle program may be good exercise to increase aerobic endurance, but it does not necessarily increase lower extremity strength needed for a specific lifting task. In this instance, squats and lunges may be a more appropriate choice. An example of detailed task analysis in prescribing exercise is presented in the section on functional activities.

Before initiating treatment, it is helpful to set the number of treatments per week and the number of weeks of treatment. Having a definite end point increases patient compliance and gives a framework to both the patient and the physical therapist in which to achieve goals and a behavioral change.

Treatment contracts are extremely helpful. These include the pain behaviors to be eradicated, goals, length of treatment, and limits on the number of times the patient can cancel or not show for treatment (Appendix 6.1). If a patient is motivated, a contract helps facilitate progress. If the patient is not motivated, displays an attitude detrimental to others in the group, systematically arrives late, or does not show up for appointments, the contract allows the physical therapist to discharge the patient.

Behavioral Modification Techniques

Abnormal illness behaviors such as fear avoidance and pain behavior need to be addressed because they maintain the vicious cycle pain patients are trapped in.

The operant behavioral approach to pain treatment involves having patients set their own functional goals and rewarding the accomplishment of each goal (positive feedback). It also includes ignoring pain behaviors such as grimacing, rubbing, sighing, and moaning (no feedback). Because patients are not being rewarded for expressing their pain, the pain behaviors gradually disappear.

Chronic pain syndrome patients need to learn to overcome their fear of activity and reinjury by increasing their activity levels gradually. This can be accomplished by a quota-based exercise program and education.

Case Example

The patient is a 39-year-old female who injured her back in a motor vehicle accident 14 months ago. After the accident, she was unable to bear weight on her left leg and was told by her physician to "stay off her leg." She complied with this advice and did not bear weight on the leg for 1 year and used bilateral crutches. She is referred with a diagnosis of possible reflex sympathetic dystrophy. The patient is encouraged to start bearing weight on her left leg. When she is able to bear enough weight on her left leg to hold her standing balance without leaning on her crutches, the next goal is use of only a cane within 2 weeks. Thus, this patient must increase her time ambulating with one crutch from no hours to 5 hours in 15 days. Increasing her ambulation time with one crutch by 20 minutes per day allows her to achieve this goal.

A home quota program allows the therapist to monitor the patient's compliance. The physical therapist can ask the patient to perform the number of exercises scheduled for that day. If the patient is unable to perform the preset number of repetitions in the clinician's office, questions can be asked about whether the patient is actually performing exercises at home. Addressing noncompliance is often a simple matter of clearing up the misconception that exercise harms the patient and providing an explanation of the importance of the home program. Patients should be told they must adhere to the program daily so they can achieve the goals they have set for themselves. If they have difficulty performing all exercises at once, they can split up their exercise routine into smaller sessions during the day. When patients understand these concepts and are compliant with them, they often report a great sense of achievement. Frequent positive feedback is very important. These patients are battling with their fear of movement and reinjury. For them, performing even five sit-ups can be a major achievement.

The cognitive-behavioral approach challenges dysfunctional beliefs. For example, patients may believe they are unable to lift more than 10 lbs. This belief is easily challenged by having the patient lift more than this without adverse effects. Showing patients that a belief is wrong is very therapeutic. Challenging dysfunctional beliefs should be done throughout the treatment process (see also Chapter 9). Repeated exposure to avoided activities has been shown to be effective in reducing fear and anxiety about them (Dolce et al. 1986). In fact, it has been shown that chronic pain levels stay the same or decrease despite significant increases in activity levels (Fordyce et al. 1981, Linton 1985, Rainville et al. 1992, Geiger et al. 1992, Dolce et al. 1986).

Behavioral treatment is most successful when done in groups. Having patients exercise with other patients who have pain provides positive reinforcement because patients come into contact with others who continue to function and exercise despite their pain. Patients realize that they are not the only ones who have pain and have others to talk to about their pain experiences and functional goals. They also receive feedback from the people they are exercising with. This feedback can be about pain behaviors other patients recognize as dysfunctional. Patients often point out to another patient that his or her behavior or belief is unhealthy. They support each other through the exercise sessions and provide positive feedback when a patient is clearly progressing or attaining a goal. This bonding between patients can be extraordinarily helpful to the patient's progress and to the amount of fun patients have while participating in physical therapy sessions.

Exercise

Perceived personal control over pain is associated with less distress and disability. The sense of personal control or internal locus of control can be strengthened by actively encouraging patients to take greater responsibility for their care. Physical exercise is of great value in addressing the need of patients to have control over their pain. Creating a normal health club or gym atmosphere provides patients with a positive environment associated with health and fitness and puts patients on a partnership level with the physical therapist.

In chronic pain syndrome patients, two sources of impairment may be identified: a primary impairment due to documented organic pathology and secondary impairments resulting from the physical and emotional consequences of painful experiences (such as inactivity and general psychophysiologic deconditioning).

Deconditioning results in decreased muscle strength and endurance, increased joint stiffness, postural strain, and loss of cardiovascular fitness, leading to activity intolerance. These impairments independently contribute to the perception of pain and inability to perform functional activities. The focus of physical therapy treatment is to improve functional ability and to help the patient achieve the goals set prior to treatment (see the section on functional goal setting). Treatment must target function to ensure carry over from the clinic to the patient's life. The impairments that interfere with the patient's ability to function and the eradication of behaviors that contribute to them need to be addressed. Specific tools to help patients achieve their goals include behavioral management techniques (see the section on behavioral management), of which progressive quota-based exercise is central, both at a patient's home and in the clinic.

A specific program is developed for each patient, addressing that patient's specific impairments and functional needs. This can be a difficult and challenging task, as it requires knowledge of tissue behavior, anatomy, and kinesiology and arthrokinematics. As stated previously, hands-on treatment can be detrimental to a chronic pain syndrome patient because it reinforces disability behavior and prevents the patient from taking responsibility for his or her own management of pain. It is easier to mobilize a joint than to invent an exercise that will allow the patient to self-mobilize it; however, physical therapists must advocate self-mobilization in the same way they do self-stabilization. The initial session with the patient is used to establish a home exercise program and the exercises the patient will perform in the treatment program. Baseline values are set for aerobic exercise (time on the treadmill, time on the bike, use of upper extremity ergometer) by telling the patient to "do as much as you can." The patient is progressed in a quota-based manner to aerobic exercise for 20–25 minutes at 60–75% of his or her maximal heart rate. Baseline values are set for weights and repetitions. Quotas are set at this time to increase the number of repetitions and weights per physical therapy session. Some therapists prefer to set a target for the program—for example, "at the end of the program you should be able to perform this exercise with x amount of weight and x repetitions"—and quotas are set accordingly. A daily, gradual progression of exercises disconnects patient's pain from function and lets the physical therapist know that the patient is exercising within the boundaries of his or her physical abilities, without doing damage to the tissues through overuse.

Although the program is individualized for each patient, each physical therapy session includes the same components: aerobic conditioning, muscle strength and endurance training, stretching, lifting, body mechanics/ ergonomics, sufficiently alternating to prevent muscle fatigue from one specific group, and review of the home-based quota exercise program. Most patients benefit from bridging and upper, lower, and diagonal abdominal; latissimus dorsi; rhomboids; quadriceps; and back extension exercises, as these exercises address muscle groups commonly used in most functional activities. Additional exercises are specific to the patient and his or her functional goals.

Patients are actively encouraged to record the amount of weight and repetitions used for each exercise at home and to take an active part in the documentation of their progress. Flow sheets are helpful for this as they can easily show progress being made (see Chapter 7).

Always inform the patients that the pain initially will worsen and that they are likely to be sore from exercising for at least the first week or weeks. After the initial increase of pain comes the sense of being able to carry out an exercise program, which will begin to erode the fear associated with movement.

Although the focus of treatment is on function and not on pain, an open mind must be kept when listening to patients. It is rare, but occasionally patients do develop new signs and symptoms consistent with new pathology and acute pain. Reevaluation and consultation with the referring physician may be appropriate.

Functional Activities

Patients should set their own goals so that treatment can be geared toward the functional goals they wish to achieve. Such a functional activity is then broken down in parts, which become part of the treatment program. It cannot be emphasized enough that in all treatment as described below, the focus is on functional restoration. Therefore, exercises should be performed in closed-chain and weight-bearing positions to simulate activities of daily living and the physical demands of functional tasks.

For example, lifting from floor to chest requires an ability to squat, bend at the hips, stabilize the upper body, and flex the arms. Preparation for this activity includes performing squats with weights combined with hip flexion and resisted arm flexion while standing with the scapulae adducted and the back and abdominal muscles co-contracted.

Lifting overhead requires scapular stabilization, full flexion of the upper extremities, and the ability to stabilize the spine and step forward. Exercises used to prepare for performing this activity include lunges; strengthening of the rhomboids and serratus anterior; strengthening and flexion of the upper, middle, and lower trapezius; and flexion of upper extremities against pulley resistance while stabilizing the lumbar and cervical spine.

Walking requires aerobic fitness, leg and trunk muscle endurance, and trunk rotation. Trunk muscle endurance and rotation can be strengthened using alternate arm extension against pulley resistance while standing. Treadmill walking simulates functional movement and increases leg endurance and aerobic capacity. Treadmill speed can be increased until normal walking speed has been achieved.

Most people need to perform activities that involve bending and rotation during their daily activities. Lumbar spine physiologic movement consists of flexion, sidebending, and rotation to the same side. This can be easily simulated with pulleys or with handheld weights.

Movement analysis is a challenge to physical therapists. Explaining to the patient that the purpose of the exercises is to achieve functional movement patterns helps ensure greater compliance with the exercise program, which leads to greater ability to perform functional tasks.

Physical impairments that interfere with functional ability should be addressed. Because joint pathology is thought to have an inhibiting influence on its surrounding musculature (Young 1987), care must be taken to restore normal strength and endurance of the musculature and to reestablish normal ROM of the joint.

Normalizing Range of Movement.   To establish normal ROM, joint hypo- and hypermobility, muscle tightness, and muscle weakness should be addressed.

Treatment of Joint Hypomobility
Active mobilization exercises play an integral role in the treatment of chronic pain patients. Self-mobilization exercises require specific starting positions or aids such as bolsters, belts, or pulleys. For example, mobilization of the upper cervical spine can be achieved by fixating the cervical spine on a roll-up to C3 in extension. The patient is then asked to tuck in the chin. This results in improved flexion of C0–C2. Another example exercise is alternating arm extensions with pulleys while standing. The patient is asked to follow the extending arm with the eyes and head. The result is a general increase in spine rotation. This exercise also simulates the functional movement of trunk rotation with walking and reaching behind. The principles of

medical exercise therapy as described by Oddvar Holten are helpful in self-mobilization of patients (Gustavsen and Streeck 1993). For example, if the goal of treatment is to improve thoracic extension, sidebending to the right and rotation to the left, then the lumbar spine should be positioned in extension and left sidebending (by putting a wedge under the left buttock). Thus, when introducing left rotation to the thorax, the lumbar movement becomes nonphysiologic, resulting in lumbar fixation (Gustavsen and Streeck 1993). An anteriorly rotated ilium can be self-corrected by maximally flexing the involved side in the direction of the axilla on the same side or by performing a strong isometric hip extension contraction (DonTigny 1993). Proprioceptive neuromuscular facilitation techniques (Sullivan and Markos 1987) can be incorporated easily, as they are based on functional movement patterns. Diagonal patterns can also be performed with pulleys or with weights.

Treatment of Joint Hypermobility
Stabilization training includes retraining the musculature to control and stabilize the painful joint. Exercise promotes the necessary strength, coordination, and endurance to maintain the joint in a stable and safe position during loading, mobility, and weight-bearing activities. Stabilization training optimizes the capacity of the joint to absorb loads in all directions while it minimizes direct strain and stress on individual tissues. It eliminates repetitive microtrauma to the joint and limits progression of muscle imbalance (Sweeney et al. 1990). Stabilizing the lumbar or cervical spine has become popular as a treatment of herniated disc disease or internal disc disruptions and is discussed further in the section about traction. In the case of a hypermobile spinal joint, physiologic movements can be used to avoid excessive movement across the hypermobile joint. For example, if the L5–S1 joint is hypermobile, the patient can be asked to exercise using pulleys with the legs spread apart, the spine extended, and weight mostly on the right leg. Sidebending to the right is associated with rotation to the left, resulting in movement in the midlumbar spine (Gustavsen and Streeck 1993).

These exercises are more difficult in the cervical spine. Care must be taken when exercising patients with cervical hypermobility with pulleys. Any movement with the upper extremities puts some force across the cervical spine. The patient must maintain co-contraction (optimal posture) at all times to avoid increased hypermobility.

Hypermobility of the sacroiliac joint is difficult to treat, as there are no muscles crossing the joint to stabilize. It may be necessary to stabilize this joint with a sacroiliac belt after making sure correct alignment is achieved with self-mobilization before having the patient engage in exercise. Commonly used exercises include resisted adductor and abductor exercises, gluteal and abdominal strengthening, and resisted internal and external hip rotation.

Stretching
Because muscle imbalance can be a precipitating factor in the development of both muscle and joint pain, it must be addressed. Janda (1986, 1988) observed that certain muscles respond to a given situation (e.g., pain, impaired afferentation by a joint) with tightness and shortening, whereas others respond with inhibition and weakness. Muscle responses seem to follow

some typical rules—the development of tightness, weakness, or both may be considered a systematic and characteristic deviation in the functional quality of these muscles. The final result of this deviation is a general imbalance within the whole muscular system (Jull and Janda 1987; Janda 1986; Evjenth and Hamberg 1984). Fine muscle coordination is needed to prevent damage to a joint, especially during fast movement; thus, balanced muscle coordination may be the best protection of our osteoarticular system.

Stiff or shortened muscles are often activated in movements in which they would otherwise take no part (Evjenth and Hamberg 1984). When this occurs, a changed sequence of activation of the muscle in the movement pattern follows, spiraling the patient further into a continuous cycle of weakness, tightness, abnormal movement patterns, and pain. Treatment consists of stretching the short musculature and strengthening the weak muscles. Normal posture will be sought, resulting in normal bony alignment and normalized stresses across the joints. Because shortened muscle is thought to inhibit the antagonist, Janda (1986) and Evjenth and Hamberg (1984) recommend stretching the tight muscles before strengthening the antagonist muscles. Khalil et al. (1992) investigated the effectiveness of systematic stretching of the lumbar paravertebrals, quadratus lumborum, tensor fascia femoris, gluteals, internal rotators of the hip, abdominals, trunk rotators, and hamstrings as an add-on treatment for chronic low back pain patients. When compared with a control group that completed the same rehabilitation program without the stretching, the stretching group showed a significantly greater decrease in pain. The stretching group also showed significantly greater increases in static back extensor strength and electromyographic output of the trunk paraspinal muscles. Back ROM in flexion and extension as well as SLR increased significantly compared with the control group.

Muscles are most safely and easily stretched when warmed up. Warming up can include an aerobic exercise or contraction against resistance. Since the shortened muscle inhibits its antagonist, the shortened muscle should be stretched before strengthening of the antagonist. A muscle should be stretched by applying a slow, static load for 15–20 seconds. Each muscle should be stretched three to five times for maximal benefit (Smith 1994).

Normalizing Muscle Strength and Endurance.   Although aerobic and strength and endurance training have been discussed at length in Chapter 4, a short review follows: Increased muscle strength, or muscle hypertrophy, is achieved by high-intensity, short-duration exercise. First, neuronal adaptation occurs by increased efficiency to recruit motor neurons. Second, an increase in myofibrillar protein occurs after about 6 weeks of exercise. The physiologic stress induced by lifting or holding a certain weight is proportional to the percentage of maximal strength involved. Increasing muscle strength enables the patient to perform such tasks with less physiologic stress.

Endurance exercise is the term used to describe two types of exercise. The first type is exercise targeted to increase maximal aerobic power or cardiovascular functioning by exercising patients at 65–85% of their maximal heart rate (e.g., treadmill walking or biking). Aerobic exercise is thought to have beneficial effects on pain perception and mood. Increased aerobic capacity supplies the patient with the energy needed to perform functional tasks. The second type is low-intensity, long-duration exercise targeted to increase the aerobic capacity of the muscle so that the muscle can sustain contraction for prolonged periods of time without fatigue. This improves neuromotor control and coordination and thus prevents injury to noncontractile structures during prolonged activities.

Numerous studies of the optimal amount of repetitions and weight for maximum strength and endurance gains have been conducted. No precise amount of resistance or number of repetitions has been conclusively demonstrated to be optimal, however. An overview of training systems has been provided by Sanders and Sanders (1985). Perhaps the most clinically useful directions are given by Holten in his pyramid training method. Exercising at a low number of repetitions (1–5) but at high resistance produces maximal strength by improving intramuscular coordination. Training at 8–12 repetitions and at a resistance intensity of 40–60% of maximal strength improves strength by increasing muscle mass. Training at high repetitions (15–30 or more) and at a low resistance of 20–40% of maximal strength improves muscle endurance (Weineck 1993, Olson and Svendsen 1992).

Instruction in Biomechanics

Once patients have normalized their ROM, muscle strength and endurance, and aerobic capacity, instruction in correct execution of functional movement patterns (e.g., lifting, reaching, getting up from a chair) and ergonomic instruction (e.g., positioning at the work site) should begin. Occupational therapists are skilled at teaching these tasks. Working with an occupational therapist, if one is available, is successful in reinforcing the carry-over from what the patient has learned in the clinic to the home and work environment.

Modalities

The evaluation of the patient is critical to the decision-making process on the use of modalities. The Multidimensional Pain Inventory assigns patients to one of three potential profiles: the adaptive coping, interpersonal distress, or dysfunctional profile. The dysfunctional chronic pain patient is least likely to be helped by the passive role most commonly assumed by patients receiving modalities. Modalities applied by the physical therapist should be recognized by the patient as passive treatment. The passive role is soothing and sympathetic and is therefore appropriate for patients in acute pain or for those who have recurrent pain from reinjury. It is also appropriate for pain due to cancer. Some modalities may be appropriate for patients with behavioral problems, illness behaviors, or secondary gain from pain behaviors, but only if the patient can control these themselves. For these patients, self-application of heat or ice can be therapeutic as positive reinforcement after activities. TENS application by these patients should be linked to increased functional activities. It is more advantageous if these patients are not allowed to adopt a passive role in treatment. Because the use of modalities is easy for patients to learn, it can play a role in effective treatment.

Heat

There are three theories regarding the mechanism of pain relief with heat application. The vascular theory postulates that heat application reduces pain by inducing vasodilatation, which can increase tissue blood flow up to 30 ml per 100 g of tissue (Lehmann and DeLateur 1990). The rise in blood flow effectively reduces ischemia by supplying oxygenated blood and nutrients while washing out metabolites (including those that contribute to nociception) accumulated during muscular activity.

The counterirritation theory is based on the gate control mechanism originally proposed by Melzack and Wall (1982). According to this proposed mechanism, thermoreceptor afferent input can act as a gating mechanism in the dorsal horn of the spinal cord at the spinal levels of the sensory input, which blocks pain transmission to higher centers. Also, heating of a painful part can induce whole body relaxation, which helps to inhibit painful muscle spasm or muscle tension. The means by which heating input activates a descending pain inhibitory system is not yet understood.

The third theory involves the direct influence of heat on muscle spindles and on sensory nerve conduction. When animal muscle spindles and exposed nerve endings are directly heated, a significant decrease in neuronal activity of the secondary endings and an increase in activity of primary endings and Golgi tendon organs have been measured. This produces a net inhibitory influence of the motor neuron pool that breaks the vicious circle of pain-spasm-pain (Newton 1990).

A variety of hot packs are commercially available for self-application of heat. Each type has advantages and disadvantages in terms of price, ease of reuse, temperature control, length of heating, and portability. Patients are instructed in the use of superficial heat to warm muscles before stretching and exercise, for relaxation, and for transient pain reduction. Once patients are instructed in the safe use of superficial heat, including the appropriate use of toweling to prevent burns, there is little clinical justification for including heat application as part of physical therapy treatment in the clinic. Patients may be invited to use heat independently before or after a treatment session.

Many therapists apply ultrasound as a heating modality. It has additional benefits because it penetrates to structures such as joints, muscle, and bone. It has been shown in experimental studies to stimulate tissue regeneration and bone growth (Dyson et al. 1968, Duarte 1983) and increase pain threshold and collagen extensibility (Alyea et al. 1956, Gersten 1955). In a meta-analysis of 22 studies on the effect of ultrasound application in the treatment of musculoskeletal disorders, however, no significant effect of ultrasound on pain reduction was found (Gam and Johannsen 1995).

Cold

Cold therapy can be delivered in two basic forms: cold packs or ice massage. Cold packs are commercially available or can be made at home with crushed ice, ice cubes, or bags of frozen vegetables. Cold packs are useful for postexercise soreness, inflammation, and transient reduction of pain (symptomatic relief). In ice massage, ice is rubbed directly over the skin until numbness is felt. Ice massage delivers cold to a more pinpointed area with greater efficiency than a cold pack and may also provide more effective counterirritant therapy for pain relief. Patients are instructed in the safe use of ice massage, the warning signs of frostbite, and the four stages of normal ice massage (cold, burning, aching, and numbness). Ice massage is useful for relaxation, transient pain reduction, and treatment of local inflammation. Cold application for pain relief can achieve peripheral or central responses. Brief, intense cold most likely produces peripheral receptor adaptation (Cattell and Hoagland 1931). The counterirritation discussed in the section on heat therapy also applies to cold therapy. Brief, intense cold (vapocoolant spray) can slow conduction velocity in C fibers carrying nociceptive input to the spinal cord. This action and receptor adaptation may be the mechanism of the trigger point therapy advocated by Travell and Simons (1983).

For every 1°C decrease in intramuscular temperature, a decrease of 1.2 m per second in motor nerve conduction velocity (Lehmann and DeLateur 1990) and a 2-m-per-second drop in sensory nerve conduction velocity has been recorded (Buchthal and Rosenfalck 1966). When tissue temperature is reduced by more than 10°C, a cold-induced vasodilatation follows the more immediate vasoconstriction effect of cold. This reversal continues as a cycling of vasoconstriction-vasodilatation, permitting tissue temperature to be kept somewhat constant, although lower than precooled temperatures. This is termed the *hunting response* and is noted primarily in areas of skin where arteriovenous anastomoses are found (ears, nose, fingers, toes) (Michlovitz 1990). Prolonged cold can also produce vasodilatation in deeper muscle tissues and stimulate profound hyperemia after withdrawal of the cold (Clarke et al. 1958).

The choice between using heat or cold for pain should take into account several factors. Heat decreases pain and induces relaxation. Therefore, it may have a counterproductive sedative effect if used before exercise. It increases tissue extensibility, which is advantageous when addressing stiff joints through self-mobilization and stretching. It decreases overall stiffness of musculoskeletal tissues. It may result in edema and should be used carefully if swelling is already a component of the patient's problem.

Cold decreases pain and swelling; however, it increases overall stiffness and decreases tissue extensibility. Some patients have a profound aversion to cold and experience anxiety with its use. This is counterproductive to most physical therapy goals. The therapist should choose a modality based on the patient's preferences and convenience for self-treatment. The emphasis is not on pain relief, but on using the modality as a method of coping with pain. It should be possible for a patient to learn to safely apply a modality as a specific part of the total pain rehabilitation program.

Electrical Stimulation

Electrical stimulation treatment ranges from low- to high-volt electricity and includes TENS, and interferential therapy. The two principal therapeutic effects of electrical energy are the generation of heat and the stimulation of neural tissue. It is most commonly used for pain, edema, muscle spasm reduction, and stimulation of muscle contraction. The passage of electrical current causes the dissipation of heat. The application of an external electrical field can cause ionic currents to flow in neural tissue. In the resting state, there is a potential difference of approximately 0.1 V across a neural membrane. If this potential is reversed for at least 20 microseconds, the neuron will be stimulated and an action potential propagated. Different types of neural tissues propagate impulses at different speeds. This factor and the differing stimulus duration requirements mean that for each type of neural tissue there is an optimum frequency at which the maximum response will be elicited. The optimum frequency for sympathetic nerves is 0–5 Hz; for parasympathetic nerves, 10–150 Hz; for motor nerves, 10–50 Hz; and for sensory nerves, 20–80 Hz.

Transcutaneous Electrical Nerve Stimulation.   TENS is based on the early work of Melzack and Wall (1965), whose theory suggests that the peripheral stimulation of large-diameter cutaneous afferent nerve fibers could block pain sensation at the spinal cord through the gate control mechanism. Based on this theory, devices were developed that allowed for stimulation of approximately 100 Hz, which was perceived by patients to be comfortable.

Stimulators have been developed that produce a more noxious stimulus of approximately 2 Hz. This is thought to stimulate the small-diameter afferent fibers, facilitating production of endogenous opiates and producing pain relief through the descending pain-inhibiting pathway (Pomeranz 1976). Other proposed mechanisms of pain relief through TENS treatment include (1) pain relief by restoring an artificial afferent input in a deafferented area (Frampton 1994) and (2) pain relief by direct mechanical inhibition of a sensitized, abnormally firing nerve ending after injury (Wall and Gutnik 1974). TENS has been shown to produce pain relief of skin and fascia but does not seem to affect deeper structures (Ishimaru et al. 1993).

TENS electrode placement and size and the selection of waveform is critical to successful pain relief. A free TENS trial of about 3 weeks is allowed by most companies that rent TENS units so that the clinician can attempt several electrode placements and stimulation parameters.

Several companies now offer high-frequency TENS, which operates at a frequency of 5,000 Hz and more easily overcomes the natural skin impedance barrier.

Case Example

A 63-year-old male treated with cryotherapy 7 weeks ago for a grade V prostate adenosarcoma begins to experience excruciating pain in his perianal area and deep pelvic pain. He rates his pain as 10 out of 10 and is unable to sleep or perform occupational and daily living activities. He is seen by a physician specializing in pain who prescribes him pain medication that reduces his pain to four out of 10. He is then referred for a TENS trial and management. Two electrodes are placed on his low sacral area and two in the S3 distribution on the inside of his thighs. The frequency is set to 150 Hz, random modulation, a clearly perceptible, but nonpainful intensity. This is successful in reducing the pain to one out of 10 immediately.

Three months after the initiation of TENS treatment, this patient still experiences significant pain relief due to his TENS and is able to decrease the amount of opioids he is taking to control his pain.

Electroacupuncture.   A technique using low-frequency, high-intensity current that produces stimulation similar to acupuncture is termed *electroacupuncture*. Stimulation is usually applied at distant acupuncture points. Conventional TENS is usually applied as high-frequency, low-intensity current and is applied near the site of painful stimulation. Electrodes are placed surrounding the pain site. With extensive areas of pain, there may be a need for dual channels to surround the area. If electrodes are not tolerated in the region near the pain, electrodes can be placed at the vertebral level corresponding to the spinal nerves innervating the painful area. Occasionally, contralateral electrode placement over the same distribution of peripheral nerve can be effective.

One of the benefits of electroacupuncture stimulation is the promotion of healing. There is considerable evidence that the cellular mechanism involved in tissue regeneration is accompanied by and may depend on the flow of an electrical current through the cells of the wounded tissue (Becker and Selden 1987). The Electro-Acuscope was developed to assist in wound healing and is good for more superficial tissues.

Microcurrent Electrical Nerve Stimulation.   Microcurrent electrical nerve stimulation has also been developed for promotion of wound healing. These devices produce a stimulating current approximately 1,000 times weaker than conventional TENS.

Interferential Therapy.   Interferential current of 4,000 or 5,000 Hz applies weak electrical current in two perpendicular directions so that the effects converge on a deeper area of tissue. Proposed mechanisms of pain relief include the following:

1. Gating in the dorsal horn by afferent input on myelinated A beta fibers.
2. Nociceptor transmission in the dorsal horn is inhibited by activation of nociceptive A delta fibers, which can provoke impulses in pain suppression systems traveling down the spinal cord.
3. Interferential current causes physiologic block in which high-frequency stimulation above 50 Hz could cause a temporary block in A delta and C nociceptive fibers. This would occur at frequencies around 80–100 Hz, whereas pain suppression systems would be activated at frequencies in the 10- to 25-Hz range. Both frequencies may be found at different stages of the interferential current cycle (Low 1994).
4. Increased blood flow in ischemic pain.
5. Placebo effect.

High-Volt Galvanic Stimulation.   High-voltage, pulsed galvanic stimulation has been recommended for wound healing, muscle stimulation, and pain control. It has a twin-pulse waveform with a very rapid rise and fall so that the high voltage lasts only a few microseconds. Average current is therefore small and relatively comfortable. The voltage applied can be from 0 V up to 500 V, and the double pulse frequency can vary from 2 Hz to 100 Hz. As a pain relief stimulation, the high frequency presumably stimulates the pain gate and the low frequency can modulate pain through endogenous opioid release.

Biofeedback. Biofeedback uses electrodes to measure the background electrical activity in muscle tissue. It has been used effectively in chronic pain to help patients reduce muscle spasm and overactivity of muscles. It is most effective in cases of low back pain, headache, or neck pain that is a result of postural adjustments resulting in overuse patterns (Janda 1986, 1988). Relaxation of muscle in the paravertebral group is difficult to achieve voluntarily, especially in the upright position. Biofeedback can assist the patient's voluntary efforts by providing a clear picture of muscle use and relaxation. In the presence of chronic pain, the sensation of muscle contraction is distorted and even masked. The electromyographic output can be used as a replacement for this poor sensory feedback (Morgan 1988). In a study of chronic pain patients, the combination of relaxation training and electromyographic biofeedback was associated with reductions in pain, depression, distress, and interference in function that was sustained over a follow-up period of 6 months (Spence et al. 1995).

Massage
Whether chronic muscle tension causes chronic pain or is a by-product of it has not been determined. Massage can be an effective tool in decreasing muscle sensitivity and therefore improving function. Massage can reduce pain by increasing local circulation and by stimulating A beta fibers. Several types of massage can be used each for specific purposes.

Ischemic Compression Massage. Ischemic compression massage applies sustained pressure to the trigger point with sufficient force and duration to inactivate it (Travell and Simons 1983). On release, the skin is blanched and then shows reactive hyperemia. To apply ischemic pressure, the muscle is first stretched to the verge of discomfort. As the discomfort tends to abate, pressure is gradually increased. If the patient tenses the muscle to protect the trigger point, the pressure is too much. This process is continued for up to 1 minute with as much as 20–30 lbs of pressure.

Transverse Friction Massage. In established scarring within a muscle, pain can be caused with contraction of this muscle due to adhesions that diminish muscular mobility. Such adhesions need to be "teased apart" by transverse friction massage (TFM). TFM attempts to break up the scar area and allow pain-free, normal mobility by preventing the scar from becoming adhered to the surrounding tissues. Deep transverse friction causes stimulation of nociceptive A delta fibers and mechanoreceptor A beta fibers. Therefore, pain modulation is thought to arise both from presynaptic inhibition (gate theory) and descending inhibition.

TFM applied to a lesion within the a muscle is performed transversely across the muscle fibers with the muscle in a relaxed and shortened position. The aim is to fully broaden the muscle and break down adhesions between adjacent muscle fibers. Tendons are placed under tension. The duration of treatment can be 10–20 minutes (Palastanga 1986).

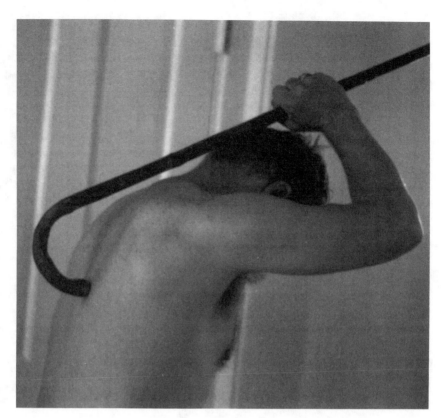

FIGURE 6.1
Use of a cane for self-massage.

Self-Massage. Self-massage is an active pain-control modality when it is incorporated into a patient's independent regimen. Self-massage may be administered by the use of a cane (Figure 6.1), umbrella handle, Theracane (a commercial device for trigger point massage), or tennis balls using the body weight as counterpressure. The patient may press a tennis ball against a trigger point and apply ischemic pressure or slowly rotate the ball around the painful area. Two tennis balls in a sock are used for neck pain and headache (Figure 6.2).

Traction

Traction applied constantly or intermittently can alter the pressure around discs or decrease the muscle tone by inducing a long-term stretch of paraspinal muscles (Myrenberg et al. 1990). Patients with signs of root compression traditionally benefit most from traction; however, it has been applied in cases of lumbago, sciatica, and rhizopathia. The following effects can be achieved with traction (Eggertz 1986):

- Opening of the intervertebral foramen
- Enlargement of the intervertebral disc space
- Separation of the intervertebral joints
- Stretching of a tight or painful capsule

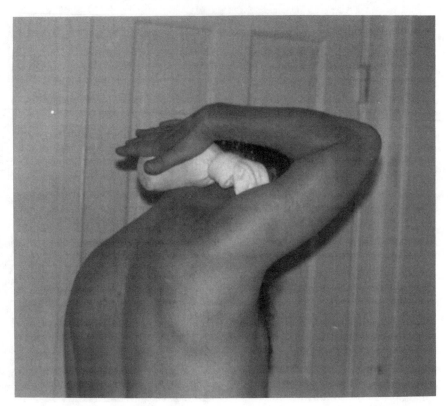

FIGURE 6.2
*Self-massage with
two tennis balls
in a sock.*

- Release of entrapped synovial membrane
- Freeing of adherent nerve roots
- Production of a central vacuum to reduce herniated disc material
- Tension of the posterior longitudinal ligament to alter the form of the herniated disc
- Improved blood flow to ischemic tissue
- Alteration of pressure within the spinal canal and across the dura mater

Intermittent and constant traction has also been indicated in the treatment of cervical syndrome, a condition in which pain and muscle spasm originate from irritation of cervical nerve roots at the exit point from the intervertebral foramen (DeLacerda 1986).

Traction of the lumbar spine is applied with the patient in supine or sidebending position. The computer-aided traction table known as Auto-traction is a specialized form of traction (Lind 1974). This form allows the initial patient assessment to be conducted so that the patient has total control of table manipulation. The patient finds the position of minimal pain for the final application of the traction force. Static traction is a passive force applied in a pain-free position for 25–35 minutes. The usual traction force is 250–300 Newtons (up to 60 kg). In their study of 200 low back pain patients, Myrenberg and Lundeberg (1989) outlined conditions that produced optimal success with this treatment. One to five sessions were usually sufficient. Back pain of greater than 10–12 months' duration was not improved as much by use of traction. The smaller the area of pain was, the greater the chance of improvement. Greater improvement was seen in pain if it was described as dull, aching, or stabbing. Patients with postural and temporal variation of pain responded better to treatment, as did patients who had asymmetric pain with passive movement assessment.

Cervical traction may be applied with the patient seated or in supine position. The supine position appears to be more effective in achieving a greater intervertebral separation. Patients must support their heads when they are seated, which may be counterproductive to muscle relaxation. Also, the angle of application can produce different effects. The angle of cervical flexion is of greater significance than the traction angle, which can vary depending on the type of halter applied to the patient. The amount of posterior intervertebral separation and elongation is associated with increasing cervical flexion (Colachis and Strohm 1965).

The most frequently recommended traction force for long-duration traction is 2.27–4.54 kg. For short-duration cervical traction, 9.0–11.3 kg of force has been found to produce a measurable posterior separation of cervical vertebrae between C2 and C7. In supine position, a cervical traction force of up to 13.6 kg applied at an angle of 24 degrees with contraction and relaxation phases of 7 seconds each was found to produce vertebral separation both anteriorly and posteriorly (Colachis and Strohm 1966).

Although the use of traction has clear benefits, the evidence that cervical traction induces soft tissue relaxation and increased blood flow is still controversial (Weinberger 1976).

Setting Limits

Emotional disturbances such as crying and outbursts of anger disrupt physical therapy sessions, other patients, and communication between patients and the therapist. A person demonstrating such behavior may not retain the material that he or she is being taught. The physical therapist should tell the patient that such behavior is disruptive to the physical therapy sessions and that the psychological counseling sessions should be used to deal with anger (Sanders 1991). The patient needs to understand that his or her anger is "displaced" onto the therapist and that misdirected anger is a sign that the patient is not ready to take responsibility for pain management. The therapist should help the patient recognize that the pain was not caused by the therapist and that it is not the therapist's responsibility to stop the pain (Sanders 1991). Clarifying the goals of treatment, (re)focusing on functional goals, and reinforcing gains already made in physical therapy sessions will help dissipate emotional disturbances.

The term *difficult* is used to describe patients with behaviors that are beyond the norm and undermine treatment. In minor cases, the difficult patient may stimulate a sense of uneasiness. In severe cases, caregivers may feel fear and hate. The difficult patient makes any treatment plan more difficult. The team's ability to cope with this hardship will be an important factor in the final treatment outcome. Treating a difficult patient forces the physical therapist to examine many factors. The patient's past psychosocial history, the team's history with the patient, and its ability to cope with this patient should be taken into account.

Some difficult patients directly inspire strong negative feelings in caregivers. Other difficult patients are identified indirectly because a struggle among the caregivers occurs. When there is substantial controversy among members of the treatment team, particularly with personal overtones, the team should still attempt to present a united appearance to the patient. The patient's best interest is served only if the treatment team is functional.

Patients may be extremely independent or dependent, active or submissive, engaging or impossible to connect with, and idealizing or devaluing of their caregivers. Some patients may even be enraged, violent, impulsive, and physically and emotionally threatening. Individual members of the treatment team may be made to feel like adored insiders (all good) or thankless scapegoats (all bad). Setting team members against each other is termed *splitting* and is a common behavior of the difficult patient.

These demanding patients may have extremely low self-esteem. They often feel at risk for imminent shame and humiliation. Confronting them only increases the possibility for shame and humiliation and may promote further demands. While working with such patients, it is best to give them frequent and varied reminders that they deserve and will receive the best and most thoughtful care.

The clinician who rushes into a case with disdain for prior management and offers alternatives that inspire the patient's effusive gratitude is likely to soon be on the receiving end of disdain. In these cases, the physical therapist should work in a manner that offers solutions without disrupting the relationship of the primary management team with the patient. The patient's sense of enormous vulnerability and the team's sense of hopelessness should be recognized. Placing blame on or embarrassing or humiliating the patient or the staff almost never results in long-term gain.

Team unity is critical to managing the difficult patient. Unity is largely a function of goodwill and communication. Frequent team meetings connect key representatives of the treatment team. Since it is usually impossible to meet with the entire team, there should be a mechanism for disseminating the plan between shifts and clinicians. Negotiating the overall treatment plan is the collective job of the team and the patient. Contingencies for possible outcomes should also be agreed on by the team and patient. Agreements should be clear and are best placed in writing. Contracts are a simple and effective means of avoiding future confusion about the plan. Written contracts offer the patient the opportunity to review and consider the information over time.

Setting limits is important in managing the difficult patient. Some patients may not believe they are cared about until someone responds to their outrageous behaviors. Such patients are usually frightened, impulsive, and very perceptive. Limit setting should not be used as an excuse for punishment. As soon as the potential for misbehavior is noted, patients must be advised of the consequences of violent behavior, threats, or imminent harm. Acts or threats of violence or self-injury must be met with an immediate and effective response to protect the patient and others. Psychiatric assistance is helpful in these situations.

Limits may be set by patients as well. Patients may have a history of physical abuse that precludes certain physical therapy modalities. The use of electrical stimulation may be appropriately refused by a patient who has been tortured in his or her childhood with electrical shocks.

Extreme care should be taken with survivors of political torture because many behaviors, examinations, or treatments may be threatening to them. Severe pain is a common long-term outcome of torture (Hough 1992). Some of the psychiatric patients referred to physical therapy have physical and sexual abuse histories that approximate torture.

Response to Patient Questions

Egan (1995) developed a clinical aid to ensure consistent responses to patient questions. Patients, particularly difficult ones, are often frightened and uncertain about treatment. Caregivers should assure the patient of the following:

1. The caregiver has expertise and experience in helping other people with similar problems turn their lives around.
2. The caregiver has confidence in each individual's unique strength and ability to rehabilitate himself or herself.
3. The caregiver understands the great difficulty of the patient's present situation and has a vision of a brighter, more productive future for the patient.
4. The caregiver has faith in the effectiveness of the treatment program.

Table 6.1 lists examples of reassuring answers to a patient's questions.

Efficacy of Treatment

Evidence in the literature indicates that an active rehabilitation approach is effective in returning patients to work and in decreasing sick time, medication use, visits with health care providers, and numbers of surgeries.

Fordyce et al. (1981) investigated the correlation of observed pain complaints with the amount of prescribed exercise performed by 25 chronic pain patients exercising to their level of tolerance. The exercises most frequently prescribed were walking, climbing stairs, riding on a fixed bicycle, and performing partial sit-ups. Patients were instructed to perform repetitions until pain, weakness, or fatigue caused them to stop. Results indicated that the more exercises were performed, the fewer pain behaviors were exhibited.

A group of 73 patients with chronic low back pain entered the functional restoration program of the Productive Rehabilitation Institute of Dallas for Ergonomics (PRIDE) between August 1983 and January 1984 (Mayer et al. 1986). Ninety percent of these patients were receiving worker's compensation, and 66 completed the program. Patients participated in a 3-week rehabilitation program for 58 hours per week. The physical rehabilitation component of the program consisted of specific exercises, training, education, and work simula-

TABLE 6.1 Possible responses to patient statements

Patient statement	Possible response
I can do everything else; why do I have to do that?	This program has been proven effective as a whole. It has been carefully constructed to maximize gains for your entire body.
I have a cold. I cannot go to physical therapy.	If you are sick, this is a good chance to practice doing what you need to do even though you are not feeling well; many people continue to work with a cold. You need to take advantage of all the time you are here. (After determining symptoms are not indicative of a serious health problem.)
I am going to do the best I can, but I am not sure I can handle the quotas you set.	I will not set quotas you cannot meet. This program has been specifically designed for you. The quotas will be gradually increased so that you can meet them.
I am tired. This is too much. I hurt too much to go to therapy.	After many years of experience, we find that this program is the best way to handle reconditioning. This is a very intensive program, and our experience has shown that, to get the most out of the time and the money you spend here, the speed we have chosen is optimal. We want to do the best we can for you in the time that you are here.
I hurt worse than when I came. I feel more anxious.	You have been disabled and inactive for a long time; we expect that coming into the program and working as hard as you have been would increase your pain temporarily. It is a very common response and will pass as your body becomes used to the demands you are making on it.
My pain is getting worse—it's 10 out of 10, stabbing, and pinching.	What kind of things do you usually do to make the pain less noticeable? Try using the techniques you have learned to manage your pain. You can expect the pain to increase some with activities. I think it is great you are able to do so much even though it hurts. This is good practice for the times you are out of the program and have a flare-up. Make a list of the things you can do to decrease pain.
I don't know what to do. Please tell me what I should do.	I think this is a decision you can make for yourself. What do you think you should do? Sit down, make a list of possible solutions, pick one, and try it. You can handle this on your own. You are the one who has to live with the decision; don't give anybody else the right to decide for you.

SOURCE: Adapted from K Egan. "What to say when . . .": a strategy for responding to patients' questions and complaints. Am Pain Soc Bull 1995;5:7.

tion/hardening to enhance spinal mobility, trunk strength, endurance, cardiovascular fitness, lifting capacity, positional tolerance, and ability to perform activities of daily living. Psychological intervention involved a multimodal pain management program of behavioral pain management training; cognitive behavioral skills training; and individual, group, and family counseling.

After 3 weeks, the patients entered a follow-up phase in which they returned to the clinic 2 hours per day for up to 4 days per week until they reached maximal benefit or returned to work.

Eighty-two percent of the 66 patients returned to work, and 6% returned to a full-time training program. Significant improvement was reported in spinal flexion, extension strength, ROM, and lifting capacity.

Mayer et al. (1987) compared 116 patients treated in a functional restoration program with 72 untreated patients in a follow-up survey 2 years' post-treatment. The 72 untreated patients had been denied entrance into the program by their insurance carrier. Analysis demonstrated that 87% of the treatment group was actively working, whereas only 41% of the untreated patients were. Twice as many untreated individuals had additional spine surgery compared with those treated. The untreated individuals had a five times higher rate of visits to health professionals in the second year. Also, treatment group reinjury rates were no higher than those in the general population, whereas untreated patients had a higher than average reinjury rate.

Hazard et al. (1989) studied a 1-year treatment program of functional restoration with behavioral support of patients disabled for an average of 19 months without evidence of surgically correctable disease. Ninety patients were studied and 64 entered the program. The 26 other patients were the control group. After initial testing, patients were treated 53 hours per week for 3 weeks. Physical therapy intervention included two daily sessions of stretching integrated with relaxation and dynamic strengthening of back extensor, abdominal, and lower extremity muscle groups. Progressive weight training for all major muscle groups and general endurance and coordination training with arm and leg cycling, walking, and recreation were conducted daily. Physical and occupational therapy was conducted for 5½ hours per day. After 3 weeks, a follow-up program of 1–2 days per week for approximately 3 weeks incorporated psychological, physical, and occupational therapy.

One year after study entry, 81% of program graduates had returned to work, 40% of program dropouts had, and only 29% of the control group had. Program graduates showed significant improvements in self-assessed pain, disability, and physical capacities after 3 weeks of treatment.

Saal and Saal (1989) reported that after treatment 11 of 14 patients receiving worker's compensation for an initial diagnosis of sciatica returned to work. Treatment included ice application, TENS, traction, nonsteroidal anti-inflammatory drugs, epidural steroid injections, a lumbar stabilization program, and instruction in body mechanics. The lumbar stabilization program began with postural control exercises and progressed to basic and advanced exercises. Once the patient was able to perform three sets of 15 repetitions, the exercise was advanced. This program was combined with stretching, self-mobilization, and aerobic exercise.

Cassisi et al. (1989) contacted 61% of 236 patients referred to an intensive, 4-week, inpatient treatment program. The average time elapsed between follow-up and referral was 22.5 months. The patients were grouped into five categories: (1) patients treated at the program (36), (2) patients denied program entrance by insurance (30), (3) patients who refused to participate (46), (4) patients who were treated in other programs (14), and

(5) patients who dropped out of the program (14). Group demographics were similar. The patients in the first group demonstrated significantly lower rates of subsequent health care utilization.

Mitchell and Carmen (1994) reported on a prospective, randomized, multicenter trial of the functional restoration approach. The exercise component consisted of physical exercise and a functional simulation program developed in an occupational gymnasium. The physical portion emphasized mobility, strength, endurance, and flexibility. Pain relief was usually attained by applying ice followed by active and passive stretching. Equipment designed to work specific muscle groups in sequence to diminish fatigue and promote mobility and strengthening of various muscle groups in harmony was used. At the beginning of treatment, a goal was established for each individual. The number of repetitions and the amount of resistance appropriate for each person's capability and work requirement were adjusted accordingly. The exercises included lifting, working above head level, stair climbing, carrying weights over a measured distance, and lifting while twisting. Patients were randomized either to the treatment group or to the primary care provider for further supervision (control group). The treatment program was 8 weeks, with 40 days of 7-hour treatments. A program was also offered in which the 40 treatment days were spread over 12 weeks. The control and the treatment group included 271 patients each. At the end of 12 months of follow-up, 79% of the treatment group worked full time, whereas 78% of the control group did. There was no statistical difference in outcome between the 8- and 12-week programs. When the patients in both the treatment and control group were divided into subsets based on the month of the accident, a comparison revealed savings in the treatment group in the days lost from work, the wage-loss benefits costs, and total costs. The cost of permanent disability awards were also less for the treatment group.

Kellett et al. (1991) investigated the effects of an exercise program on sick leave due to back pain in 111 employees of Scandinavia's major producer of kitchen units. Criteria for inclusion in the study were self-reported current or previous back pain, written commitment to participate in the exercise program during working hours, and a willingness to exercise at least once a week outside working hours for 1½ years. The group was divided into an exercise group of 58 subjects and a control group of 53 subjects. The number of sick-leave days attributable to back pain and the number of episodes of back pain were recorded during the intervention period and compared with data recorded before intervention. There were no significant differences between mean ages in the groups. Exercise included a warm-up, gentle stretching exercises, alternate strengthening and cardiovascular fitness exercises, and 10 minutes of lectures on causes and treatment of back pain. Each exercise session lasted 30–35 minutes and was followed by 5–10 minutes of relaxation. Attendance averaged 77% at each session. The participants kept a diary of their activities, including their exercise outside of working hours. Cardiovascular fitness of both the exercise and the control groups was tested using a computerized exercise bicycle before and after the program. Dropout rate was 36% in the exercise group and 9% in the control group. After the program, sick days attributable to back pain decreased 51.2% in the exercise group and increased 65% in the control group. There was no significant difference between the number of back pain episodes reported by both groups. Eighty-one percent of the exercise group reported subjective improvement in their back pain.

The operant-conditioning behavioral approach (progressive quota setting) was described in a study by Lindstrom et al. (1992). The purpose of the study was to determine if this approach restored occupational function in industrial workers who had nonspecific low back pain for 8 weeks. The study compared traditional medical care alone and in combination with a gradually increasing activity program. Patients in the activity group returned to work significantly earlier than the patients in the medical care–only group. The average duration of sick leave in the next year was significantly less for the activity group. The individually graded exercise program included endurance and strength training, lifting exercises, walking, jogging, swimming, group gymnastic exercises, and fitness exercises on a bicycle ergometer.

Edwards et al. (1992) reported that 55% of 54 patients with chronic low back pain returned to work after a 4-week intensive physical treatment program. The program consisted of weight-resisted trunk and limb muscle exercises based on the Daily Adjusted Progressive Resistance Exercise method. In addition, stretching exercises and their aquatic variations, aerobic exercise, a strenuous walking program, and a functionally appropriate work program were performed.

These studies reached the same basic conclusions. In these studies, patients are treated with a combination of stretching, strengthening, endurance, and aerobic exercise. Work-specific and functional tasks are often incorporated in the program. The number of hours per day and number of days per week of program participation vary across programs. Some programs have more behavioral support than others, but even the programs without behavioral support seem to have good results. The range of those returning to work after these exercise programs is 55–87%, a percentage that far exceeds any other single approach studied for returning chronic pain patients to work.

Most of the published research on outcomes of chronic pain treatment has been done on inpatient or outpatient treatment conducted 5 days a week for 4–6 weeks. Whether outcomes are the same when patients are treated less intensively is unknown. It could be argued that treating patients two to three times a week places a larger responsibility on the patient to carry through with their home programs and to integrate their newly regained functional ability and pain management techniques in their home environment. This could lead to greater success. It can also be argued, however, that a more intensive treatment program is required to achieve a behavioral change. More research is needed to establish the treatment time and duration needed to achieve optimal results in a cost-effective manner.

References

Alyea WS, Rose DL, Shires EB. Effect of ultrasound on threshold of vibration perception in a peripheral nerve. Arch Phys Med Rehabil 1956;37:265.
Becker RO, Selden G. The Body Electric, Electromagnetism and the Foundation of Life. New York: Quill-Morrow Publications, 1987.

Buchthal F, Rosenfalck A. Evoked action potentials and conduction velocity in human sensory nerves. Brain Res 1966;3:1.

Cassisi J, Sypert G, Salamon A, Kapel L. Independent evaluation of a multi-disciplinary rehabilitation program for chronic low back pain. Neurosurgery 1989;25:877.

Cattell M, Hoagland H. Response of tactile receptors to intermittent stimulation. J Physiol 1931;72:392.

Clarke RSJ, Hellon RF, Lind AR. Vascular reactions of the human forearm to cold. Clin Sci 1958;17:165.

Colachis SC, Strohm BR. A study of traction forces and angle of pull on vertebral interspaces in the cervical spine. Arch Phys Med Rehabil 1965;46:220.

Colachis SC, Strohm BR. Effect of duration of intermitted cervical traction on vertebral separation. Arch Phys Med Rehabil 1966;47:353.

DeLacerda FG. Cervical Traction. In G Grieve (ed), Modern Manual Therapy in the Vertebral Column. Edinburgh: Churchill Livingstone, 1986;680.

Dolce JJ, Crocker MF, Moletteire C, Doleys DM. Exercise quotas and anticipatory concern and self efficacy expectancies in chronic pain: a preliminary report. Pain 1986;24:365.

DonTigny R. Mechanics and treatment of the sacroiliac joint. J Manual Manipulative Ther 1993;1:3.

Duarte LR. The stimulation of bone growth by ultrasound. Arch Orthop Trauma Surg 1983;101:153.

Dworkin SF, Von Korff M, LeResche L. Epidemiologic studies of chronic pain: a dynamic-ecologic perspective. Ann Behav Med 1992;14:3.

Dyson M, Pond JB, Joseph J, Warwick R. The stimulation of tissue regeneration by means of ultrasound. Clin Sci 1968;35:273.

Edwards B, Zusman M, Hardcastle P, et al. A physical approach to the rehabilitation of patients disabled by chronic low back pain. Med J Aust 1992;156:167.

Egan K. "What to say when . . .": a strategy for responding to patients' questions and complaints. Am Pain Soc Bull 1995;5:7.

Eggertz AMK. Auto-Traction: A Non-Surgical Treatment of Low Back Pain and Sciatica. In G Grieve (ed), Modern Manual Therapy. Edinburgh: Churchill Livingstone, 1986;796.

Evjenth O, Hamberg J. Muscle Stretching in Manual Therapy (Vols I & II). Sweden: Alfta Rehab, 1984.

Fordyce W, Fowler R, Lehmann JF, DeLateur B. Some implications of learning in problems of chronic pain. J Chron Disord 1968;21:179.

Fordyce W, McMahon R, Rainwater G, et al. Pain complaint-exercise performance relationship in chronic pain. Pain 1981;10:311.

Fordyce W, Roberts A, Sternbach R. The behavioral management of chronic pain: a response to critics. Pain 1985;22:113.

Frampton V. Transcutaneous Electric Nerve Stimulation and Chronic Pain. In PE Wells, V Frampton, D Bowsher (eds), Pain Management by Physical Therapy (2nd ed). Oxford: Butterworth-Heinemann, 1994;117.

Gam AN, Johannsen F. Ultrasound therapy in musculoskeletal disorders: a meta-analysis. Pain 1995;63:85.

Gatchel RJ. Occupational low back disability. Why function needs to "drive" the rehabilitation process. Am Pain Soc J 1994;3:107.

Geiger G, Todd DD, Clark HB, et al. The effects of feedback and contingent reinforcement on the exercise behavior of chronic pain patients. Pain 1992;49:179.

Gersten JW. Effect of ultrasound on tendon extensibility. Am J Phys Med 1955;34:362.

Greenhoot JH, Sternbach RA. Conjoint Treatment of Chronic Pain. In A Jacox (ed), Pain Source Book for Nurses and Other Health Professionals. Boston: Little, Brown, 1977;295.

Gustavsen R, Streeck R. Training Therapy. Stuttgart, Germany: Georg Thieme Verlag, 1993.

Hazard R, Fenwick J, Kalich S, et al. Functional restoration with behavioral support. A one year prospective study of patients with chronic low back pain. Spine 1989;14:157.

Hough A. Physiotherapy for survivors of torture. Physiotherapy 1992;78:323.

Ishimaru K, Shinohara S, Iwa M, et al. Effects of electric acupuncture and transcutaneous electric nerve stimulation on the deep pain threshold in human subjects. J Kyoto Pref Univ Med 1993;102:189.

Janda V. Muscle Weakness and Inhibition (Pseudoparesis) in Back Syndromes. In G Grieve (ed), Modern Manual Therapy of the Vertebral Column. Edinburgh: Churchill Livingstone, 1986;197.

Janda V. Muscles and Cervicogenic Pain Syndromes. In R Grant (ed), Clinics in Physical Therapy of the Cervical and Thoracic Spine. New York: Churchill Livingstone, 1988;152.

Jull G, Janda V. Muscles and Motor Control in Low Back Pain. In L Twomey, J Taylor (eds), Physical Therapy of the Low Back. New York: Churchill Livingstone, 1987;253.

Kellett K, Kellett D, Nordholm L. Effects of an exercise program on sick leave due to back pain. Phys Ther 1991;71:283.

Khalil T, Asfour S, Martinez L, et al. Stretching in the rehabilitation of low back pain patients. Spine 1992;17:311.

Lehmann JF, Delateur BJ. Cryotherapy. In Lehmann JF (ed), Therapeutic Heat and Cold (4th ed). Baltimore: Williams & Wilkins, 1990;590.

Lind GAM. Auto-traction. Treatment of low back pain and sciatica. Linköping, Sweden: University of Linköping; 1974. Thesis.

Lindstrom I, Ohlund C, Eek C, et al. The effect of graded activity on patients with subacute low back pain: a randomized prospective clinical study with an operant conditioning approach. Phys Ther 1992;72:279.

Linton S. The relationship between activity and chronic pain. Pain 1985;21:289.

Low J. Electrotherapeutic Modalities. In PE Wells, V Frampton, D Bowsher (eds), Pain Management by Physical Therapy (2nd ed). Oxford: Butterworth-Heinemann, 1994;177.

Mayer T, Gatchel R, Koshino N, et al. A prospective short term study of chronic low back pain patients utilizing novel objective functional measurement. Pain 1986;25:53.

Mayer T, Gatchel R, Mayer H, et al. A prospective two year study of functional restoration in industrial low back injury. JAMA 1987;258:1763.

Mayer T, Gatchel R. Functional Restoration for Spinal Disorders: The Sports Medicine Approach. Philadelphia: Lea & Febiger, 1988.

Melzack R, Wall PD. Pain mechanisms: a new theory. Science 1965;150:971.

Melzack R, Wall P. The Challenge of Pain. New York: Penguin Books, 1982.

Michlovitz SL. Cryotherapy. The Use of Cold as a Therapeutic Agent. In SL Michlovitz (ed), Thermal Agents in Rehabilitation (2nd ed). Philadelphia: F.A. Davis, 1990;68.

Mitchell R, Carmen G. The functional restoration approach to the treatment of chronic pain in patients with soft tissues and back injuries. Spine 1994;19:633.

Morgan D. Concepts in functional training and postural stabilization for the low back injured. Top Acute Care Trauma Rehabil 1988;2:8.

Myrenberg M, Lundeberg T. Computer aided traction treatment in patients with low back pain. Pain Clinic 1989;3:5.

Myrenberg M, Lundeberg T, Odeen I. Effect of traction treatment on EMG activity during walking in erecti spinae in patients with low back pain. Pain Clinic 1990;3:69.

Newton RA. Contemporary Views on Pain and the Role Played by Thermal Agents in Managing Pain Symptoms. In SL Michlovitz (ed), Thermal Agents in Rehabilitation (2nd ed). Philadelphia: F.A. Davis, 1990;38.

Olson J, Svendsen B. Medical exercise therapy: an adjunct to orthopaedic manual therapy. Orthop Pract 1992;4:7.

Palastanga N. The Use of Transverse Frictions for Soft Tissue Lesions. In G Grieve (ed), Modern Manual Therapy. Edinburgh: Churchill Livingstone, 1986;819.

Pomeranz B. Naloxone blockade of acupuncture analgesia: endorphin implicated. Life Sci 1976;19:1757.

Rainville J, Ahern D, Phalen L, et al. The association of pain with physical activities in chronic low back pain. Spine 1992;17:1060.

Saal J, Saal J. Nonoperative treatment of herniated lumbar intervertebral disc with radiculopathy. An outcome study. Spine 1989;14:431.

Sanders P. Breaking the cycle of chronic pain. Clin Manage 1991;11:72.

Sanders M, Sanders B. Mobility: Active-Resistive Training. In JA Gould III, GJ Davies (eds), Orthopaedic and Sports Physical Therapy (Vol 2). St. Louis: Mosby, 1985;228.

Shutty MS, DeGood DE, Tuttle DH. Chronic pain patients' beliefs about their pain and treatment outcomes. Arch Phys Med Rehabil 1990;71:128.

Smith C. The warm-up procedure: to stretch or not to stretch. A brief review. J Orthop Sports Phys Ther 1994;19:12.

Spence SH, Sharpe L, Newton-John T, Champion D. Effect of EMG biofeedback compared to applied relaxation training with chronic, upper extremity cumulative trauma disorders. Pain 1995;63:199.

Sternbach RA. Mastering Pain. A Twelve Step Program for Coping with Chronic Pain. New York: Ballantine, 1987;107.

Sullivan PE, Markos PD. Clinical Procedures in Therapeutic Exercise. Reston, VA: Reston Publishers, 1987.

Sweeney T, Prentice C, Saal J, Saal J. Cervicothoracic muscular stabilization techniques. Phys Med Rehab 1990;4:335.

Travell JG, Simons DG. Myofascial Trigger Point Manual. Baltimore: Williams & Wilkins, 1983.

Wall PD, Gutnik M. Ongoing activity in peripheral nerves. The physiology and pharmacology of impulses originating from a neuroma. Exp Neurol 1974;43:580.

Weineck J. Training Methods. In R Gustavsen, R Streeck (eds), Training Therapy (2nd ed). New York: Thieme, 1993.

Weinberger LM. Trauma or treatment: the role of intermitted traction in the treatment of cervical soft tissue injuries. J Trauma 1976;16:377.

Young A, Stokes M, Iles JF. Effects of joint pathology on muscle. Clin Orthop 1987;19:21.

Functional Restoration
Treatment Agreement

Patient:	John Doe
Date of birth:	2/15/50
Date:	6/8/96

Welcome to the pain management program. For the next 4 weeks, you will be a participant in a multidisciplinary, intensive, rehabilitation-oriented treatment program. This treatment agreement will orient you to the program and its services.

The program is designed to condition you so that you can return to a normal physical, social, and emotional level of function. Treatment is directed at helping you learn how to live with your current pain and change actions and attitudes (behaviors) associated with the pain. During the evaluation phase, the staff identified aspects of your behaviors with you that communicate to others that you are in pain. These behaviors include the following:

- Complaining about pain
- Depending on others to do activities of daily living such as household cleaning and getting medicine
- Shaking or rubbing leg
- Having to stand up after 10 minutes of sitting
- Limping

You and the treatment team understand that the focus is on a decrease in attention to pain, complaints of pain, and behaviors related to pain. Entering this phase of treatment assumes that you have completed all necessary diagnostic tests. If other acute medical problems are present, the program medical director and your primary care physician will assist with any necessary additional evaluation.

The goal is to increase your ability to do certain activities to a normal level. The specific goals established by you in conjunction with the treatment team and your family are listed here.

Work goals (all related to returning to the restaurant business)	**Target date**
Start looking for a location	
Outline a business plan	
Establish work capacity demands (e.g., lifting, bending, time on feet)	
Start practice work at brother's restaurant	

Exercise goals
Standing and working 4 hours per day
    with 10-minute breaks
Lifting 50 lbs from the floor
Home repair (e.g., painting)
Exercycle
    Starting: 5 minutes; goal: 25 minutes
Walking
    Starting: 10 minutes; goal: 60 minutes
Sitting
    Starting: 30 minutes; goal: 60 minutes
Lifting weights from knee to chest:
    Starting: 10 lbs; goal: 25 lbs

Recreational activity goals   **Target date**
Riding a bicycle
    Starting: 5 minutes; goal: 90 minutes
Fishing
Use a small boat

Medication goals
Eliminate hydrocodone bitartrate (Vicodin)
    use with a reduction schedule

ADL goals
Effective reaching for showering
Use hands for more than 30 minutes
    (yard work)
Improve dexterity (cooking tasks)

Social and emotional goals
Improve mood, reduce Beck Depression
    Inventory score to <10
Improve relaxation skills, reduce Burns
    Anxiety Inventory score to <10

ADL = activities of daily living.

Please notify us of any upcoming visits to another physician or health care provider. Avoid missing any appointments. If you miss two consecutive appointments or a total of three appointments, we will assume that we cannot assist you and your participation in the program will end.

With your permission, we also will arrange occasional meetings with any other members involved in your care (e.g., rehabilitation counselors or nurses) and will ask that you participate.

You will need to bring your program book including your treatment plan and exercise graphs to all appointments.

We look forward to working with you.

_____   _____
Patient   **Date**

_____   _____
Family member   **Date**

_____   _____
Pain program staff/Primary therapist   **Date**

SOURCE: Developed by R Kulich, PhD, New England Medical Center Pain Management Program.

Management of Selected Syndromes

Harriët Wittink, Joanna R. Allan,
Theresa Hoskins Michel, and Lisa Janice Cohen

Headaches

The International Headache Society (IHS) classifies headaches into 13 different categories (IHS 1988). The types often treated in physical therapy are migraine (with or without aura), tension-type headache (with or without muscle involvement), and acute and chronic post-traumatic headache. Many patients assume they have migraines if they have severe headaches, but tension-type, post-traumatic, and other headaches can also be severe and disabling. Physical therapists treating headaches should become familiar with the IHS classification system.

Diagnosis

It is preferable to obtain a precise diagnosis from the patient's referring physician, but the diagnosis of headache without a specific classification is still common. A precise diagnosis helps the physical therapist to determine treatment objectives and prognosis. If the precise diagnosis is unknown, treatment results should not be adversely affected because treatment of headache is largely based on the signs and symptoms of the patient. It will, however, be more difficult to explain the role of physical therapy treatment in the total care of the patient's headache.

Muscle pain is an important component of headaches (Lance 1993). A musculoskeletal evaluation of the head, neck, and shoulder girdle areas and a postural evaluation should be done on headache patients. Evaluation should include palpation of all soft-tissue areas, particularly the muscles of the head and face (Kendall et al. 1993). Passive range of motion (ROM) testing should also involve accessory movement testing of the joints of the cervical spine. The presence of muscle guarding in passive and accessory movement should be classified as mild, moderate, or severe.

A brief evaluation of the temporomandibular joint area should be included. The patient should be asked if he or she has pain when chewing hard fruits or tough meat or has habits such as clenching or grinding the teeth. Assessment of the active range of mandibular motion and palpation of temporomandibular joints and pterygoid, temporal, and masseter muscles should be completed.

The patient's headache may be reproduced during the evaluation. For example, palpation of both temporal muscles may reproduce a patient's temporalis muscle headache. It would be unusual to reproduce a migraine headache. A migraine headache patient is likely to experience tenderness of cervical muscles on palpation, mild loss of active ROM, and muscle guarding with passive movement, however.

Common Headache Types in Physical Therapy

Tension-Type Headache

Tension-type headache is characterized by a bilateral, dull ache across the frontal and temporal areas (IHS 1988). The pain may radiate posteriorly or start as a dull ache in the upper trapezius or cervical paraspinal areas and radiate forward. Patients often describe the headache as feeling like a tight band around the head. These headaches may occur as often as several times a week and are typically mild to moderate in intensity and last several hours (IHS 1988). They can become severe or constant when a patient is under additional psychosocial stress, is very symptom-focused, or is overusing painkillers or muscle relaxants.

Patients with tension-type headache with muscle involvement have tightness and tenderness of facial and pericranial muscles on palpation (Corrigan and Maitland 1983). This type of headache is generally triggered by muscle overuse. Patients often assume the overuse is due to overactivity with poor posture, such as working for long periods at a computer. Such conditions may produce upper back and neck pain that can be referred from the upper trapezius muscle to the temple and behind the eye (Evjenth and Hamberg 1984). Overuse of the facial muscles due to habits such as frowning and clenching the teeth may also contribute to these headaches. These habits typically occur in response to everyday stressors. Patients are often confused about why they have headaches because they do not feel they are under any undue stress. It is helpful to explain that the overuse of facial muscles is as common an occurrence as poor posture.

Physical therapy can significantly decrease the severity and frequency of these headaches by using soft-tissue and joint mobilization techniques and by teaching correct, relaxed posture; home stretching and strengthening exercises; the use of pain control modalities; and biomechanical and ergonomic principles. Tension-type headaches are usually chronic, so an important part of treatment is providing the patient with a comprehensive home exercise program that should become a lifelong routine.

A number of patients may respond to physical therapy treatment alone, but many do better with a combination of behavioral medicine and physical therapy. Behavioral medicine treatment typically consists of general relaxation and stress management training. If patients seen in physical therapy are not improving at the expected rate, have continued difficulty relaxing facial and pericranial muscles, or are complaining of psychosocial stressors, the physical therapist should contact the referring physician to suggest an evaluation by a psychologist or mental health counselor.

Migraine

Migraines are a genetic disorder and occur twice as often in women as in men. They are triggered by a variety of factors, including hormonal changes, diet, environment, overactivity, stress, irregular sleep patterns, and lack of exercise. They usually start at puberty and decrease in frequency, severity, and duration after menopause. Migraines are typically unilateral, although they may shift sides. They are usually experienced as a throbbing, pounding pain in one temple and behind the ipsilateral eye. They occur one to several times a month (Corrigan and Maitland 1983).

Physical therapy cannot cure migraines, but it can help a great deal by promoting regular aerobic exercise and alleviating secondary myofascial problems of the head and neck that can increase the frequency, intensity, and duration of migraines. The secondary muscle tenderness, increased tone, and muscle guarding in the facial, neck, and shoulder girdle muscles appear to be due to the patient bracing the head, neck, and shoulder girdle during severe migraine pain. This pain can last for 24–48 hours (Corrigan and Maitland 1983). Migraine patients frequently have rigid posture, especially of the head, neck, and upper back.

In migraine with aura, pain is preceded by a visual aura that lasts approximately 20 minutes. The aura is characterized by zigzag lines and black spots that radiate progressively outward from the center of a homonymous field defect called the *scintillation scotoma* (Mumenthaler 1990). Physical therapy treatments cannot change the frequency, intensity, or duration of the aura.

Headache Associated with Substance Abuse

When patients with tension-type or migrainous headaches overuse pain medicines, their headaches can become more frequent or even constant with moderate to severe pain and no discernible headache trigger. These headaches typically do not respond to any other form of treatment until the patient has completed detoxification.

Acute or Chronic Post-Traumatic Headache

Acute or chronic post-traumatic headache is associated with head trauma, often from a motor vehicle accident. The pain is usually either frequent or constant and is often accompanied by dizziness in the acute stages. These headaches usually respond slowly to treatment. It is best if they are treated as early as possible after the trauma. Use of an interdisciplinary team consisting of a physician, psychologist, and physical therapist is appropriate. Successful physical therapy will only partially decrease this type of headache, since it is not just due to myofascial damage.

Physical therapists can decrease these headaches by using soft-tissue and joint mobilization techniques and by teaching correct, relaxed posture; home stretching and strengthening exercises; the use of pain control modalities; and biomechanical and ergonomic principles. Patients often discontinue home practice because they are discouraged by their slow progress. They should be informed that much of the treatment is preventative and that without it the headaches will worsen. These headaches improve on a weekly or monthly basis, although they improve more rapidly in the first few months after the trauma that causes them.

Cervicogenic Headache

The pain of cervicogenic headache is referred from the neck and tends to respond well to physical therapy. It is characterized by neck and occipital pain that radiates to the temporal region, frontal region, or both and is either unilateral or bilateral. Examination of the neck should reproduce the headache. This would occur from palpation of the neck and shoulder muscles, accessory movement testing of upper cervical joints (C0–C3, possibly C4), or palpation of the C2 nerve as it passes through the suboccipital musculature. The patient should be given a preventative home program of exercise to maintain improvement.

Cluster Headaches

These headaches are more rare than other types and occur mostly in men. They occur in clusters, often at the same time in each year. The patient may then have no headaches for months at a time. They are characterized by severe, brief periods of unilateral facial pain, head pain, or both and are accompanied by unilateral parasympathetic nervous system signs such as weeping and eye redness. They generally respond well to medical treatment such as oxygen administration, but a patient may be referred to physical therapy with secondary muscular problems of the neck or face that have occurred due to muscle bracing against the pain of the headache.

Treatment

Goals

Most headaches are chronic conditions. Therefore, treatment modalities may provide only temporary relief unless the patient is also instructed in a comprehensive home program involving muscle conditioning exercises and postural and ergonomic concepts. The goals of treatment for headache involve sympathetic pain relief; resolution of treatable impairments such as decreased ROM, muscle strength and endurance; and instruction regarding preventative measures.

1. Immediate relief of symptomatic pain. Good relief is possible with neck pain, headaches due to referred neck pain, and acute headaches. Chronic tension-type and post-traumatic headaches are only slightly diminished in intensity by pain control modalities and soft-tissue techniques. The aggregate effect of these treatments can be beneficial,

however. Immediate relief should be expected for the secondary neck pain of migraine.

Techniques for relief of symptomatic pain include hot and cold therapy, ultrasound, electrical stimulation, and small-amplitude joint mobilizations (Hertling and Kessler 1990). The patient should be taught the home use of hot and cold therapy and self-massage for daily symptomatic relief. Some patients find neck-relaxing exercises provide symptomatic relief.

2.   Restoration of normal ROM. Many headache patients have at least a mild to moderate decrease in cervical spine and shoulder girdle active ROM often associated with forward head posture. Restriction in ROM is usually due to increased tone of suboccipital, cervical paraspinal, and upper trapezius muscles. It can progress to the point of limiting functional activities such as driving. Limited passive and accessory movement of the cervical spine is usually associated with muscle guarding due to increased muscle tone of the small intervertebral muscles, rather than with ligamentous restrictions. Exceptions are seen in post-traumatic headache, headache patients who have separate neck problems (e.g., osteoarthritis), and patients with active restriction of neck motion who are experiencing secondary joint stiffness, however.

Techniques that decrease muscle tone are highly effective at restoring normal ROM. Pain control modalities, soft-tissue techniques, and small-amplitude joint mobilizations that reflexively relax muscles are effective. If ligament tightness is present, larger amplitude joint mobilizations should be used (Hertling and Kessler 1990).

3.   Increase in muscle strength and endurance. Patients often exhibit mildly decreased muscle strength of pericranial, paraspinal, interscapular, and upper-extremity muscles. This is usually much more pronounced in patients with post-traumatic headache. Occasionally, patients may complain of subjective weakness that is part of their pain experience and be very motivated to do resisted exercises. These patients may present with severely increased muscle tone and guarding and often experience more functional gains by learning local muscle relaxation and relaxation during movement and then progressing to relaxed neck and upper extremity exercises. Headache patients typically present with the tendency to over-recruit, using more than the necessary muscle work for any activity. Habits such as hunching shoulders, bracing the neck, and frowning while using a computer typify this problem. Before being taught resisted exercises, they need to be taught to do gentle, active exercises.

4.   Patient understanding of preventative measures. Patients should be instructed in neck and back care, postural correction, and biomechanical and ergonomic principles.

Methods

Heat and Cold Application

The application of heat and cold is very valuable for symptomatic relief of all headaches. In order for them to be fully effective, patients must be taught to use these modalities at home on a daily basis. It is also beneficial to use one of these modalities in office sessions to relax muscles or decrease pain sufficiently so that soft-tissue or joint mobilization can be performed. Heat and cold are also helpful in decreasing post-treatment soreness.

Migraine patients benefit particularly from the use of ice massage or cold packs applied to the forehead or neck during severe migraine pain. Ice massage has been found to increase pain tolerance with long-term use. This massage can be used on areas other than the affected muscles, and good results have been achieved with use of the acupuncture hoku point between the thumb and index finger.

Because the use of heat not only relieves pain but also relaxes muscle, it should be used daily when muscle tenderness and increased tone are present even if there is no symptomatic relief from pain. Tension-type headache patients benefit from the soothing, relaxing effects of moist heat applied to the affected muscles. This treatment should be applied one to three times daily. A warm bath, shower, or sauna may occasionally be substituted. Patients will need education about the effects of heat so they are motivated to continue it in the absence of pain relief.

Heat therapy can be used for 20–30 minutes and cold therapy for up to 10 minutes per application. It is advisable to wait an hour or more between applications. Contraindications for use of heat and cold include broken areas of skin and decreased skin sensitivity and circulation to an area.

Electrical Stimulation
Electrical stimulation can be useful for patients who are very symptom focused or whose muscles are reacting in an oversensitized manner to soft-tissue techniques.

Soft-Tissue Techniques
All soft-tissue techniques should be performed gently, for short periods, and with frequent assessment because severe headaches frequently develop suddenly and persist for long periods.

Occasionally, when massage and stretching techniques to increase ROM progress slowly because the assessing movement reproduces pain, it is helpful to decrease assessment within the session and focus on assessment of movement 12–24 hours after the session. This should be done only when previous assessment has provided a good understanding of the effects of the treatment and the patient is a good historian. Any change in treatment would then be accompanied by assessment within the session.

Massage.   Because headache patients tend to overuse the muscles of their head, face, and neck, the muscles frequently become tender and oversensitive to touch and movement. Massage is a very important modality for headache patients because it is effective at decreasing both muscle tension and tightness. It is also very effective for symptomatic relief of local tenderness. By loosening tight muscle fibers and working on trigger points, massage can effectively reduce referred pain.

It is often helpful to precede massage with the use of heat or cold to relax muscles and increase pain tolerance. Soreness due to massage can be decreased by following the massage with heat, cold, or small-amplitude joint mobilizations. If treatment soreness is significant and lasts more than 1 hour, the massage is too vigorous or the patient should be reevaluated. In some cases of post-traumatic headache and tension-type headache, muscles have become so oversensitized to touch that several treatments of gentle electrical stimulation and joint mobilization are necessary before massage can be performed. The presence of secondary gain factors or chronic pain syndrome should also be considered in these cases.

Massage to the facial muscles, particularly the temporal muscles, can prevent, lessen, and stop muscle tension headaches involving the frontal and temporal regions and lessen the throbbing pain of a severe migraine. Signs and symptoms are common in this region because of the patient's tendency to brace, clench, or grind the jaw. The suboccipital area is also important because muscle tightness builds up due to the forward head position and muscle tone is high due to bracing of the head and neck against pain and stress.

There are a wide variety of massage techniques. Facial muscles respond well to gentle, circular finger-and-thumb kneading massage. Suboccipital muscles respond to both circular and transverse finger and thumb kneading. This should be done deeply but gently. Cervical and upper trapezius muscles respond to a range of techniques. Deep thumb kneading to areas of increased tone and tenderness is particularly helpful, especially when palpation of these areas refers pain to the headache area. When muscles are oversensitized or the patient has a low pain tolerance or difficulty relaxing, slow, deep techniques are useful.

Muscle Stretching Techniques.   Headache patients typically present with tight, shortened pericranial muscles. Muscle stretches are effective for suboccipital, cervical paraspinal, and upper trapezius muscles. They are particularly helpful if used with gentle hold-relax techniques to promote relaxation (Evjenth and Hamberg 1984).

Joint Mobilization Techniques

Vigorous joint mobilizations can quickly increase local pain and provoke a headache. Small-amplitude techniques performed gently and with frequent assessment are the most helpful to treat headache. Techniques to mobilize the typically hypomobile upper cervical spine include manual traction; passive cervical rotation; and unilateral pressures to C1/2, C2/3, and C3/4, particularly end-of-range oscillations. It is especially beneficial to apply unilateral pressure anteriorly or posteriorly with the patient's head rotated away from the pain. Transverse and central pressures to the upper cervical spine may be of additional benefit. A large-amplitude, gentle transverse pressure to both sides of the midcervical area and gentle large-amplitude oscillations help to relax the small muscles of the upper cervical spine and reduce treatment soreness from the use of end-of-range oscillations.

Case Example

A 69-year-old male has a 15-year history of headaches not classifiable (IHS 1988) and an additional diagnosis of cervical spine osteoarthritis. He has moderate to severe headaches in the right occipital region that wake him and last 1–2 hours until he is able to fall asleep again. They usually occur 5 days per week. He occasionally experiences a mild, dull ache in the same area during the day and frequently experiences a mild, dull ache bilaterally in the suboccipital area. The patient has cardiac problems and wonders if this stress could be contributing to his headaches. He states that he practices stress management and relaxation and is interested only in physical therapy.

On examination, he has a 50% decrease in cervical spine ROM consistent with osteoarthritis, but more limited upper cervical forward bending that reproduces his headache. Cervical backward bending reproduces his headache and neck pain. He has moderately increased muscle tone in his frontal and temporal muscles and severely increased muscle tone in his suboccipital, cervical paraspinal, and upper trapezius muscles. His right suboccipital area is tender to palpation, but this does not reproduce his headache. He is severely hypomobile on accessory joint testing of the cervical spine, with particular restrictions of forward bend at C2/3 and C3/4. He tends to avoid neck and upper thoracic movements by holding his back rigidly and turning at the lower thorax.

He receives six treatments of massage to the frontalis, temporalis, suboccipital, and cervical paraspinal muscles. Manual traction is administered four times as end-of-range oscillations to suboccipitals and then cervical paraspinals. Joint mobilization includes central pressures to C2, C3, C4, and C5 and unilateral pressures to C2/3 and C3/4 on the right. Large-amplitude cervical rotation mobilization to both left and right is also performed as a treatment for limited active ROM due to cervical osteoarthritis.

He is taught a home program of postural and biomechanical correction, neck stretches, and thoracic rotation. He finds that the relaxed neck exercises lessen his headache, and he performs them when woken at night.

At the end of treatment he has one mild nocturnal headache every 1–2 weeks that does not prevent him from falling asleep again. His active cervical forward bending and rotation increases to 75%. Two further sessions are scheduled, but the patient decides to discontinue treatment and continue with home exercises. At 1-month follow-up, the patient's psychosocial stressors have significantly increased, and his headaches have increased to two to three times per week but are lessened or stopped by the exercise program. The patient decides to continue without further treatment, stating that his increased stress is short term, and that he is very satisfied with and committed to his home exercise program.

Relaxation Techniques

Overused muscles have a higher baseline muscle tone because they are required to contract often without sufficient relaxation. They develop the tendency to contract when movement is occurring elsewhere in the body, leading to pain and fatigue. This problem can be identified by palpating the suboccipital muscles while the patient is moving the arms or legs. Muscle over-recruitment can lead to tension-type and cervicogenic headaches and plays a role in the neck pain that accompanies migraines.

There are many techniques to relax muscles locally. These include soft-tissue techniques, gentle manual traction, and hold-relax techniques.

Case Example

The patient is a 41-year-old female who has had bilateral, frontal tension-type headaches with muscle involvement (IHS 1988) for 10 years. She has decreased the frequency and duration of episodes with relaxation training using biofeedback. She is referred for a physical therapy evaluation, however, because she continues to have almost constant, bilateral neck pain that is particularly severe in the suboccipital area. Her neck pain can become severe and trigger a frontal headache.

On examination, the patient has a significant forward head position and moderately increased muscle tone of the frontalis, temporalis, suboccipital, paraspinals, and upper trapezius muscles. These muscles are not tender on palpation, and her headache is not reproducible. Her active and passive ROM is within normal limits with the exception of reduced active cervical rotation to the right that is not associated with any pain or muscle guarding.

The patient is taught postural correction, relaxed neck and postural exercises, and self-massage. The self-massage provides symptomatic relief, but the exercises tend to increase her neck pain. Assessment shows that she performs the exercises with significant shoulder bracing and a rigidly held neck with elevated chin. She is asked to discontinue the exercises temporarily and receives four sessions of localized muscle relaxation for the trapezii, cervical paraspinal, and suboccipital muscles. She is taught to keep these muscles relaxed while exercising her arms and legs. She is also taught to perform gentle neck retraction. The patient gradually learns to locally relax her posterior neck muscles and home exercises are reintroduced. After six treatment sessions, the patient has improved her posture, is able to relax her shoulder girdle effectively, and has decreased her overuse of the suboccipital muscles. She now has only occasional, mild neck pain that does not trigger headaches. She continues with relaxation training and feels better able to relax her neck and shoulders. She now has an average of one brief, mild headache per week.

This patient is seen for two 1-month follow-up sessions focusing on localized relaxation because of initial difficulty maintaining improvement between sessions. She continues to improve.

Self-Management

Because most headaches are chronic problems, physical therapy treatment should teach the patient to manage the condition on an ongoing basis. Patients should be instructed about the use of pain control modalities, a comprehensive exercise program, and postural correction. Patients should be taught the home use of hot or cold therapy and self-massage. Patients may have tried heat or cold, but discontinued use because their effect was only temporary. They should be reminded that the aggregate effect is beneficial.

Self-Massage

If patients develop good massage skills, they can stop or significantly lessen a tension-type headache and provide good relief for migraine and post-traumatic headache. Patients must be taught to do self-massage in a relaxed position (e.g., reclining with arms fully supported by cushions or pillows to promote shoulder relaxation). If necessary, they can reduce the amount of muscle work by performing the massage unilaterally and alternating sides. Patients typically maintain a forward head position and should be instructed to relax the neck and head by bringing the elbows up in a supported position. They should be taught finger massage with a gentle pressure and release that promotes relaxation of the arms as well as the affected muscles.

Case Example

The patient is a 45-year-old female who has had migraine without aura for many years and presents with an almost constant, dull ache in her right temporal area. She also complains of bimonthly migraines involving pain behind the left eye that radiates into the left temporal area. The dull ache varies in intensity from mild to severe, and the patient thinks that an increase in severity occasionally precedes a migraine. She can achieve slight relief by steady finger pressure onto the left temporalis, which she performs in a forward head posture with significant grimacing.

On examination, she has moderately increased muscle tone of the frontalis and cervical paraspinal muscles and severely increased muscle tone of the temporal and upper trapezius muscles. Palpation of the right temporalis reproduces her dull pain but does not trigger a headache. She has a significant forward head posture and mildly decreased ROM of cervical spine in forward bending and right rotation. Passive and accessory movements are within normal range, although suboccipital muscle guarding creates a slight hypomobility of the upper cervical spine on passive movement testing.

Relief of the dull ache is achieved with therapeutic massage, but the ache recurs between sessions despite a home program of postural correction and relaxed neck exercises that improve her posture and increase her cervical spine active ROM to within normal range. The patient is taught self-massage to the temporal, frontal, suboccipital, and cervical paraspinal muscles. She performs a home program of application of moist heat to the forehead and neck and a 5-minute massage to the temporales and suboccipitals (twice a day) and to frontalis and cervical paraspinals (once a day). She treats her left temporal and migraine pain with a cold pack followed by self-massage to the left temporalis.

The patient reports significant improvement in the dull ache and no longer rates the pain as severe enough to record on her monthly headache chart. At 1-month follow-up, she reduces her home program to heat and massage to temporalis and suboccipital muscles (once a day), frequent posture correction, relaxed neck exercises (once a day), and treatment with cold and massage for a migraine. She states that she feels better able to lessen her migraines and that their duration and intensity have decreased.

Exercise

It is important to evaluate whether nonaerobic and aerobic exercise increases or decreases intensity, frequency, duration, or has no effect on headaches in the individual patient. When exercise relieves headache, it can be integrated into the treatment program.

Case Example

The patient is a 35-year-old male who has had chronic tension-type headache with muscle involvement for 5 years. The pain occurs daily, starting in the late morning and increasing in intensity during the day. The patient has had a trial of relaxation training and continues to practice it even though he has found that sitting still increases his mental and physical tension. He reports that using the treadmill for 20 minutes decreases his headache slightly. He is given ROM exercises that restore a mild loss of active movement but do not change his headaches. He is instructed to increase his treadmill use. Exercising 20 minutes daily decreases the frequency, intensity, and duration of his headaches by 60%.

Relaxed Active Exercise

Relaxed active exercise promotes localized relaxation. Performance of relaxed movement can be promoted by teaching diaphragmatic breathing and instructing patients to lower their shoulders slightly during the exercise. Two exercises are outlined below. The first relaxes the neck.

1. Lower the chin slightly by looking at the knees.
2. Lower the chin toward the chest.
3. Roll the chin slowly around to one shoulder and pause.
4. Tuck the chin in slightly again and roll forward and down to return to the middle.
5. Without pausing, repeat in the other direction.

The second relaxes the shoulder girdle.

1. Roll both shoulders forward slowly 10 times and pause.
2. Repeat backward.

The number of repetitions of both exercises should depend on an assessment of the patient's muscle reactivity and pain tolerance.

Patients typically do exercises quickly in a jerky and uncoordinated manner. Precise instruction on breathing and gentle guidance through the movement should be provided. Instructing the patient to lower the shoulders during movement is helpful. The patient frequently is unaware that his or her shoulders are hunched and it will take time to correct this habit.

If a patient cannot develop the skill of relaxed movement despite physical therapy instruction, he or she may have an inability to generally relax and could benefit from a referral to behavioral medicine for relaxation training and stress management.

Stretching

It is useful to alternate stretching exercises with relaxed active exercises to prevent muscle over-recruitment. The following exercise combines neck retraction and forward bend to correct a forward head position and stretch out tight suboccipital muscles, which are both involved in migraine and tension-type headache.

1. Lower the chin slightly by looking at the knees.
2. Lower the chin toward the chest and hold for a slow count of five.
3. Repeat three times.

The next exercise stretches tight muscles of the shoulder girdle.

1. Interlace the fingers above the head.
2. Push the arms slightly back and up.
3. Feel a gentle stretch in the arms, shoulders, and upper back and hold for 5 seconds.
4. Lower arms, pause, and repeat three times.

It is extremely important that stretching exercises are done slowly and gently. A full set of stretches including neck retraction, forward bend, neck rotation, neck side bend, and shoulder girdle retraction should be performed once to twice daily.

Strengthening Exercises

Once the patient can perform exercises in a relaxed, coordinated manner, strengthening exercises can be added to the regimen. It is best to start with active exercises using body weight as resistance and progress to the use of rubber bands or free weights as possible. Teaching resisted head movements to strengthen pericranial muscles is useful in promoting localized relaxation.

Strengthening exercises can be alternated with stretch or relaxed active exercises to promote relaxation and prevent muscle over-recruitment. If patients wish to use equipment for resisted exercise, they need to be given good postural and ergonomic instructions and have developed the skill of relaxation during movement to prevent the triggering of headaches.

Aerobic Exercise

When aerobic exercise increases headaches, it is usually because the exercise is being performed with poor body mechanics or over-recruitment. Initially, it is important to evaluate whether the patient has the required muscle strength, ROM, balance, and coordination for the chosen activity. Jogging with a forward head position or swimming breaststroke with excessive neck extension are examples of how neck muscle tone can be increased and lead to localized or referred pain.

Migraines can decrease in frequency, intensity, and duration with regular aerobic exercise, but migraine patients typically overdo exercise. Simple instruction in pacing and body mechanics can prevent triggering of headaches. If the patient has difficulty with pacing, he or she may need a referral to behavioral medicine for general relaxation training and stress management.

Case Example

A patient with migraine with aura finds her migraines are triggered after 5 minutes of jogging. After correction of her forward head posture and instruction on pacing, her migraines are triggered after 10 minutes and are less severe. She is advised to experiment with different types of exercise and joins an aerobic class. She finds that this does not trigger her headaches. She had not enjoyed jogging but ran because she thought it was good for her. She often ran competitively against a partner. She finds the aerobic class relaxing and fun, a factor that may contribute to the cessation of exercise-triggered headaches.

Postural Correction

Headache patients usually present with a forward head posture and an elevated and protracted shoulder girdle. They may have a flattened cervical spine with a level chin position or an increased cervical lordosis with an elevated chin. Migraine patients often present with a flattened thoracic spine and a rigid, erect posture with spinal muscle guarding. Tension-type headache patients often present with an increased thoracic curvature.

Typically, patients correct their posture with maximum muscle effort. They need to be guided into sitting and standing with a relaxed posture so that muscle tone is not further increased. Patients also tend to forget to practice posture correction. It is helpful to ask patients to correct their posture for 1 minute once an hour, rather than to ask them to remember a correct posture at all times. Regular repetitions develop good habits at a pace that should not cause new muscle strains.

Postural correction instructions should be as simple as possible to follow. Patients should perform postural stretches such as bilateral arm elevation. They should also be advised to take regular breaks to stretch and walk around if their occupation involves a lot of time in one position or activity. They should be instructed on the response of muscles and ligaments to prolonged positioning.

Patients need instruction about correct sleeping positions, particularly if they read in bed. Tension-type headaches often start in the early morning and are associated with anticipatory tension or a buildup of muscle tension from the previous day that does not dissipate with sleep.

Headache Management Principles

The physical therapist should remember several principles of sound headache management:

1. Assess and discuss with the patient the role of physical therapy in his or her treatment. It may be the primary treatment or a small part of a multidisciplinary approach.

2. When a multidisciplinary approach is required, communicate effectively with the other clinicians involved. Help the patient to be aware of the importance of the team approach and that individual treatments are not cures in themselves, but pieces that fit together to ensure effective, long-term headache control.

3. Monitor the patient's weekly or monthly headache diary. This diary should record frequency, duration, intensity, and possible triggers of

headaches. Without daily assessment recorded on a long-term basis, improvement in headaches cannot be assessed.

4. Choose specific objective findings such as ROM to assess pre- and post-treatment goals. A patient can improve objectively but not subjectively or vice versa, which has implications for the team's approach.

5. Focus on long-term headache management. Most headaches are chronic problems and patients need self-management strategies to prevent or lessen their pain problem.

Neck Pain

Neck (cervical spine) pain is a common occurrence. Trauma, overload, or poor posture is responsible for many cases. Spinal degeneration may be either a causative or contributing factor. Trauma superimposed on degeneration may result in a complex clinical picture (Rossi 1994).

The cervical spine and musculature not only have to stabilize and balance the head, but also are exposed to virtually constant traction from the hanging upper limbs. The shoulder and neck muscles are activated during all movements of the upper extremity in space (Janda 1988).

Anatomy

The upper extremities are actively suspended by the levator scapulae and the upper trapezius. Holding a weight in the upper extremities or active elevation of the scapula initiates a brisk response by the levator scapulae (De Freitas et al. 1980) and the upper trapezius (Bearn 1961) and therefore places an increased load on the head and neck. De Freitas et al. (1980) demonstrated high activity in the levator scapulae and rhomboid muscles during free movements with manual submaximal resistance against arm abduction or flexion.

Inman et al. (1944) identified a force couple in each muscle that is composed of upper and lower segments that produce upward rotation of the scapula. For the serratus anterior, the levator scapulae was considered to be the upward force unit. Within the trapezius, the upper segment displayed consistent action in both abduction and flexion. The reduced participation of the lower trapezius leaves the scapula free to move anteriorly (Inman et al. 1944). To attain maximal scapular rotation, both the trapezius and the serratus anterior must be active. Clinically, a disruption of normal force couple action is often seen; with a weak serratus anterior, the levator scapulae becomes overactive to compensate. A weak lower trapezius is compensated for by an overactive upper trapezius. As a result movement patterns become abnormal (e.g., shrugging the shoulders when elevating the arms). This can lead to the neck and shoulder pain seen often by physical therapists.

Pathophysiology

Habitual postures can lead to neck pain. Harms-Ringdahl (1986) demonstrated that the extreme flexed neck position leads to neck pain within 1 hour.

Work with an abducted arm leads to increased activity in the trapezius, the cervical erector spinae, and the thoracic erector spinae/rhomboid muscles (Schuldt 1988) and subsequently to muscle fatigue and pain.

Therefore, upper extremity movement will necessarily exert forces on the neck and head. Evaluation and treatment of neck pain therefore must include evaluation of the interscapular muscles and the "suspension mechanism" of the upper extremities, the trapezius and levator scapulae. Any dysfunction in these muscles can contribute to neck pain.

Subtle changes in postural muscle activity can have important functional consequences. The recommended level for maintained static muscle work is 2% of a maximum voluntary contraction (MVC), and the suggested acceptable limit is 5% (Jonsson 1982). At this level of static contraction, the energy yield to the muscle is most likely aerobic. At a higher MVC level (e.g., as that generated by poor posture), pain, and significant increases in sick leave due to musculoskeletal complaints occur (Ashton-Miller et al. 1990). This may be due to the anaerobic energy supply to the muscle, which results in a buildup of lactic acid and decreased contractile strength. An MVC of higher than 30% results in a decrease of blood flow in the muscle, provoking an even greater energy crisis (Astrand and Rodahl 1986).

This appears to be confirmed by Larsson et al. (1988), who documented a decreased level of high energy phosphates and the presence of ragged-red fibers, a finding suggestive of mitochondrial damage in biopsies taken from the upper part of the trapezius in patients with static work-related chronic myalgia with clinical findings suggestive of myofascial pain. In a 1990 study, Larsson et al. (1990) measured the blood flow in the painful upper part of the trapezius and found that the myalgia correlated with reduced local blood flow. Therefore, addressing work postures and ergonomics to reduce static muscle activity must be a part of the treatment of patients with neck pain.

Exercise

Correct dispersal of segmental movement of the cervical spine depends on the balanced relationship between the head, cervical spine, and thorax and dynamic muscular control. Total movement of the cervical spine is the composite of segmental motion of all the cervical vertebrae and the first three thoracic vertebrae. The majority of rotation occurs in the upper three cervical segments. Movement patterns on a poor postural base contribute to repetitive microtrauma of the cervical structures, including the facets, discs, ligaments, articular capsules, and muscles. These poor patterns of movement contribute to habitual overuse at isolated motion segments and minimize normal movement at others. Habitual dysfunction at isolated segments may generate bony hypertrophy, ligamentous laxity, and breakdown of disc and facet articulations. This dysfunction can perpetuate itself in a cycle of pain, muscle imbalance, and postural abnormality.

The most common postural abnormality involves the forward head position, elevation and protraction of the shoulders, rotation and abduction of the scapulae, and a variable degree of winging of the scapulae. This abnormality is usually associated with the "proximal syndrome," or "shoulder-crossed syndrome" (Janda 1988), a muscle imbalance characterized by tightness and weakness of upper body musculature. The following is a list of the muscles that are typically tight or weak in this syndrome:

Tight	Weak
Sternocleidomastoid	Serratus anterior
Pectoralis major and minor	Lower and middle trapezius
Levator scapulae	Rhomboids
Upper trapezius	Neck flexors
Suboccipital muscles	Suprahyoid
Masseter	Mylohyoid
Temporalis	
Digastric	

This altered posture likely stresses the craniocervical junction as well as the cervicothoracic junction. Muscles such as the upper trapezius, levator scapulae, and sternocleidomastoid not only play a role in the development of neck pain, but also in the development of cervicogenic headache. The forward head position also plays a role in the development of temporomandibular dysfunction and the development of facial pain (Janda 1986b). Furthermore, the alteration of the position of the glenoid fossa results in altered biomechanical forces across this joint, leading to increased muscle activity of the upper trapezius, levator scapulae, and the rotator cuff.

Treatment of the cervical spine must therefore include restoration of normal muscle balance; postural retraining; flexibility, strength, and endurance exercises; and instruction in proper body mechanics. The following studies suggest that exercise has an important role in the treatment of neck pain.

Highland et al. (1992) investigated the effect of full-range isometric contractions on strength and ROM in 90 subjects at eight equidistant positions in a device that constrained all motion with the exception of cervical flexion and extension. The patients participated in an 8-week program. Training consisted of two sessions per week for 4 weeks and one training session per week for 4 weeks. All patients showed significant reduction in their perception of pain as well as significant gains in strength and ROM of the cervical spine. Berg et al. (1994) examined whether neck resistance training could increase strength and reduce pain in workers with neck pain. Seventeen women exercised twice weekly for 8 weeks. Each session (12 minutes) consisted of three sets of 12 repetitions of resisted rotation, flexion, and extension using hydraulic dampers. Resistance was set individually and increased every second week. After training, neck strength had increased significantly with significantly reduced perceived neck pain.

Exercise promotes the necessary strength, coordination, and endurance to maintain the cervical spine in a stable and safe position during loading, mobility, and weight-bearing activities. Exercise training optimizes the capacity of the cervicothoracic muscles to absorb loads in all directions while minimizing direct strain and stress on individual cervical tissues, thus reducing repetitive microtrauma to the cervical segments.

Training the upper, middle, and lower trapezius; serratus anterior; and rhomboids provides scapular stability and thus indirect stability for the cervical spine. Dynamic stabilization exercises superimpose extremity movement on stable spine positions and can be performed with or without aids such as balls, bolsters, pulleys, and weights (Saal and Saal 1989).

Saal and Saal (1989) report having patients perform three sets of 15 repetitions per exercise before the patient is progressed to the next exercise. This endurance exercise ensures motor learning that is thought to establish a motor pattern that becomes automatic, rather than conscious.

Sweeney et al. (1990) provide an excellent treatment outline for cervical stabilization.

Ergonomics

Factors considered to increase the static level of activity or fatigue in neck and shoulder muscles include excessive horizontal distance between work object and the worker, high position of the work objects, high work table surface, narrow constraints on the sitting posture, postures with flexed shoulder joint, postures with abducted arms, and postures with flexed neck (Schuldt 1988). The duration of each contraction (i.e., the interval between muscular contractions) is thought to be of major importance, as is the duration of the whole work process.

Schuldt (1988) investigated neck muscle activity and load reduction in sitting postures and found that it is possible to reduce neck and shoulder muscular activity significantly by choosing a sitting position with the trunk slightly inclined backwards and with the cervical spine vertical. In addition, muscle activity of the neck and shoulder was reduced by using forearm support and avoidance of arm abduction.

Tan and Nordin (1992) make the following recommendations for ergonomic adjustments of the sitting workplace:

1. The distance between the eye and the object worked on should be 12 inches. This is considered normal for reading a book or a computer screen.
2. Work should be done at the same height as the elbows.
3. The work surface should be arranged so that everything is within easy reach.
4. The chair should have a back support below the shoulder blades with well-designed lumbar support, swivel, rollers, and arm rests for support. The seat height should be low enough for the feet to be resting comfortably on the floor.

Those involved in primarily static work are also advised to take small breaks to delay muscle fatigue and avoid abnormal postures such as cradling the phone or sleeping on the stomach.

Case Example

The patient is a 64-year-old female who has had total body tightness and stiffness for many years, mainly in her neck and shoulders. She also complains of daily headaches. Her previous history includes a lumpectomy 5 years ago for breast cancer followed by radiation. Interventions for her pain included splint therapy for her temporomandibular joint dysfunction, which was thought to be associated with her headaches, and physical therapy in which she was instructed in a general stretching program.

Pain   On a 10-point pain scale, the patient rates her headache as five on average, three at best, and eight at worst. She describes her neck pain as stiffness. Her pain is decreased by stretching and heat and increased by all physical activities.

Function   The patient is an artist and makes small statues, which requires her to be in a sitting position, working with her arms overhead. She is able to sustain this for 10 minutes. She occasionally goes for a walk. She performs her stretching exercise daily. Her social functioning is decreased due to her discomfort and headaches.

Multidimensional Pain Inventory Profile   The patient is classified as an adaptive coper.

Physical examination   Posture is remarkable for forward head and thoracic kyphosis with internally rotated shoulders. Cervical, lumbar, and hip ROM is normal. Manual muscle testing of both upper and lower extremities is 5/5. Interscapular strength is 4/5. Pectorales major and minor are tight. Reflexes and sensation are normal. Palpation reveals diffuse musculoskeletal tenderness of the neck and shoulders.

Aerobic fitness   The patient is in the "low-fit category" for her age group.

Pain behaviors   This patient has no verbal or nonverbal pain behaviors.

Patient goals   To sustain overhead positions for 1 hour at a time as necessary for her work. To decrease the frequency and average intensity of her headaches.

Assessment   The patient has muscle imbalance, poor aerobic capacity, and insufficient muscle endurance to sustain overhead work.

Plan   Aerobic conditioning; stretching of the pectorales; endurance training of the serratus anterior, rhomboids, and lower and middle trapezius; postural training; patient education; independent stretching; walking program; and transition into an independent health club program, three times per week for 6 weeks.

Treatment contract goals

1. Walk for 20–30 minutes each day, starting at 10 minutes and increasing by 5 minutes per week.
2. Work with arms above head. Start at 10 minutes a day, with a goal of 60 minutes continuously.

Treatment

1. The patient is instructed on correct posture and building in short breaks during her work. Working on a lower table is discussed; however, the patient feels that this would interfere with the quality of her work.
2. The patient's stretching program is reviewed and specific stretches are added for the pectorales, levator scapulae, and suboccipitals.
3. Instruction in a home walking program, starting at 10 minutes per day, increasing by 5 minutes per week to achieve a goal of a 30-minute walk per day in 1 month.

4. Instruction in a rubber band home exercise program is given, including exercise for the upper trapezius, rhomboids, serratus anterior, and lower trapezius (using diagonal patterns) starting at five repetitions each, adding one repetition per exercise per day to a maximum of 25 repetitions per exercise to increase interscapular muscle endurance.

5. The physical therapy program consists of a quota-based program of treadmill walking; upper-extremity ergometer exercises; pulley exercises for the rhomboids, latissimus dorsi, and serratus anterior; proprioceptive neuromuscular facilitation pattern of flexion; external rotation and abduction to increase endurance of upper trapezius, rhomboids, serratus anterior, and lower trapezius using the pulleys in standing; and abdominal exercises while sitting to increase interscapular muscle endurance and improve trunk stabilization.

After eight sessions the patient's pain decreases from an average of five to three and her work tolerance increases to 1 hour. She is independent in her home exercise and stretching and walking program.

She is seen for a total of 15 sessions. At this time, she has no more headaches. Her interscapular strength is normal, her posture is improved, and she is able to work continuously for several hours. She joins a health club and performs her exercises there two to three times per week. At follow-up 6 months later, she is headache free and independent in her health club program.

Case Example

The patient is a 45-year-old male who underwent neck surgery after a work injury 3 years ago. His injury occurred with a heavy lift and he experienced immediate right arm and hand numbness with neck pain. Surgeries included an anterior cervical discectomy at C5/6 2 years ago and an anterior cervical discectomy and fusion at C4/5 1 year ago. Both surgeries were unsuccessful in alleviating his pain and numbness.

Electromyography shows mild chronic denervation of the left C5 and the right C6 nerve roots. His computed tomography scan shows marked narrowing of the neural foramen at C4/5 that is worse on the left than on the right.

Previous treatment included two courses of physical therapy with ultrasound, electrical stimulation, and soft-tissue mobilization. This treatment was not helpful in decreasing his pain or improving his function.

The patient has been diagnosed with bipolar affective disorder. He sees a psychiatrist for treatment.

Pain The patient complains of neck pain that radiates into the back of his skull, shoulders, shoulder blades, and right arm in the triceps area. He states his pain is constant and rates it as a seven to eight on average on a 10-point scale. His pain intensity is four at best and eight at worst. His pain is increased by walking and standing for more than 10 minutes and sitting for more than 30 minutes. His pain is eased by changing positions. His sleep is interrupted by his pain.

Function   The patient owned his own business, but closed it 2 years ago due to his sense of inability to take care of it. He has not worked since. He does not socialize because he feels he is poor company. All of his functional activities are limited due to his pain.

Multidimensional Pain Inventory Profile   The patient is classified as dysfunctional.

Physical assessment   Posture is unremarkable. Cervical spine ROM is 50% in forward bending, backward bending, and rotation and is reported to be painful. Side bending is 20% in both directions with pain.

Flexion of both shoulders is 135 degrees.

Manual muscle testing is 5/5 in the left upper extremity and 4/5 in the right upper extremity. Deep tendon reflexes in the right biceps and brachioradialis are decreased. He has decreased sensation to light touch and pinprick in his right thumb and lateral index finger.

He has significant tenderness and pain in the right upper quadrant musculature with palpation.

Aerobic fitness   The patient's fitness is very low for his age group.

Pain behaviors   The patient exhibits moderate verbal and nonverbal (grimacing, bracing, and guarding) pain behavior.

Patient goals   Pain relief, increased general function, re-establishing business.

Assessment   Patient has chronic neuropathic pain, superimposed by myofascial pain and chronic pain syndrome. Impairments include decreased cervical spine and shoulder motion, fear, related lack of movement, and activity intolerance due to deconditioning.

Plan   Functional restoration three times a week for 6 weeks, behavioral medicine group and individual treatment, and a treatment contract are included in the treatment plan for this patient.

Treatment contract goals

1.   Decrease behaviors that communicate to others that you are in pain (e.g., crankiness, decreased socialization, reduced activity participation, complaining, grimacing, and moaning).
2.   Return to work. Plan the re-establishment of former business.
3.   Bike 10 minutes with a goal of 30 minutes.
4.   Improve flexibility to better reach behind back in the shower.
5.   Floor-to-chest lifting starting at 5 lbs, with a goal of 50 lbs and 20 repetitions.
6.   Lifting 5 lbs overhead with a goal of 15 lbs and 20 repetitions.
7.   Walking for 20 minutes with a goal of 60 minutes.
8.   Eliminate down time required after exercise.
9.   Prepare to make the transition to an independent health club program.

Treatment

1.   The patient is educated regarding pacing and use of heat, cold, and self-massage with tennis balls for independent pain management after activities and exercise.

2. Home stretching exercises for latissimus dorsi, upper trapezius, scalenes, and levator scapulae are assigned. Five repetitions of each are performed three times per day. The patient is instructed in a walking program that begins at 20 minutes and increases by 1 minute per day to 60 minutes by the sixth week.

3. Lifting is an essential part of work for this patient. Lifting requires strength in the quadriceps, gluteals, trunk stabilizers, interscapular muscles, and arms. The patient is instructed in bridging, sit-ups, and back extension exercises. He starts with 10 repetitions of each and adds two repetitions per day until he reaches 30 repetitions. After this, the level of difficulty of each exercise is increased. These exercises are part of his home exercise plan.

   Exercises done in physical therapy include quota-based pulley exercises for rhomboids, serratus anterior, and latissimus dorsi; abdominal and multifidi exercises while standing; diagonals in flexion, external rotation, and abduction; and lifting simulation. Squatting and lunging exercises are performed with 5-lb weights. Five additional pounds are added per week until 25-lb weights are used in each hand.

4. The patient is instructed in proper lifting techniques starting with five repetitions, increasing by seven lifts per week.

5. The patient bicycles 20 minutes at 25 W on his first visit and is progressed to 30 minutes at 90 W in 1 month.

At the sixth week, all physical therapy goals are met.

Chronic Back Pain

Studies from Canada, Sweden, and the United States show that back pain is the first or second most prevalent pain complaint in the general population (Raspe 1993). Fortunately, 90% recover within a few months with or without treatment. For those who remain in pain and are disabled and unable to work beyond these initial months, the functional prognosis is grim. *Less than 50% of people who are disabled by their pain for more than 6 months ever return to work, and reemployment is almost never achieved after 2 years of disability (Waddell 1992).* The functional restoration approach and aggressive exercise with a focus on function have been demonstrated to be highly effective (see Chapter 6).

More frequent exercise is associated with a stronger belief in personal control over back pain (Harkapaa et al. 1991). Similarly, the successful attainment of functional goals has been associated with increased self-efficacy. The challenge for the physical therapist is to determine how much exercise is required for the patient to achieve functional goals.

Anatomy

The abdominal muscles provide stability to the trunk. Posteriorly, the abdominal muscle group becomes contiguous with the thoracolumbar fascia, which sheaths the bundles of erector spinae muscles. The lateral abdominal muscles are therefore in a position to assist and enhance the role of the erector spinae. The superficial lamina of the thoracolumbar fascia is composed primarily of the aponeurosis of the latissimus dorsi. The gluteus maximus inserts into the external fascia of the sacrum, which connects with the thoracolumbar fascia. The paired contralateral external and internal obliques can provide a very strong rotary movement because of their long-movement arm of force. Therefore, they are more important in trunk rotation movements than the multifidus (Liemohn 1990). Snijders (1994) maintains that biomechanical studies indicate that the stability of the sacroiliac joint is important in treatment of low back pain. The hamstrings are capable of tensing the sacrospinal and sacrotuberal ligaments. Contraction of the gluteus maximus and the oblique abdominal muscles increases compression of the sacroiliac joint, thus providing stability.

Pathophysiology

Although the mechanism of muscle insufficiency associated with low back pain is not well understood, it is commonly believed that the passive structures of the spine are increasingly stressed with increasing functional muscle insufficiency. Nicolaisen and Jorgensen (1985) performed studies of isometric trunk extensor performance and found that patients with low back pain had significantly shorter endurance than controls. Despite the difference in muscle endurance, there were no differences in isometric back muscle strength between patients and controls. In a subsequent study (Jorgensen and Nicolaisen 1987), they found that back muscles have a relatively longer endurance capacity than other muscle groups. They attributed this to the fiber composition of the back muscles—largely slow-twitch, oxidative fibers. They also found that people with earlier attacks of back pain had less endurance capacity, but similar strength in their back muscles. They interpreted this to mean that the composition of back muscles in the patients was dominated by a greater proportion of easily fatigable, type II fibers.

Andersson et al. (1989) reported on a study in which a triaxial dynamometer was used to measure torques and angular positions and velocities while the subjects, who were in upright positions, moved through an extension/flexion arch repeatedly until fatigued. As the muscles fatigued, ROM increased in the secondary planes of motion, indicating diminishing control and coordination of the fatigued neuromuscular system (Andersson et al. 1989).

Roy et al. (1989) developed the computer-aided Back Analysis System using electromyographic spectral measurements to quantify lumbar muscle function. This technique reliably discriminates back pain patients from normal controls. They observed higher rates of fatigue in the low back pain group as compared with the control group, whereas isometric muscle strength was similar for both groups.

Explanations for this observation included a greater proportion of type II fibers in low back pain patients than control subjects or high precontraction metabolite levels in low back pain patients resulting from persistent muscle spasm and prolonged muscle tension.

Based on these studies, there seems to be evidence that lack of trunk muscle endurance plays an important role in chronic low back pain. A problem often cited is that measurement is difficult as various trunk muscles seem to have distinctly different fiber composition and function.

The innervation and function of the erector spinae and the multifidus muscle are so different that they cannot be classified as a single unit. Considerable individual variation exists among individuals in the fiber-type distribution of these muscles.

The predominance of type I fibers in both the erector spinae (Johnson et al. 1973) and the multifidus (Kalimo 1989) is consistent with their function of maintaining spinal posture and stabilizing the trunk.

Mattila et al. (1986) studied the multifidus muscles from patients with lumbar disc herniation and cadaver controls. They found that the type II fibers were markedly and selectively smaller than the type I fibers in both groups and that the internal structure of type I fibers showed so-called targetoid, or moth-eaten, changes. Zhu et al. (1989) took biopsy material from the fast-twitch fatiguable erector spinae in patients with lumbar disc herniation. They found (1) angulated and selective atrophy of type II fibers with a higher ratio of type IIb fast-twitch fatiguable to IIa intermediate fibers; (2) more marked atrophy of type II fibers with increasing age and duration of symptoms; and (3) moth-eaten fibers, central cores, and internal nuclei. They attributed these findings to muscle disuse and denervation as immobilization increases the ratio of type IIb to IIa. Endurance training decreases the ratio of type IIb to IIa.

Kalimo et al. (1989) found significant selective type II atrophy in the multifidus muscle, not only in patients with disc prolapse, but also in controls. They attributed this to deconditioning and a sedentary lifestyle.

Thus, many of the major back muscles have a preponderance of type I fibers. Given their postural function, this is not surprising; however, individual variability is considerable. Researchers concluded that the changes seen in both the muscle fatigue and the muscle fiber-type studies are likely a result of deconditioning (see Chapter 5). Since the back muscles are mostly built for and need endurance to function, an argument can be made that aggressive endurance training is the treatment of choice in the rehabilitation of a patient with back pain.

Exercise

In the spine, the health of the joints depends largely on repeated low stress movements (Twomey 1992). The intervertebral joints and the facet joints require movement for the proper transfer of fluid and nutrients across the joint surfaces (Frank et al. 1984). In the same way, the intervertebral disc depends largely on movement for its nutrition (Bogduk 1986). The anatomy of the back and tissue behavior (see Chapter 5) support the argument made earlier for treating back pain patients with an aggressive endurance training program with a focus on the erector spinae, multifidi, latissimus dorsi, gluteals, abdominals (oblique), and hamstrings.

One of the goals of exercise training is adequate dynamic control of lumbar spine forces in order to eliminate repetitive injury to the intervertebral discs, facet joints, and related structures.

Normal posture that includes elimination of muscle imbalances needs to be maintained. The most common postural abnormality in back pain seen is the one in which the patient presents with hyperextension of the knees, increased lumbar lordosis, and a protruding abdomen. This tends to be a result of a distinct pattern of muscle imbalance in which the following muscles are either tight or weak (Janda 1986a):

Tight	Weak
Hamstrings	Abdominals
Rectus femoris	Gluteals
Hip flexors	Multifidi
Gastrocnemius	Rotatores
Soleus	
Back extensors	
Piriformis	
Quadratus lumborum	

Tightness of the hip flexors, for example, results in an inability to extend the hip sufficiently for walking, resulting in increased anterior rotation of the ilium and therefore increasing stresses across the lumbar spine. Insufficient pelvic stabilization due to weakness of the gluteus medius and minimus and abdominal muscles results in similar increased stresses across the lumbar spine. The development of trigger points in the gluteus medius and minimus can refer pain into the leg, simulating sciatica (Travell and Simons 1992).

The goal of back stabilization exercises is development of the ability to maintain a simultaneous contraction of the abdominal, buttock, and back extensor muscles. Exercises such as the "dead bug" are helpful. Other exercises include bridging with both feet on a ball, partial sit-ups, lying prone on a ball while alternating arm and leg raises, and pulley exercises performed standing with a pelvic tilt and both knees slightly bent. The difficulty of these exercises is increased by changing from a sitting to standing position or from straight plane to diagonal patterns and incorporating rotations.

Ergonomics

Andersson et al. (1989) proposed that factors contributing to low back pain include physically heavy work, static work postures, frequent bending and twisting, lifting and forceful movements, repetitive work, and vibration. Sustained postures, bent postures, and prolonged sitting also have been associated with low back pain. Job dissatisfaction, blue-collar work, and depression have been associated with the occurrence of low back pain. Depression, low activity levels, significant pain behavior, and negative beliefs regarding the ability to function despite pain have been associated with the occurrence of chronic disability.

An excellent review on the assessment of an individual's capacity for work in relation to the physical effort requirements of a job is provided by Rodgers (1988).

Lifting instruction is essential. Patients should not lift objects that are too heavy or lift without a secure foothold. The weight should be held close to the body, and foot position should turn with the weight (the spine should not twist with the weight). The low back should be held in lordotic position.

Case Example

The patient is a 43-year-old female who weighs 320 lbs and presents with complaints of low back pain and pain in the back of her legs. The onset of her pain was insidious about 1 year ago.

Magnetic resonance imaging of her lumbar spine shows minimal intervertebral disc space narrowing between L3–L4 and a grade I spondylolisthesis of L4–L5. She was treated with physical therapy about 6 months ago that included hot packs, ultrasound, knee-to-chest exercises, and quadriceps strengthening. This did not help her pain or function.

Her past medical history is significant for chronic renal failure, hypertension, hypothyroidism, and schizophrenia. She is under the care of a psychiatrist, and her schizophrenic symptoms are controlled. She takes numerous medications.

Pain   The patient describes piercing pain in the middle of her low back and aching pain in the back of her legs. She rates her average pain as eight on a 10-point scale. At best, there is no pain. She rates her worst pain is an eight. Her pain is increased with walking and decreased by sitting and lying down.

Function   The patient is single and lives alone. She was very functional until about 1 year ago. She was volunteering 20 hours per week and would walk 15 minutes to her volunteer work. She stopped volunteering and walking due to her pain. She no longer goes to the grocery store or pharmacy due to the pain of walking. She has difficulty performing housekeeping chores. She has begun to sleep 12 hours per night and to lie down in the afternoon for several hours due to her pain.

Multidimensional Pain Inventory Profile   The test is invalid (this occurs in cases where no profile can be established).

Physical examination   Patient is morbidly obese. Posture is remarkable for a forward bent position of the trunk on the hips that she claims eases her leg pain. Pelvic symmetry cannot be palpated.

ROM of the lumbar spine is essentially normal with forward bending with fingertips to the shins. Extension, rotation, and sidebending of the lumbar spine are within normal limits and do not cause pain. ROM of both hips is within normal limits.

Manual muscle testing of both lower extremities is 5/5. Hip flexors are 3/5.

Straight-leg raising is 50 degrees due to hamstring tightness and is negative for radicular pain. Sensation and deep tendon reflexes are normal. No muscle spasm is palpated in the lumbar spine. The sciatic notch is not tender. Gait is abnormal with small step length. The patient uses a cane for support.

Aerobic fitness   This could not be assessed due to the patient's medication use.

Pain behaviors   Verbal pain complaints about pain and abnormal posturing are present.

Patient goals   To decrease pain; to be able to walk to the grocery store (20 minutes).

Assessment   The patient has chronic mechanical low back pain, superimposed with chronic pain syndrome. Impairments include pain with walking, hip flexor weakness, hamstring tightness, abnormal standing posture, and activity intolerance due to deconditioning.

Plan   Functional restoration sessions are completed two times a week for 6 weeks, with careful monitoring of the patient's blood pressure. Borg's Rating of Perceived Effort is used to monitor intensity of cardiovascular exercise. Behavioral medicine group treatment is included.

Treatment contract goals

1.   Decrease behaviors such as walking bent over, complaining about pain, needing to sit down constantly, and lying down during the day.
2.   Physical therapy goals include walking for 1 minute and gradually increasing the amount of time until able to walk 20 minutes to the grocery store. Also, improve flexibility of hamstrings from 50 degrees to 70 degrees in straight leg raising and improve posture until a normal upright position is maintained.

Treatment

1.   The patient is educated in the use of heat and cold after walking and in using transcutaneous electrical nerve stimulation (TENS) while walking for independent pain management.
2.   The patient begins a 1-minute quota-based home walking program that is increased 1 minute every 2 days to 20 minutes by the sixth week.
3.   A home program for stretching of the hamstrings and back extensors and a quota-based strengthening program of the gluteals and abdominals are also begun.
4.   Exercises performed in physical therapy sessions include review of the home program and appropriate progression of number of repetitions as set by the quota schedule. Quota-based squatting exercise, abdominal exercises with pulleys, and latissimus dorsi exercises with pulleys are also performed. Her blood pressure remains stable during exercise.
5.   Finally, treadmill walking is included to increase aerobic capacity. At the first visit the patient is able to walk for 4 minutes at 0.5 mph with a 1-minute break. Her blood pressure remains stable and the rate of perceived exertion is 14.

In the second week of treatment, the patient is redirected in her home program because she is not following the quota-based program and is only walking occasionally. Use of the TENS unit is discontinued because she does not think it is helpful. In the sixth week, she is walking on the treadmill for 22 minutes at 0.7 mph with three short rests and stable blood pressure. Rate of perceived exertion is 11. She is independent in her home program and is performing 25 repetitions of all her exercises. Her posture is now normal and she walks to the grocery store without a cane. She continues to complain of pain and plans to see an acupuncturist for this.

Case Example

The patient is a 35-year-old man complaining of chronic low back pain. He was diagnosed with a grade II spondylolisthesis 11 years ago after a work-related injury and underwent decompression and stabilization with a fusion 9 years ago. For 2 years he was pain free, but then his pain returned. It steadily increased until 3 years ago, when he underwent further stabilization using pedicle screws that actually made the pain worse.

Previous interventions have included epidural steroid injections without pain relief, seven admissions to the hospital for pain control and medications, and 14 separate courses of physical therapy.

Other medical history includes a C5–6 disc bulge, bilateral carpal tunnel syndrome, right ulnar nerve entrapment, and irritable bowel syndrome.

Pain   The patient complains of constant low back pain that radiates into the right leg and down the posterior thigh and calf into the great toe. During periods of extreme pain it radiates into the posterior left thigh and lower leg as well. He rates his average pain as eight on a 10-point scale. At best, it is a five, and at worst, an eight. He describes his pain as shooting with severe cramping. Coughing and sneezing increase his pain as do all physical activities. Sitting and walking aggravate the pain the most. His pain is decreased with medications and temporarily decreased with cold and heat.

Function   The patient is a computer scientist and is required to sit throughout the day. He has not worked for 3 years but still has a position available to him with his former employer. He is married and has two children he believes he is unable to take care of due to his pain. He spends the day on the couch, reading occasionally. He does not socialize, exercise, or engage in recreational activities.

He is able to sit for 5 minutes and stand and walk for 10 minutes. His sleep is interrupted due to his inability to tolerate a particular position for any length of time.

Multidimensional Pain Inventory Profile   The patient is classified as dysfunctional.

Physical examination   Posture is abnormal with right leg bent. Patient claims it makes his pain worse to straighten his leg. Pelvis is level. The left shoulder is elevated. Lumbar spine ROM is limited to 25% in all directions and is painful. Flexion, extension, and sidebending to the left increase his right leg pain. Hip ROM is limited in all directions due to significant muscle guarding. He is unable to flex his hips beyond 45 degrees due to muscle guarding and reported severe pain. In prone position, he is unable to extend his thighs due to pain. Flexion of the knees in the prone position is limited to 90 degrees due to rectus femoris shortness. He is able to stand on his toes and heels. With manual muscle testing he has give-away weakness in all muscle groups in both lower extremities. Abdominal strength is 3/5. Straight leg raising is 20 degrees bilaterally due to muscle guarding and is negative for radicular pain. The Achilles reflex is absent on the left. Sensation is decreased in the entire left leg. Palpation with the patient in supine position does not reveal muscle spasm in his back or buttocks. Sciatic notch is not tender. Sacroiliac testing is negative. All Waddell signs are positive (see Table 4.1).

Gait is abnormal with decreased step length and decreased weight bearing on the right leg. Knees remain flexed throughout the gait cycle. The patient ambulates with a cane in the left hand.

Aerobic fitness   The patient was unable to achieve steady state on either bike or treadmill, so this could not be measured.

Pain behaviors   The patient remains standing throughout the interview with significant guarding, inappropriate illness signs, verbal pain complaints, moaning, sighing, and rubbing.

Patient goals   To decrease pain.

Assessment   The patient has chronic neuropathic back pain with superimposed myofascial pain and chronic pain syndrome. Impairments include decreased trunk and hip flexibility, muscle imbalance, abnormal movement patterns, fear-related lack of movement, and activity intolerance due to deconditioning.

Plan   The patient will participate in a functional restoration program, behavioral medicine group and individual treatment, and will have a treatment and medication contract.

Treatment contract goals

1. Decrease behaviors that indicate to others that you are in pain such as slow walking, reclining, complaining, and using medications.
2. Formulate a plan for returning to work by the tenth day of the program.
3. Progressively increase time sitting until in the third week you are able to sit for 60 minutes.
4. Lift and carry 20 lbs as necessary for grocery shopping by the third week.
5. Walk for 60 minutes by the fourth week.
6. Increase trunk and hip flexibility to normal ranges by the sixth week.
7. Increase trunk and leg strength to normal by the sixth week.
8. Increase aerobic capacity.

Treatment

1. The patient is educated on pacing and the use of heat and cold after exercise and sitting and self-massage for neck and shoulder pain.

2. The patient is instructed in a home stretching program for gastrocnemius, hamstrings, rectus femoris, hip flexors, and back extensors; a quota-based strengthening program for the gluteals, abdominals, and back extensors; a quota-based program to improve sitting tolerance to 6 hours per day; and a walking program with a goal of 60 minutes of walking by the third week.
3. Exercises in physical therapy include review of the home program, squatting with hand-held weights, abdominal exercises, multifidus exercise, latissimus dorsi exercise with pulleys, and ball exercises.
4. Biking is used to increase aerobic capacity.

By the end of the second week, the patient is able to walk for 30 minutes and sit long enough to watch a movie or eat a meal. He feels he is unable to increase his sitting tolerance in a straight-backed chair beyond 30 minutes as this consistently increases his pain. Ergonomics are discussed. The patient finds a recliner that does not increase his pain and allows him to perform his work duties. By the fourth week he is able to walk 60 minutes per day without his cane. At the sixth week, he is able to sit enough to work for a day without an undue increase in pain. His back ROM improves to 80% in all directions and his hip ROM is within normal limits. Trunk and extremity strength improve to within normal limits. He is independent in his home exercise and decides to engage in a swimming program to further increase his aerobic capacity, strength, and endurance. He is off his diuretic patch and not taking any pain medications. At 6-month follow-up, he is working full-time and swimming three times a week.

Fibromyalgia

Fibromyalgia is characterized by widespread pain in all four quadrants. The cause and pathophysiology of fibromyalgia are unknown, although changes in central pain modulation due to an aberrant serotonin metabolism, nociceptive sensitization secondary to a disturbed microcirculation, and central sensitization (Henriksson 1994) have all been hypothesized as possible causes (Figure 7.1). Diagnosis follows specific criteria: 11 or more tender points at 18 possible sites, defined by palpation at approximately 4 kg with the thumb pulp over the following nine paired locations (Wolfe et al. 1990):

1. 2 cm below lateral epicondyle of the elbow
2. Insertion of nuchal muscle into the occiput
3. Intertransverse ligaments of C5–C7
4. Upper border of the trapezius
5. Supraspinatus, medial aspect, just above the scapular spine
6. Pectoralis, over upper border of second rib about 2 cm from sternum
7. Upper gluteal area, just below iliac crest in outer quadrant
8. Insertion of muscle into greater trochanter
9. Medial condyle of femur, about 2 cm above joint line on the anterolateral aspect of the bone

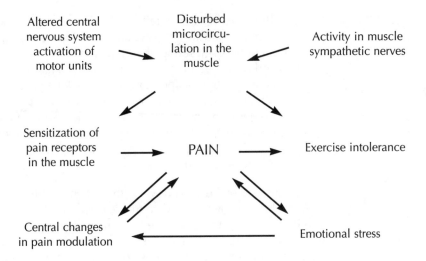

FIGURE 7.1
A model for the pathogenesis of pain and exercise intolerance in fibromyalgia. (Redrawn with permission from S Mense. Fibromyalgia. Can J Physiol Pharmacol 1991;69:676.)

McCain (1986) evaluated aerobic fitness in a group of women with fibromyalgia and found that 84% had below average physical fitness levels based on their maximum oxygen uptake. He concluded that fibromyalgia patients are commonly aerobically unfit and that deconditioning may contribute to symptomatology. McCain (1988a, 1988b) found that aerobic exercise was effective in reducing perceived pain and improving psychological profiles.

Case Example

The patient is a 48-year-old female complaining of pain all over her body. She fell in the parking lot at her workplace 3 years ago and injured her back. X-rays and magnetic resonance imaging were negative at the time of injury. She reports that the pain "spread" to her entire body in the subsequent 2 years and that she was diagnosed with fibromyalgia last year. She also complains of fatigue. She receives workers' compensation and has secondary litigation pending against the owners of the parking lot.

The patient has been diagnosed with irritable bowel syndrome and chronic fatigue syndrome.

Pain She rates her average pain as eight on a 10-point scale. At best, her pain is an eight and, at worst, a 10. Her pain is made unbearable by all physical activities and decreased only by medication.

Function The patient has not worked since her injury. Until 6 months ago, she was performing some housework and occasional grocery shopping. For the past 6 months, she has been bedridden. Her husband dresses her for appointments with health care providers. She showers every third or fourth day with help from her husband. Her husband performs all the housework, grocery shopping, and meal preparation and works full-time.

Multidimensional Pain Inventory Profile   The patient is classified as dysfunctional.

Physical examination   The patient asks to lie down during the interview due to her pain. She is transferred with her husband's help from her wheelchair to a table. She stays in a fetal position during her interview. When asked to sit up, she does so with great difficulty. Examination is conducted with the patient seated. Posture is remarkable for slumped sitting with forward head, thoracic kyphosis, and forward flexed trunk.

ROM of both shoulders is limited to 80 degrees of flexion and abduction. ROM of the elbows, wrists, ankles, and knees is within functional limits. Neck ROM is 50% in all directions. She reports that all these movements cause pain. Assessment of strength of both lower and upper extremities is not possible due to patient's complaint of pain with all muscle contractions. Sensation and reflexes are normal.

Aerobic fitness   This could not be assessed.

Pain behaviors   The patient exhibits severe verbal and nonverbal pain behaviors, including sitting in a wheelchair, lying down during the interview, lack of cooperation with physical assessment, moaning, sighing, grimacing, and narcotic dependence.

Patient goals   To decrease pain and be able to play with her grandchild.

Assessment   The patient's impairments include pain and associated symptoms; loss of general strength and endurance; loss of shoulder, neck, and hip ROM; fatigue; and activity intolerance.

Plan   The patient will participate in a functional restoration program, behavioral medicine group and individual treatment, and will develop treatment and medication contracts.

A treatment contract with functional goals is established. After a very lengthy discussion, however, she refuses to sign her medication contract that is designed to decelerate her narcotics use after the second week of the program. She is asked to reconsider and return in 1 week if she changes her mind. The patient refuses because she feels she cannot survive without her medication. The team refers her to her primary physician for medication management. Treatment is delayed until this issue is resolved.

Case Example

The patient is a 26-year-old male complaining of fatigue, nausea, dizziness, and headaches. He sustained a whiplash injury from a motor vehicle accident 6 years ago. The patient was wearing a seatbelt and did not lose consciousness. He reported feeling some soreness immediately and that he was taken to a local emergency room. X-rays were negative for fracture or dislocation of cervical spine. He was sent home with muscle relaxants and was told to follow up with his primary care physician. He reported a gradually increasing frequency and severity of headaches with nausea and dizziness over the next 6 months that required him to drop out of college and return to live with his mother. Medical management of his headaches included muscle relaxants and narcotics.

The patient began to complain of increasing fatigue, loss of concentration, and diffuse soreness approximately 4 years ago. Tests for Epstein-Barr, Lyme disease, hepatitis, or other infectious disease were negative. The patient was eventually diagnosed with fibromyalgia with chronic fatigue and headaches.

Pain   Patient rates current pain as seven on a 10-point scale. He rates it five at best and 10 at worst. Pain is described as a diffuse, deep, throbbing ache of the shoulders, back, hips, and knees. His fatigue is described as "numbing" and "wearing." His headache is sharp, stabbing pain over both temples and the back of the head. The pain follows no temporal pattern. Increased headache severity is accompanied by nausea and dizziness. The headaches occur 1–2 times per week for 2–12 hours. His muscle ache is constant, with significant flare-up accompanied by fatigue.

Pain worsens with activity, damp weather, and trying to read or concentrate. It is relieved by rest and medication.

Function   The patient has not worked or studied in the past 5½ years. On good days, he is in bed 12–15 hours; on bad days, he is in bed all day. He gets out of the house only for medical appointments and depends on his mother for transportation, meals, and laundry. He is able to sit for 30 minutes, stand for 5 minutes, and walk one block with shortness of breath.

Multidimensional Pain Inventory Profile   The patient is classified as dysfunctional.

Physical examination   The patient displays forward head posture with significantly increased thoracic kyphosis with loss of all other spinal curves and left shoulder girdle elevated. He has pain on palpation of suboccipital muscles, upper and middle trapezius regions, shoulders, chest wall, paraspinals, and bilateral piriformis at the sciatic notch. He has decreased muscle tone and atrophy of the shoulder girdle and paraspinals and tightness of the pectoralis and latissimus dorsi. Cervical spine ROM is limited to 50% with pain.

Aerobic fitness   The patient's aerobic capacity is poor for his age group.

Pain behaviors   The patient exhibits marked verbal and nonverbal pain behaviors, with rubbing, sighing, moaning, and frequent position changes.

Patient goals   To live independently, have no pain, and have more energy.

Assessment   The patient has chronic pain syndrome. Impairments include postural abnormality, decreased neck ROM, decreased muscle strength and endurance, and activity intolerance due to perceived pain and deconditioning.

Plan   Physical therapy sessions will be conducted twice a week for 10 weeks focusing on a self-management and a graded functional restoration approach incorporating education, exercise, and pain control.

Treatment contract goals   The patient will be able to tolerate being up and somewhat active for 8 hours a day. He will learn independent use of pain control modalities and follow a structured, independent, daily home exercise program.

Treatment

1. The patient is taught pain control modalities including ice massage and self-massage.
2. The patient is given a structured, quota-based exercise program beginning with five repetitions of chin tucks, shoulder squeezes, shoulder shrugs, diagonals, and sitting pelvic tilts. The patient is instructed to increase by one repetition every 3 days until he is able to perform 10 repetitions twice a day.
3. A mirror for cuing is used to improve the patient's posture.
4. Patient's limited cervical ROM is improved with diagonals, head and neck movements, and contraction and relaxation techniques in the supine position.
5. Strengthening exercises are added in the fourth week, including a rubber band exercise program for upper quadrant musculature.
6. Flexibility is addressed within the home exercise program. Stretches for the pectoralis, upper trapezius, and levator scapulae are added.
7. Aerobic fitness is increased with an ergometer and treadmill program.

After three sessions, the patient experiences a significant pain flare-up and cancels appointments for several weeks. When the patient returns to therapy, the program is reinstated. Patient's progress is slow due to multiple complaints and extreme somatic focus. He requires frequent redirection within and between sessions. After 6 weeks of therapy, the patient remains somatically focused but is showing some improvement in pain and independent program compliance. He makes a transition to conditioning and stretching groups for his last 4 weeks of therapy. At the end of treatment, all goals are met, with the exception of tolerating 8 hours of active time per day. He remains inconsistent with this due to his excessive somatic focus. It is recommended that the patient seek behavioral medicine treatment for his excessive somatic focus.

Neuropathic Pain

Damage to a peripheral nerve results in profound changes in nociceptive input and transmission. The normal pathways for pain sensation and perception no longer function normally, resulting in abnormal peripheral discharges and consequent central nervous system alterations. The alterations due to peripheral nerve lesions makes it extremely challenging to appropriately intervene. The pain experienced in these cases is called *neuropathic pain.*

Severance or crush injury to peripheral nerve can cause the cessation of all input from that part of the periphery to the dorsal horn. This is called *deafferentation* and results in the spontaneous firing of dorsal horn neurons (Davar and Maciewicz 1989). The frequency of these spontaneous firings increase. Dorsal horn transmission interneurons have been found to be firing almost continuously 3 weeks after an injury (Loeser and Ward 1967), apparently due to the loss of inhibitory input from the periphery. Peripheral mechanoreceptor discharge from damaged nerve endings may drive hyperexcitable central pain signaling neurons found in the dorsal horn (Roberts 1986). One approach to treatment, therefore, is the restoration of inhibitory afferent input to the dorsal horn by artificial stimulation techniques. Electrical stimulation such as TENS may be used to provide peripheral input along nerve pathways that are intact. Alternative forms of stimulation such as light touch (massage), proprioception, vibration, or heat may also be considered.

The pain of neuralgia is described as constant, searing, and burning, with accompanying allodynia. There may be occasional shooting pain as well. These sensations are typical of deafferentation hyperexcitability and central nervous system sensitization due to spinal neurons engaging in ectopic spontaneous firing. These wide-dynamic range interneurons in the dorsal horn now recognize all stimuli as nociceptive when sensitized (Kramis et al. 1996). TENS can be especially appropriate in these cases because the stimulus can be selected to stimulate only A beta myelinated fibers using the appropriate strength-duration curves for those fibers and avoid the stimulation of C and A delta fibers. This approach is based on the notion that TENS treatment can restore the usual inhibitory influence to the dorsal horn of these A beta fiber inputs. Postoperative incision–site neuralgias respond especially well to TENS. Massage or heat may be impossible because touching the affected part is not tolerated due to the allodynia created by sensitization of interneurons.

Patients often prefer to wear tight clothing to prevent the summation of stimuli from increasing their already significant pain. Patients with hyperalgesia or allodynia may be helped by protecting the painful area from this summation by wearing elastic stockings, gloves, or even tape. Creams that numb the area (e.g., lidocaine or capsaicin) may be helpful as well.

The patient with phantom limb pain is truly a challenge. Phantom limb pain is due to pain memory, usually from a preamputation painful extremity. Amputation obviously removes all peripheral afferent input from the missing body parts, but the dorsal horn cells and others higher in the central nervous system fire spontaneously to produce a perception of pain in the same pathway where once there was a volley of pain input. Restoration of peripheral afferent input to the dorsal horn with stump stimulation procedures is the treatment most often attempted. Desensitization of stump tissues can be done with massage, tapping, fluidotherapy, touch, and pressure. TENS is also an obvious option. Stump wrapping and wearing of the prosthesis will also obviously help to restore afferent stimulation and promote functional use of the limb.

Painful neuromas can occur after amputation or other causes of transected nerves. Sprouts of regenerating afferents of all sizes begin to discharge spontaneously. Neuromas are also likely to be found in nerve entrapment injuries (e.g., carpal tunnel syndrome and nerve stretch or crush injuries). These sprouting neurons in neuromas are abnormally sensitive to all mechanical, sympathetic, and thermal stimuli and to chemical nociceptive substances. They can frequently become sensitive to sympathetic stimulation due to the acquisition of adrenergic receptors on the sprouting neurons. (Sato and Perl 1991). When this occurs, sympathetically maintained pain may result. Causalgia and reflex sympathetic dystrophy (now known as complex regional pain syndrome [CRPS]) are two clinical entities described within the number of sympathetically maintained pain syndromes.

In the acute phase of sympathetically maintained pain (CRPS with sympathetic involvement), the initial injury that precipitates the condition is usually quite trivial and often does not involve nerve damage (Schwartzman 1993). For this reason, it may be ignored by health care providers or treated with icing, taping, protective covering, or casting, depending on whether it involves fracture, soft-tissue damage, hematoma, or inflammation. As the tissues begin to heal, the patient continues to protect the injured body part by nonuse and splinting. The pain of the acute injury is altered by time and becomes characterized by exquisite sensitivity to touch. Patients refuse to use their body part, since any light touch stimulus causes dramatic pain. A hand or a foot held in a protective posture and not used will exhibit shortened muscles and tendons and weakening of these functional units.

CRPS appears initially as discoloration, trophic changes with shiny skin surface, and growth of hair on extensor surfaces. In stage I, the acute phase, the pain and hyperalgesia is localized to a peripheral nerve distribution or body segment. The skin is dry, red, and warm. Within approximately 3 months it becomes cold, cyanotic, and sweaty. There is usually some local edema and muscle spasm. In stage II, muscles atrophy, and there is x-ray evidence of osteopenia. Pain is described as diffuse, deep, and is usually felt in a distal extremity rather than being localized to a single nerve. Movement, anxiety, and distress make pain worse. Stage III, the atrophic stage, involves severe contractures and osteoporosis. There may be edema, hypothermia, and increased hair growth with thickened nails. Muscle spasm, fixed joint limitations and subluxations, and even pathologic fractures are characteristic. As the problem progresses, the pain spreads, leading to hyperalgesia, allodynia, and hyperpathia in a wider, more generalized pattern. At this stage of illness a movement disorder is usually seen, characterized by difficulty initiating movement, weakness, tremor, spasms, dystonia, and increased reflexes. Fascia become thickened, and atrophy of muscle, cartilage, and soft tissue becomes evident (Raja and Hendler 1990).

The earlier the diagnosis and intervention, the more likely the success. Early physical therapy treatment often involves desensitization techniques such as tapping, stroking, and massaging the skin of the affected area. Patients wear gloves or socks with rough inside surfaces to become habituated to the sensory input. Simple functional activities must be initiated as soon as possible. Using functional activities with loaded joints may help patients with CRPS to overcome the painful condition. Additional functional progress must be stressed in order to correct imbalance of muscle, improper use of muscle, and to restore normal muscle length and postural alignment.

In chronic CRPS, the patient becomes much more dysfunctional, and it is more difficult to reverse the pain and restore function. Serial sympathetic ganglionic blocks and physical therapy treatment to restore function have been effective. In patients who have intractable pain and experience no relief with medication or blocks, physical therapy should attempt to decrease the sympathetic nervous system's activity with relaxation techniques such as Jacobson's progressive relaxation, imagery, meditation techniques, tai chi, gentle rocking on a Swiss ball or in a rocking chair, deep diaphragmatic breathing, and massage. Biofeedback, hypnosis, acupuncture, stress management, behavioral modification, and TENS can also be helpful.

There are additional clinical examples of neurogenic pain disorders that may need physical therapy treatment, including spinal cord injury; vascular accidents affecting thalamic nuclei and parietal cortex; and peripheral neuropathies due to diabetes mellitus, alcohol, and other neurotoxins. Findings on pathophysiologic mechanisms suggest new pharmacologic interventions and stimulation techniques that may prove more effective than previously available treatments.

Case Example

The patient is a 25-year-old male complaining of severe left foot pain and sensitivity. His leg was initially injured at work when a tree rolled onto it. This resulted in an unstable, comminuted, closed fracture of the left distal tibia and fibula. He underwent a closed reduction that day and had surgery 2 days later for placement of an intermedullary nail in the left tibia. He was hospitalized for 1 week and discharged with instructions to not bear weight on the injured extremity. He began physical therapy 1 month later for progressive gait training, ROM improvement, and exercise. After five visits, he was able to bear normal weight on the leg without an assistive device. His doctor approved his return to light-duty work approximately 2½ months after the injury. He was informed that light-duty work was unavailable. He continued his rehabilitation for an additional 17 visits with a progressive increase in complaints of left lower leg, ankle, and knee pain. His gait became increasingly antalgic. His frustration and anger increased, and he was discharged to pursue a home exercise program because no signs of progress were evident.

X-rays indicated incomplete union and he had an autogenous bone graft about 7 months after the injury. Physician follow-ups over 3 weeks revealed decreased sensation of the foot; decreased active movement of the toes; and complaints of difficulty sleeping, ankle swelling, and donor site inflammation.

He is referred again to physical therapy 1 month after the bone graft.

Pain Patient experiences marked hyperalgesia with palpation of the foot and first toe. Pain is severe and rated by the patient as nine on a 10-point scale and 10 when touched.

Function The patient is living with his father and has not worked since his injury. He is unable to perform his previous activities, such as hunting, fishing, and hiking, and is unable to walk any distance except with crutches. He is nonweight-bearing on his left leg and unable to tolerate a sock or shoe on the left foot. He has difficulty carrying things due to his crutches. The patient is unable to sit for more than 15 minutes and needs to keep his leg elevated. His social life is much decreased.

Multidimensional Pain Inventory Profile   The patient is classified as dysfunctional.

Physical examination   He has minimal edema of the left foot, limited active ankle ranges, and generalized decreased strength of the ankle. With light touch and palpation he has significant hyperalgesia and allodynia of dorsal, lateral, medial and the entire plantar surfaces of the foot. Surgical scar is healed but very sensitive.

Aerobic fitness   The patient's aerobic fitness is moderate for his age group.

Pain behaviors   The patient exhibits extreme muscle guarding and grimacing.

Patient goals   To decrease his pain and to be able to walk again without crutches.

Assessment   The patient is a thin, pale man with chronic neuropathic pain and sympathetic nervous system signs of dysfunction. Impairments include loss of muscle strength, shortening of muscle, and tight joint structures in the foot with loss of ROM. The patient exhibits fear of touch and movement with consequent activity intolerance.

Plan   Treatment will focus on increasing weightbearing, decreasing sensitivity of the foot and toes, improving active ROM in the foot, and strengthening the ankle and foot muscles. A functional restoration session will be attended three times a week for 8 weeks. The patient will make a treatment contract and participate in a behavioral medicine group and individual treatment.

Treatment contract goals

1. Decrease behaviors that communicate to others that you are in pain such as not wearing a sock and shoe, not placing foot on ground, guarding, and grimacing.
2. Formulate a plan for returning to work and talk to your employer.
3. Learn self-desensitization through massage, tapping, and use of textured fabrics.
4. Perform closed-chain activities such as stepping on scale or balance board.
5. Bear weight on compliant surfaces while sitting or standing.
6. Lift 80 lbs from the floor to your chest for 20 repetitions.
7. Walk for 30 minutes.
8. Bike for 30 minutes.

Treatment

1. Education includes self-management of pain, desensitization with self-massage using tennis balls or textured substances, and information on pacing.
2. Instruction is given in foot stretching exercises and a walking program.
3. The patient lifts weights and rides a bicycle for general reconditioning using proper lifting techniques and full weightbearing on both feet.

All physical therapy goals are met by the eighth week.

References

Andersson G, Bogduk N, DeLuca CJ, et al. Muscle. In JW Frymoyer, SL Gordon (eds), New Perspectives on Low Back Pain. Park Ridge, IL: American Academy of Orthopedic Surgeons 1989;14.

Ashton-Miller JA, McGlashen KM, Herzenberg JE, Stohler CS. Cervical muscle myoelectric response to acute experimental sternocleidomastoid pain. Spine 1990;15:1006.

Astrand P-O, Rodahl K. Neuromuscular Function. In P-O Astrand, K Rodahl (eds), Textbook of Work Physiology. Physiological Bases of Exercise (3rd ed). New York: McGraw-Hill, 1986;117.

Bearn JG. An electromyographic study of the trapezius, deltoid, pectoralis major, biceps and triceps muscles during static loading of the upper arm. Anat Rec 1961;140.

Berg H, Berggren G, Tesch P. Dynamic neck strength training effect on pain and function. Arch Phys Med Rehabil 1994;75:661.

Bogduk N. Cervical Causes of Headache and Dizziness. In G Grieve (ed), Modern Manual Therapy of the Vertebral Column. Edinburgh: Churchill Livingstone, 1986.

Corrigan B, Maitland GD. Practical Orthopedic Medicine. London: Butterworths, 1983.

Davar G, Maciewicz RJ. Deafferentation pain syndromes. Neurol Clin 1989;7:289.

De Freitas V, Vitti M, Furlani J. Electromyographic analysis of the levator scapulae and rhomboideus major muscles in movements of the upper limb. Anatomischer Anzeiger 1980;148:337.

Evjenth O, Hamberg J. Muscle Stretching in Manual Therapy, A Clinical Manual (Vols I & II). Sweden: Alfta Rehabil, 1984.

Frank C, Akesow WH, Woo SL-Y, et al. Physiology and therapeutic value of passive joint motion. Clin Orthop 1984;185:113.

Harkapaa K, Jarvikoski A, Mellin G, et al. Health locus of control beliefs and psychological distress as predictors of treatment outcome in low back pain patients: results of a three month follow-up of a controlled intervention study. Pain 1991;46:3.

Harms-Ringdahl K. On assessment of shoulder exercise and load elicited pain in the cervical spine. Biomechanical analysis of load-EMG-methodological studies of pain provoked by extreme position. Scand J Rehabil Med 1986;14(suppl):1.

Henriksson KG. Have new aspects on referral of muscle pain and on hyperalgia any bearing on the pathogenesis of chronic widespread muscle pain and tenderness? Am Pain Soc J 1994;3:13.

Hertling D, Kessler RM. Management of Common Musculoskeletal Disorders: Physical Therapy Principles and Methods (2nd ed). Philadelphia: Lippincott, 1990.

Highland TR, Dreisinger TE, Vie LL, Russell GS. Changes in isometric strength and range of motion of the isolated cervical spine after eight weeks of clinical rehabilitation. Spine 1992;17:S77.

Inman VT, Saunders JBDe CM, Abbott LeRC. Observations on the function of the shoulder joint. J Bone Joint Surg 1944;26:218.

International Headache Society. The Classification and Diagnostic Criteria for Headache Disorders, Cranial Neuralgias, and Facial Pain. Toyen, Norway: Norwegian University Press, 1988.

Janda V. Muscle Weakness and Inhibition (Pseudoparesis) in Back Pain Syndromes. In G Grieve (ed), Modern Manual Therapy of the Vertebral Column. Edinburgh: Churchill Livingstone, 1986a;197.

Janda V. Aspects of extracranial causes of facial pain. J Prosthet Dent 1986b;56:484.

Janda V. Muscles and Cervicogenic Pain Syndromes. In R Grant (ed), Clinics in Physical Therapy. Physical Therapy of the Cervical and Thoracic Spine. New York: Churchill Livingstone, 1988;153.

Johnson MA, Polgar J, Weightman D, Appleton D. Data on the distribution of fiber types in thirty-six human muscles. J Neurol Sci 1973;19:111.

Jonsson B. Measurement and evaluation of local muscular strain in the shoulder during constrained work. J Hum Ergol 1982;11:73.

Jorgensen K, Nicolaisen T. Trunk extensor endurance: determination and relation to low back trouble. Ergonomics 1987;30:259.

Kalimo H, Rantanen J, Viljanen T, Einola S. Lumbar muscles: structure and function. Ann Med 1989;21:353.

Kendall FP, McCreary EK, Provance PG. Muscles: Testing and Function (4th ed). Baltimore: Williams & Wilkins, 1993.

Kramis RC, Roberts WJ, Gillette RG. Post-sympathectomy neuralgia: hypotheses on peripheral and central neuronal mechanisms. Pain 1996;64:1.

Lance JW. Mechanism and Management of Headache (5th ed). London: Butterworth-Heinemann, 1993.

Larsson SE, Bengtsson A, Bodegard L, et al. Muscle changes in work-related chronic myalgia. Acta Orthop Scand 1988;59:552.

Larsson SE, Bodegard L, Henriksson KG, Oberg PA. Chronic trapezius myalgia. Morphology and blood flow studied in 17 patients. Acta Orthop Scand 1990;61:394.

Liemohn W. Exercise and the back. Rheum Dis Clin North Am 1990;16:945.

Loeser JD, Ward AA. Some effects of deafferentation on neurons of the cat spinal cord. Arch Neurol 1967;17:629.

Mattila M, Hurme M, Aleranta H, et al. The multifidus muscle in patients with lumbar disc herniation. A histochemical and morphometric analysis of intraoperative biopsies. Spine 1986;11:732.

McCain GA. Role of physical fitness training in the fibrositis/fibromyalgia syndrome. Am J Med 1986;81:73.

McCain GA. A controlled study of the effects of a supervised cardiovascular training program on the manifestations of primary fibromyalgia. Arthritis Rheum 1988a;31:1135.

McCain GA, Bell DA, Mai FM, Halliday PD. A controlled study of the effects of a supervised cardiovascular fitness training on the manifestations of primary fibromyalgia. Arthritis Rheum 1988b;31:1135.

Mumenthaler M. Headache and Facial Pain. In M Mumenthaler (ed), Neurology (3rd ed). New York: Thieme, 1990;440.

Nicolaisen T, Jorgensen K. Trunk strength, back muscle endurance and low-back trouble. Scand J Rehabil Med 1985;17:121.

Raja SN, Hendler N. Sympathetically Maintained Pain. In M Rogers (ed),

Current Practice in Anesthesiology. St. Louis: Mosby–Year Book, 1990;421.

Raspe HH, Kohlmann T. The current backache epidemic. Ther Umsch 1994;51:367.

Roberts WJ. A hypothesis on the physiological basis for causalgia and related pains. Pain 1986;24:297.

Rodgers SH. Job evaluation in worker fitness determination. Occup Med 1988;3:219.

Rossi U. Cervical nonradicular pain syndromes. Int J Pain Ther 1994;4:63.

Roy SH, DeLuca CJ, Casavant DA. Lumbar muscle fatigue and chronic lower back pain. Spine 1989;14:992.

Saal J, Saal J. Nonoperative treatment of herniated lumbar intervertebral disc with radiculopathy. An outcome study. Spine 1989;14:431.

Sato J, Perl ER. Adrenergic excitation of cutaneous pain receptors induced by peripheral nerve injury. Science 1991;251:1608.

Schuldt K. On neck muscle activity and load reduction in sitt⁻ ʒ postures. An electromyographic and biomechanical study with applicat.⌐.ıs in ergonomics and rehabilitation. Scand J Rehabil Med 1988;19(suppl):1.

Schwartzman RJ. Reflex sympathetic dystrophy. Curr Opin Neurol Neurosurg 1993;6:531.

Snijders CJ. Biomechanische modellen van neck and rug klachten. De Ingenieur 1994;18:16.

Svensson H, Vedin A, Wilhelmsson C, Andersson G. Low back pain in relation to other diseases and cardiovascular risk factors. Spine 1983;8:277.

Sweeney T, Prentice C, Saal J, Saal J. Cervicothoracic stabilization techniques. Phys Med Rehabil 1990;4:335.

Tan JC, Nordin M. Role of physical therapy in the treatment of cervical disk disease. Orthop Clin North Am 1992;23:435.

Travell JG, Simons DG. Myofascial Pain and Dysfunction: The Trigger Point Manual (Vol 2). Baltimore: Williams & Wilkins, 1992.

Twomey L. A rationale for the treatment of back pain and joint pain by manual therapy. Phys Ther 1992;72:12.

Waddell G. Biopsychosocial analysis of low back pain. Ballieres Clin Rheumatol 1992;6:523.

Wolfe F, Smythe HA, Yunus MB, et al. The American College of Rheumatology 1990 criteria for the classification of fibromyalgia: report of the Multicenter Criteria Committee. Arthritis Rheum 1990;33:160.

Zhu XZ, Parnnianpour M, Nordin M, Kahanovitz N. Histochemistry and morphology of erector spinae muscle in lumbar disc herniation. Spine 1989;14:391.

8   Documentation

Lisa Janice Cohen

Documentation is used to record the course of care, ensure reimbursement, and mark changes in patient status and outcome. Ideally, documentation should provide the therapist with a framework for reassessment and treatment planning. Unfortunately, documentation is too often seen as a necessary evil completed only for the purpose of reimbursement, legal protection, or compliance with facility policy. Much physical therapy documentation is poorly written, with little standardization or logical structure. Standardization and structure, however, are especially important in documenting the care and progress of patients with chronic pain.

Documentation is a process that should begin with the initial assessment. Documentation of the assessment includes goal setting, objective data collection, and program planning. Ongoing documentation, or reassessment, clarifies the patient's reaction to treatment, the patient's status between sessions, clinical assessment of progress, and program modifications. Despite wide variations in documentation styles, the thought process underlying the documentation process should be consistent.

Documentation of Initial Assessment

The evaluation process follows a basic structure that is independent of both the patient's specific diagnosis and the format of the evaluation (narrative versus preprinted form). Therefore, the process of documenting the evaluation of a patient with chronic pain does not substantially differ from that of documenting the evaluation of a patient with a spinal cord injury or myocardial infarction. The Hypothesis-Oriented Algorithm for Clinicians (HOAC) by Rothstein and Echternach (1987) provides an excellent framework for the evaluation process. The HOAC outlines a rational, scientific process of hypothesis generation, testing, and reassessment. It attempts to codify the thought process behind physical therapy management, including initial evaluation, treatment, and reevaluation.

1. Initial data
    Chart review
        • Patient is a 72-year-old married female.
        • She has a 60-year history of headaches.
        • She presents with the following complaints:
            – Daily headache
            – Right upper and lower extremity pain
            – Right neck and upper back pain
        • Medical workup revealed:
            – Migraine and tension-type headaches
            – Chronic pain syndrome
            – Moderate degenerative changes in the spine
            – No neurologic signs or symptoms
    Patient interview
        • Her life is totally disrupted because of her pain.
        • She is dependent on her husband for care.
        • She has managed her pain with narcotics for 10 years.
        • She has had physical therapy treatment limited to use of
          modalities, which did not change her pain.
2. Problem statement
    Pain limits this patient's function.
3. Initial functional goals
    "I want to go shopping"
    "I want to cook supper for my husband"

The clinician using the HOAC begins by (1) collecting initial data through chart review and the patient interview, (2) generating a problem statement based on the patient's chief complaint and initial data, and (3) establishing functional goals with input from the patient.

The initial steps when using the HOAC with a patient with chronic pain are illustrated in Figure 8.1.

Functional Problems and Goals

The HOAC directs the clinician to obtain the patient's functional goals before the physical examination. These goals, based on the patient's perception of problems in performing life tasks, direct the therapist's choice of evaluative tools. Although this may seem backward to the clinician accustomed to performing data collection before setting goals, this process ensures a closer match between the patient's expectations and the therapist's goals.

Problems can be separated into two components: functional problems and contributing factors. The functional problems come from the patient before data collection is complete. Contributing factors emerge from physical therapy assessment of the data collected: signs, symptoms, and function.

The following questions should be asked during the initial interview to establish what the patient's functional problems are. The questions attempt to elicit specific functional problems from patients, such as "I can't work," "I can't take care of my children," and "It's difficult to go shopping."

- What are you unable to do now that you were able to do before your pain?
- What do you want to be able to do better a month from now?
- In what areas of your life does your pain interfere?

Once the patient has discussed his or her functional problems, the therapist should ask the patient about goals:

- How will you know you are better?
- What will you be able to do when you are better?
- What would you be able to do if your pain bothered you less?

The specific wording of these questions should convey to the patient that the primary treatment focus is on function rather than pain relief. If a patient cannot think of a single functional goal despite assistance from the therapist, an essential mismatch may exist between treatment philosophy and patient expectations. If this is the case, treatment based on the functional restoration paradigm will be unsuccessful, and the therapist should consider referring the patient to other types of treatment.

Ideally, the patient's functional goals will be a restatement of his or her functional problems ("I want to return to work," "I want to be able to care for my children," "I want to go grocery shopping"). The patient can then be asked to measure his or her subjective ability to do a specific functional task related to those goals on a Visual Analogue Scale:

Totally unable   Completely able

Take care of my children

Objective Data Collection and Analysis

After the physical therapist establishes functional goals, the HOAC continues with data collection and analysis. The therapist is instructed to (1) perform evaluation/data collection, (2) generate a working hypothesis, and (3) modify goals if appropriate.

Data Collection
For the patient introduced in Figure 8.1, the physical assessment findings include the following:

- Painfully limited active cervical range of motion (ROM)
- Asymmetric posture with forward head, prominent C7, excessive thoracic kyphosis, high and forward right shoulder, abducted right scapula, and posterior pelvic tilt with loss of lumbar lordosis
- Decreased mobility in right scapular region
- Pain on palpation of suboccipital muscles
- Increased density and bogginess of suboccipital muscles

- Decreased upper extremity strength
- Significant deconditioning (Patient ambulates 500 ft in 6 minutes with four rests and significant pulse increase.)

Hypothesis Generation

After the data collection, a working hypothesis is generated about the patient's pain and its effect on his or her ability to function. For the patient introduced in Figure 8.1, her inability to manage her pain and her long history of inactivity and disuse have made her unable to function in her roles as wife and homemaker. If no reasonable hypothesis can be made relating objective data to function, the therapist must consider discharge from physical therapy and referral elsewhere for treatment.

Goal Modification

The physical assessment may indicate a need to modify the original goals or add new ones. In this case, two goals have been added. First, the patient will be independent in using pain control modalities before functional activities. Second, the patient will be able to ambulate approximately ½ mile (2,500 ft) in 15 minutes with improved cardiovascular response.

An understanding of the terms *functional goals* and *contributing factors* is important for assessing the efficacy of treatment and the accuracy of the working hypothesis. A functional goal refers to a specific task, such as shopping. Contributing factors are the aspects of the patient's condition that make it difficult or impossible to perform the specific task that is now the patient's functional goal. For example, weak quadriceps and ankle dorsiflexors, poor endurance and balance, and the inability to lift 5 lb or walk more than 100 ft are all factors that contribute to the patient's inability to shop. If the clinician addresses these factors and the patient is still unable to shop, the therapist must reassess the hypothesis and look for other factors that may contribute to this inability (Table 8.1).

Program Plan

As part of the HOAC, the therapist must also develop an overall program plan that includes (1) establishing a time frame for reevaluation, (2) developing a treatment philosophy based on the working hypothesis, and (3) determining the specifics of a treatment strategy and plan.

A treatment philosophy based on the working hypothesis for the patient described in this chapter should make a positive statement about how the patient can achieve her goals. For example, "pain control strategies and gentle graded conditioning and activity tolerance training will enable this patient to improve her function," is a simple but inclusive statement of the treatment philosophy. For this patient, treatment strategies include instructing the patient in pain control modalities, proper posture, and body mechanics and increasing aerobic endurance, spinal flexibility, strength, and activity tolerance.

The treatment plan for the patient discussed in this chapter includes instruction in assisted- and self-massage techniques and independent use of superficial heat and cold for pain relief. The patient is also assigned an indi-

TABLE 8.1   Problems, contributing factors, and goals in pain rehabilitation

Functional problem	Functional goal
Patient is unable to grocery shop.	Patient will tolerate grocery shopping including pushing a cart, lifting light (<5 lbs) objects from a shelf, and walking for 30 minutes.
Patient is unable to tolerate 8 hours of active "up time" per day.	Patient will tolerate 8 hours of active "up time" per day.
Pain limits this patient's ability to perform household activities, such as cook a meal, wash dishes, or make a bed.	Patient will be able to perform household activities without being limited by pain.

Contributing factors	Goal
Patient is dependent in the use of PCMs.	Patient will independently use PCMs to decrease pain.
Ambulation is limited to 200 ft in 6 minutes with an abnormal hemodynamic response.	Patient will ambulate 1,000 ft in 6 minutes with an appropriate hemodynamic response.
Significant gait deviations (i.e., unequal stance time, decreased left push-off, Trendelenburg-type left gait, and absent trunk rotation and arm swing).	Patient will ambulate with increased symmetry and without gait deviations.
Patient lacks an independent exercise program.	Patient will be independent in performing a quota-based exercise program.
Patient demonstrates poor body mechanics in all activities.	Patient will demonstrate proper body mechanics.

PCM = pain control modality.

vidualized, quota-based exercise program and an aerobic exercise program using a stationary bicycle. She is instructed to practice proper posture and body mechanics for household tasks using visual feedback.

Following the HOAC steps thus far has enabled the clinician to complete a thorough, well-organized, and logical evaluation that completely and concisely documents goals, status, and the treatment plan.

Documentation of Progress

The HOAC continues with a framework for reassessment based on the following series of questions:

- Have the goals of treatment been met?
- If they have not, are the treatment techniques being implemented correctly?
- If they are, are the tactics appropriate for the treatment strategy?
- If so, is the strategy correct?
- If it is, is the hypothesis correct?

The reassessment framework helps the clinician to write progress notes, which are essentially periodic reassessments. Progress notes are generally written on a weekly, biweekly, or monthly basis, depending on insurance regulations, practice setting, and anticipated length of treatment. This periodic note must address whether the goals have been met. If they have, the remainder of the note can address either discharge plans or upgraded goals for further treatment. If the goals have not been met, the therapist must begin to investigate why they have not. The reassessment framework will guide the clinician's investigation.

SOAP Note

The SOAP note is a useful format for the periodic note. The acronym *SOAP* refers to the four parts of the process: (1) gathering *subjective* information, (2) obtaining *objective* data, (3) performing an *assessment*, and (4) formulating a *plan*.

Subjective Information

Any relevant information that the patient, family, or friends tell the clinician is considered subjective information. This includes information about prior level of function, pain intensity, response to treatment, and other factors that might impact treatment. The following statements are examples of subjective information:

- I used to run 3 miles every day.
- I cannot go up or down stairs because of my pain.
- My pain is getting worse and worse.
- After therapy, my pain is so bad that I have to stay in bed the next day.
- I was in a car accident over the weekend.

Subjective information can be written as direct quotes when relevant. These statements may reflect the fact that patients' perceptions of their function may be quite distorted. Information from family or friends should be included regardless of whether it corroborates or contradicts information provided by the patient.

Objective Information

Objective information is measurable or observable factual information recorded without interpretation. The current status of functional problems and contributing factors identified during the initial evaluation are included in this section (e.g., ROM, manual muscle testing, physical tolerance, gait, and balance). If rating scales are used, they must be clear and standard within the profession. Terminology such as *within functional limits* should not be used because it is not well defined. In the absence of definitive measures, statements such as "adequate shoulder range for self-care" or "limited trunk range continues to limit independent transfers" may be used. Treatment rendered is included here as well.

Objective information may be organized in several ways. In a standard SOAP note, the objective section is a freestanding narrative. This allows each reassessment to be read and interpreted as a whole. It can be difficult to follow a patient's progress over time without reading through multiple reevaluation notes, however.

Assessment

The assessment is the clinician's analysis of the subjective and objective components of the evaluation and reevaluation process. The assessment should relate the status of physical findings (contributing factors) to function. It should clearly document whether goals have been met. If goals have not been met, the assessment should address the possible reasons for this. A thorough assessment can justify discharge, continued treatment, or a change in the treatment plan. Items that are typically included in an assessment are patient tolerance of treatment, areas of progress, new goals, areas in which inconsistency between subjective and objective findings exist, clarification of major problems in relation to function, patient's level of cooperation or engagement, and recommendations for further treatment.

An example of an assessment for a patient with chronic headaches follows:

Pt. tolerated first week of treatment well without pain flare. Progress seen in use of PCMs, cervical ROM, and use of home exercise program. No change in pain report, cervical muscle tension, sitting tolerance, or daily activity time; however, significant progress was not expected in these areas. Goals remain appropriate as per initial evaluation. Pt. appears discouraged and is unable to acknowledge her gains. Pt.'s function continues to be limited by daily uncontrolled headaches that appear to be related to decreased cervical ROM and increased muscle tone and guarding. Pt. continues to be cooperative but withdrawn during therapy sessions. Pt. would benefit from continued therapy as per initial evaluation.

Plan

The plan synthesizes all of the information in the SOAP note into a course of action intended to ameliorate the problems identified in the assessment. It is critical to note when a particular plan represents a change from a previous plan of care. Information in this section may include frequency and remaining length of stay, the type of treatment to be rendered, and discharge plans.

The following is an example of a plan for a headache patient:

Continue with outpatient PT BIW x 8 weeks for functional restoration and headache management as per initial evaluation. Treatment focus will include instruction in self-cervical massage and initiation of aerobic conditioning. Plan is unchanged at this time.

Organization

The organization of a SOAP note is as important as its content. Because the note is read by a variety of people and serves many functions, it must be clear and concise. Any abbreviations used must be standard. It can be difficult to gather specific information by reading through a narrative note.

An optimal note, particularly the objective section, is organized so that information is presented in categories with items bulleted. The use of complete sentences is not necessary and may obscure the pertinent data. All information should be relevant to the treatment plan and the patient's function. Problems, goals, objective data, and plans should be stated in specific and measurable terms.

Note writing is a skill that takes thought and practice. In today's fast-paced environment, it may be difficult to set aside the time it takes to become proficient; however, as the prevalence of managed care increases, documentation will become more crucial in justifying care.

Documentation Styles

This section discusses several examples of documentation styles based on the SOAP note format. Different styles are appropriate for different practice settings. Regardless of the style, the well-written note is based on the clinical thought process described in the HOAC.

Narrative Note

Narrative notes are probably the most widely used format within physical therapy. They can be used in inpatient or outpatient settings, as daily contact notes, or periodic assessments. See Figure 8.2 for an example of a narrative SOAP note.

Flow Sheets

A flow sheet is a simple grid in which a patient's status can be recorded across time on a single page. If a patient requires long-term follow-up or has multiple functional deficits and contributing factors, it may be easier to track progress using a flow sheet. This can be advantageous to the clinician in cases in which continued insurance approval depends on objective progress. A flow sheet format also can make the assessment portion of the SOAP note easier to write. There are several types of flow sheets that are useful in documentation:

1. An objective status flow sheet is useful in an inpatient setting when stays are long and note writing is frequent (Figure 8.3).

2. Exercise flow sheets are useful for patient self-report of home exercise program compliance. An example is provided in Figure 8.4. In this flow sheet, the therapist sets a quota. The patient records the actual number of repetitions he or she has done. Information from this flow sheet can be used for patient education regarding pacing and the need for consistency.

3. Daily note flow sheets are useful in outpatient settings in which formal reevaluation documentation may be required on a monthly basis, but

S: Pt. reports increasing difficulty "keeping up" with HEP. Fearful of RTW plan.

O: Pt. seen for 5/8 scheduled sessions since last note. Rx focus remains on HEP progression, physical tolerance training, and D/C planning.

1. Physical tolerances: sitting 25–30 min, standing 15 min, walking 0.75 miles, lifting floor to waist 10 lbs.
2. HEP: inconsistently performing 12 reps of all exercises (see exercise flow sheet).
3. Pain: Pt. needs cues to use indep. PCMs. Significant relief with ice massage.
4. AROM LS: 25% limited in FB, SB bilat., ROT bilat.; 50% limited in BB.
5. Body mechanics: Needs cues to maintain neutral spine position for lifting.

A: Gains made in 1, 4, and 5. No significant change in 2 and 3. Pt. remains pain and somatically focused, fearful of movement and exercise. Pain behaviors include missed sessions and poor compliance with HEP, which increased when the RTW plan was formulated.

P: Pt./team meeting recommended to address decreased attendance/compliance and discuss RTW fears. Continue PT BIW x 4 add'l weeks; change Rx focus to work simulation according to RTW plan.

FIGURE 8.2   *Example of a narrative note. (S = subjective; Pt. = patient; HEP = home exercise program; RTW = return to work; O = objective; Rx = treatment; indep. = independent; D/C = discharge; PCM = pain control modality; AROM = active range of motion; LS = lumbosacral; FB = forward bending; SB = side bending; bilat. = bilateral; ROT = rotation; BB = backward bending; A = assessment; P = plan; BIW = twice weekly.)*

brief contact notes are required for each patient treatment session. These flow sheets lend themselves well to settings in which physical therapists and physical therapist assistants work together. The physical therapist assistant can document treatment rendered, and the physical therapist can use that information in treatment planning and reevaluation (Figure 8.5).

If flow sheets are used in narrative documentation, the therapist must reference the appropriate flow sheet within the body of the note. The flow sheet must be easily located within the medical record and clearly titled.

FIGURE 8.3
Example of an
objective status
flow sheet. (HEP
= home exercise
program; bid =
twice a day; reps
= repetitions; tid
= three times a
day.)

Problem	Date/signature	Date/signature	Date/signature	Date/signature	Goal
Pt. lacks an independent HEP	9 reps bid of all exercises	15 reps bid	20 reps bid with 5-lb weights	Goal met	25 reps bid with 5-lb weights
Poor physical tolerances	Sit 10 min; walk 1/4 mile	Sit 15 min; walk 1/2 mile	Sit 30 min; walk 1/2 mile	Sit 45 min; walk 1 mile	Sit >60 min; walk >2 miles
Unable to lift >5 lb from floor to waist	5 lb, 5 reps tid	7 lb, 5 reps tid	10 lb, 5 reps tid	15 lb, 5 reps tid	Lift >25 lb from floor to waist
Unable to control pain	Needs cues to use pain control modalities	Incorporates heat in HEP independently	Uses ice occasionally before and after PT session	Goal met	Independent use of heat and ice for pain control

FIGURE 8.4
Example of an
exercise flow
sheet. Note: In
x/y, x is the
quota, and y is
the actual number
of the exercise
performed.

Exercise	Date	Date	Date	Date	Date	Date	Date
Pelvic tilt	5/5	5/10	5/0	6/6	6/6	6/6	7/
Knee-chest	5/5	5/8	5/0	6/6	6/6	6/6	7/
Trunk rotation	5/5	5/8	5/0	6/6	6/6	6/6	7/
Abdominal curl	5/5	5/8	5/0	6/6	6/6	6/6	7/
Straight-leg raising	5/5	5/10	5/0	6/6	6/6	6/6	7/
Cat/camel	5/5	5/8	5/0	6/6	6/6	6/6	7/

FIGURE 8.5
*Example of a
daily note flow
sheet. (LS = lum-
bosacral; Ther Ex
= therapy exercis-
es; TFM = trans-
verse friction
massage; Pt. =
patient; BIW =
twice a week.)*

Objective	Date/signature	Date/signature	Date/signature	Date/signature	Date/signature
Ther Ex	Bicycle: 5 min; treadmill: 2 mph, 10 min	Bicycle: 8 min; treadmill: 2 mph, 15 min			
Massage	TFM to adherent LS scar	TFM to adherent LS scar			
Patient edu-cation	Sitting posture using lumbar support	Integration of pain control modalities into exercise pro-gram			
Assessment	Pain-focused during aerobic training; vitals unchanged indi-cating submaxi-mal effort	Remains pain-focused but compliant with increased activity levels. Scar mobility improving.			
Plan	Cont. BIW	Continue current treatment plan			

References

Rothstein JM, Echternach JL. Hypothesis-oriented algorithm for clinicians. A method for evaluation and treatment. Phys Ther 1987;66:1388.

Suggested Reading

American Physical Therapy Association. Guidelines for Physical Therapy Documentation. Alexandria, VA: American Physical Therapy Association, 1995.

Kettenbach FA. Writing SOAP Notes (2nd ed). Philadelphia: FA Davis, 1995.

9 Behavioral Medicine Assessment and Treatment

Alan Witkower

Patients seen by physical therapists may have problems related to their pain or other conditions that are best addressed by behavioral medicine specialists. Examples of such patients are discussed in this chapter. These patients represent a clinical challenge for physical rehabilitation and highlight the value of obtaining a psychological consultation to clarify the complex issues surrounding persistent pain and disability. Physical therapists can benefit by becoming aware of the nature of psychological issues in patients by adopting some behavioral principles in their approaches to patients and by knowing how to integrate psychological findings into their own assessment findings to make realistic treatment decisions for complex patients.

Case Example

A 58-year-old, married female is complaining of neck, shoulder, and diffuse back pain. She works as an office manager, and her two children have recently left home—one for college and another to enter the army. Her pain has been diagnosed as being related to degenerative disc disease and possible arthritis. She is not considered a candidate for any surgical intervention. She has had pain for approximately 10 years but reports that in the past 6 months her pain has increased considerably and is causing her significant distress and disability. She reports that after work she often returns home and goes directly to bed. She presents as extremely pain-focused with displays of excessive pain behavior such as groaning and wincing with the slightest movements. When not describing how much pain she is experiencing, the patient complains bitterly about being unappreciated by her husband. She describes her husband as insensitive to her discomfort and confides that she fears he may be losing interest in her and the marriage. At times during treatment, the patient begins to cry but generally excuses her behavior as being related to her pain or fatigue.

Case Example

A 22-year-old male who had traumatic amputation of both legs above the knees after a motorcycle accident 1 year ago has been in physical therapy for 3 months and is making very limited progress in learning to ambulate with his prostheses. He complains of phantom limb pain and diffuse back pain that limit his tolerance for weightbearing. He is prescribed a narcotic pain medication, an anti-inflammatory medication, a muscle relaxant, and an antidepressant. The patient continually complains that his physician is not providing him with enough narcotic medication to control his pain. His presentation is notable for a sad and irritable affect with frequent complaints about his previous care providers. Despite his expressed dissatisfaction with his care, he is reliable and on time to all of his appointments regardless of weather or illness. He avoids discussing his accident but does comment that he wishes he had not survived it.

Case Example

A 44-year-old male complains of low back pain. The onset of his pain followed a work-related injury in which the patient attempted to lift a heavy object and reports that he heard a "popping noise" and then felt "something let go in my back." Several diagnostic procedures have been performed, including magnetic resonance imaging, myelography, bone scans, and an electromyography. None of these procedures have shown any spinal abnormality. He has also had consultations with an orthopedic surgeon, a neurologist, a chiropractor, and most recently, a physiatrist. He is diagnosed with a severe sprain/strain. Despite reassurances that his injury is not serious, the patient expresses considerable fear of engaging in any activity that might further harm him. He has not progressed in previous courses of physical therapy but now states that he has no other alternatives because he is not a surgical candidate and his insurer refuses to cover any further diagnostic procedures. His wife accompanies him to all appointments and appears very solicitous of his needs. According to the patient, he is totally dependent on his wife for basic activities of daily living such as showering and dressing. The patient states he is extremely frustrated with his dependency but maintains that this state of affairs is preferable to "becoming paralyzed."

Behavioral Assessment

These patients are excellent examples of cases in which behavioral assessment should be included in rehabilitation. Behavioral assessment is generally indicated when a patient's pain is (1) causing significant impairment in normal functioning, (2) compromising relationships with family or friends, (3) contributing to emotional distress such as anxiety or depression, (4) resulting in the patient's overuse of health care resources, (5) creating a dependence on the use of narcotic or sedative-hypnotic medications, or

(6) significantly disproportionate to the physical findings (Kerns and Jacobs 1992, Romano et al. 1989).

Psychological and behavioral factors can contribute to the maintenance or exacerbation of a particular pain problem. A behavioral assessment only explores possible contributions to a patient's pain experience, and there is no intent to differentiate organic versus psychogenic pain. This does not, however, rule out the contribution of physiologic processes to the nociceptive element of the pain (DeGood 1988). A patient who is depressed and is abusing narcotic pain medication can still be receiving noxious input from a strained muscle. Conversely, the presence of observable and positive signs of an organic basis for the nociceptive element of pain does not preclude significant behavioral and psychological factors from influencing pain and disability. A patient with an obvious herniated disc impinging on a nerve root can still present with an anxiety disorder that may be fueling the patient's excessive "doctor shopping." A view that pain arises either in the body or mind overlooks the critical role of the patient's environment on pain and disability. A patient's adversarial relationship with the insurer over a work-related injury or the patient's overly solicitous spouse may contribute more to the course and outcome of the patient's pain and suffering than emotional or physiologic variables.

Psychosocial and behavioral assessments of patients by behavioral psychologists range from brief screening interviews to in-depth psychological evaluations. In some settings, the assessment is performed in an expedient manner to determine the appropriateness of a particular treatment program (e.g., admission to an inpatient versus an outpatient pain rehabilitation program). In this case, the assessment may involve a relatively brief interview along with a review of the patient's responses to a general pain questionnaire. After the patient has been admitted to the pain rehabilitation program, a more comprehensive psychosocial evaluation is performed. In other settings, a comprehensive psychological evaluation performed at the beginning of treatment may include (1) the completion of a battery of psychological and pain-focused instruments, (2) an extensive, structured clinical interview, and (3) psychophysiologic assessment with biofeedback instrumentation. The goals of this more comprehensive evaluation include establishing a psychiatric diagnosis and identifying psychophysiologic aspects of the pain problem and the contributions of behavioral, cognitive, environmental, and emotional factors to the pain experience (Bradley et al. 1992).

The in-depth behavioral assessment described here reflects an emphasis on a cognitive-behavioral orientation to pain that is described later in the chapter in the section on cognition and coping. The goals of the behavioral assessment include (1) understanding patients' view of their pain problem and treatment expectations; (2) delineating the behavioral, cognitive, affective, and environmental influences on patients' pain problems; (3) establishing realistic and measurable treatment goals; (4) determining appropriate treatment interventions for achieving those goals; and (5) engaging patients in a collaborative treatment approach, including physical therapy, to achieve those goals (DeGood 1988, Romano et al. 1989).

It is not surprising that patients referred to a psychologist for a behavioral assessment may be resistant and suspicious of the reason for the referral. This resistance is understandable when the patient's point of view is considered. Often, the initial perception of patients referred for behavioral assessment is that they are being viewed as "crazy" and that therapists and doctors think the pain is "all in their head." Many patients consider a behavioral assessment to be irrelevant to their pain problem, which they believe is strictly physical in nature. The patient's concern is that the referring clinician will not pursue further medical testing or intervention despite the patient's belief that there is an undiagnosed medical disorder causing the pain. Some patients believe the referral is a statement that their pain problem cannot be "fixed" by health care professionals and that they are therefore being "dumped." For patients who are involved in compensation claims or litigation, there is often concern that the legitimacy of their pain is being questioned and that they are being viewed as malingerers. Therefore, the behavioral assessment is seen by some patients as an effort to "prove" that they do not have a legitimate pain problem (Cameron and Shepel 1986, Romano et al. 1989).

A behavioral assessment is of questionable value if the validity of the patient's responses are compromised by a hostile and defensive attitude. Patients may choose to be circumspect about their answers to questions during the assessment, or they may deny any psychological distress and present a "cheerful" picture of their problems in order to suggest psychological health. It is therefore extremely important for all members of the pain rehabilitation team to consider the following referral guidelines to ensure a valid outcome and a useful experience for the patient.

1. Discuss the disrupting impact that chronic pain can have on all areas of life, including family, work, and social aspects. It may be helpful to personalize the rationale for the referral by using hypothetical examples of how others might respond to the pain problem the patient is experiencing or by discussing the range of personal problems the patient has disclosed in the course of treatment (Cameron and Shepel 1986, Romano et al. 1989). The clinician may empathize with the patient by using a statement such as "I can only imagine that if I could not play with my kids I would be very frustrated and sad." To remind the patient of the range of problems experienced, a statement such as "you have mentioned several times how discouraged you get when you can't fix things around the house or be a good partner for your wife; maybe it would help if you had an opportunity to talk with someone about how you are feeling," might be helpful.

2. The patient should be reassured that the clinician believes in the validity of his or her pain but should also be reminded that there are complex interactions between physical and psychological processes that influence pain perception, disability, and suffering. Even when a patient's pain complaints are disproportionate to the physical findings, the patient's distress and perception of pain can be acknowledged as genuine despite the lack of

physical findings (Cameron and Shepel 1986, Romano et al. 1989). Again, statements such as "I know you have been told that your back does not look that bad on the tests, but I have seen patients with a bad muscle strain like yours causing a great deal of pain that left them discouraged and frustrated also," can be reassuring to the patient.

3.   Inform the patient that he or she will be seeing a psychologist. Explain that a psychologist is interested in learning about what factors affect the patient's pain and how each person reacts to pain. Emphasize that the role of the psychologist is to help the patient identify practical solutions to problems. Reassure the patient that he or she is not being referred with the intent of having a mental illness diagnosed. If possible, describe the psychologist in a personal way or as someone who has been helpful in similar situations (Cameron and Shepel 1986). Hearing a statement such as "I have referred patients to Dr. Smith before and they tell me how helpful he has been in teaching them how to cope better with their pain," can make a difference in a patient's attitude about the referral.

4.   It is also helpful to prepare patients for the involvement of significant others or family members. Patients can generally accept the rationale that information provided to the psychologist from someone close to them will enhance understanding of their pain problem.

5.   Reassure patients that the referral does not mean you will be transferring the patient's care. Reminding patients of the multifaceted nature of their pain problem and emphasizing the benefit of a comprehensive approach can support the addition of the psychologist to the treatment team (e.g., "You and I have been making progress with your flexibility and endurance; now it may help you to learn how to transfer your gains to activities you enjoy with your family. Dr. Smith could help you find ways to become more active with your spouse and children").

Pain History

The behavioral psychologist's role is described in order for the physical therapist to have a good understanding of the way in which this team member can contribute to the pain patient's total care. For each member of the team, a good introduction is crucial in establishing rapport with a new patient. This rapport will influence the course and outcome of the subsequent assessment. In this introduction, the behavioral psychologist should address the role of the psychologist, the purpose of the psychological interview, and the issues to be covered in the interview. The interview may begin with a question about the patient's referral for the behavioral assessment. The patient should be asked what he or she was told about the reasons for referral and why he or she thinks the referral was made. The patient's responses to these questions will then allow the psychologist to clarify any misperceptions or allay any of the patient's concerns.

A pain history should be elicited after the introduction. Inquiring early on about a patient's pain permits the psychologist to establish a rapport with a patient before proceeding into areas of psychosocial functioning that may be more difficult and sensitive areas for the patient to discuss (Bradley et al. 1992, Romano et al. 1989).

Chapters 1 and 4 describe the assessment of pain from a sensory perspective, focusing on the patient's description of the intensity, location, duration, frequency, and quality of pain. It is also important for the psychologist to explore how the pain began (Romano et al. 1989). If the pain began with a traumatic event, such as a motor vehicle accident or work-related injury, it is necessary for all members of the team to understand what specifically occurred and how the patient has responded to the injury or accident since it occurred. A patient who was injured in a serious motor vehicle accident and reports that he or she cannot tolerate driving distances because of pain may also have developed a phobia about being in a car. A patient who suffered a traumatic injury at work might be reluctant to return to work, in part because of a post-traumatic stress response associated with the accident.

Assessing what was occurring in the patient's life before or during the onset of pain is particularly important if the patient reports that his or her pain began spontaneously or developed during a chronic illness (Bradley et al. 1992, Turk et al. 1983). There may be environmental or psychosocial factors that contributed to the patient's awareness of discomfort or intolerance for pain that was previously manageable. An example of this situation is a patient whose increased complaints of pain and disability due to a chronic illness such as arthritis coincide with a separation from a close family member.

The psychologist also asks patients to describe factors (e.g., weather, activity, or the menstrual cycle) that influence the intensity and daily fluctuations of the pain. Patients are also encouraged to consider what variables contribute to decreased tolerance for pain (e.g., lack of sleep, frustration, distractions, worrying) and what events usually precede or follow exacerbations of pain (Bradley et al. 1992). For example, a patient may state that her pain always seems to increase just before her spouse returns home from work. Further questioning may show that the patient's spouse has been experiencing stress at work and has a tendency to complain about work when he arrives home. This line of inquiry elicits valuable information about the patient's pain and reinforces the idea that pain is multidimensional in nature.

The pain history also includes a review of all of the previous and current treatments for the patient's pain. Often this will reveal important information about the patient's expectations of treatment and identify the patient's attitudes toward health care providers (DeGood 1988, Bradley et al. 1992). Patients often will relate a lengthy history of multiple practitioners who failed to ameliorate the patient's pain. Therefore, the patient is feeling discouraged and is likely to be skeptical of any further "promises" to help alleviate the pain. A patient who reports that previous physical rehabilitation has "made me much worse" will obviously require a thorough reeducation before further physical therapy is recommended. Some patients may state that they have had many passive modalities applied and received numerous medication trials and still did not improve. Patients may then conclude that nothing will help them because they have not been introduced to active and self-management strategies. These patients may have become dependent in previous treatment on physical therapists and physicians and believe that they must submit to the ministrations of health care providers. Closer review of the reported unsuccessful treatments such as medications and modalities may also show that the patient was not fully compliant with the recommended treatment. For example, many patients prematurely discontinue an antidepressant medication trial due to unpleasant side effects or because of the stigma attached to these medications. Other patients stop treatments because of an increase in pain and an inadequate explanation of how the treatment will benefit them. Ultimately, it is important for all team members to know in advance how a patient responded to previous treatment recommendations so the patient's responses to any of the treatment approaches recommended can be anticipated.

It is also valuable for the pain team members to have information about the patient's coping strategies (e.g., medications, resting, watching television, hot showers) that have helped the patient with the pain (DeGood and Shutty 1992). Some patients may identify coping strategies (e.g., talking to friends, taking walks, listening to music, keeping busy) that suggest they are more amenable to a self-management or behavioral approach. Some of the patient's coping strategies may become targets for intervention and change (such as medication intake); other strategies may involve behaviors that can be reinforced or increased, such as efforts to socialize and distract oneself from pain.

The interview can be supplemented with the use of a pain diary. This method provides the psychologist with more data, underscores how many variables influence pain, and provides the patient with a record of his or her responses to the pain. The pain diary was initially developed to record information on a patient's positioning during the day (i.e., sitting, reclining, standing, walking) (Fordyce 1976). It is now often modified to include additional variables such as pain intensity, medication intake, mood, tension levels, where and with whom the time was spent, use of pain control strategies (e.g., hot pack, distraction), and sleep. Patients are generally asked to fill out the diaries three to four times a day, noting how they spent the preceding period of time on an hourly basis. The pain diary therefore provides direct, immediate, and repeated data in contrast to the clinical interview, which focuses on retrospective data and relies on the patient's memory. The pain diary also provides a baseline of behaviors that will be used to develop treatment goals and measure the patient's progress. Additionally, the pain diary can be used throughout the treatment program to identify problematic behavioral patterns that interfere with progress and to document areas of improvement during treatment (Karoly and Jensen 1987).

Assessing Dysfunction and Distress

Patients expect and appreciate inquiry about their distress, since it permits them to describe how much pain they are suffering and explain how their pain has interfered with their lives. Each team member inquires into this aspect in a slightly different way. The behavioral psychologist explores how these patients were functioning in family, social, and vocational aspects of their lives before the development of pain (Bradley et al. 1992). The comparison of a patient's pre- and postpain activity level is critical in developing hypotheses regarding what consequences or variables could be maintaining pain behaviors and augmenting pain perception. For example, a patient may report that he or she can no longer assist with household activities such as doing the laundry because of pain, but the patient's spouse may report that the patient used to complain about this task before the onset of pain.

Thus, avoidance of certain unpleasant activities due to complaints of pain may be a function of negative reinforcement rather than actual pain intolerance. Patients may report that they can still perform other physical activities that require comparable physical effort. An example is a patient who claims he cannot assist with the dishes because of pain in his back when he stands at the sink, but he may report that he is able to stand at his work bench to repair a broken fixture.

During this portion of the interview, the psychologist should also note how people in the patient's environment respond to the patient's pain behavior (Turk et al. 1983). The patient should be asked how his or her spouse (or "significant other") reacts when the patient takes medication or when the patient complains about increased pain. The spouse may respond with expressions of concern and an effort to make the patient more comfortable, thus reinforcing the patient's pain behavior and reducing the likelihood that the patient will engage in well behavior. A patient might report that her spouse reacts to her complaints of pain with frustration and avoidance of the patient. In this case, the patient's emotional distress will increase and her efforts to receive validation of her pain may lead to an increase in pain behavior with health care providers. It is also possible that, for this patient, having her spouse avoid her solves a long-standing difficulty with intimacy in the marriage. Thus, her complaints will persist despite efforts by professionals to ameliorate her pain problem.

This line of questioning may also involve discussion of the patient's marital and family relationships (Bradley et al. 1992, Romano et al. 1989). Patients will be more comfortable with questions about their relationships when they have acknowledged that the pain problem has had an impact on the quality of those relationships. In some instances, the focus on pain permits a couple to become closer and spend more time with each other. This unacknowledged benefit should be addressed before rehabilitation for pain can be effective. For another couple, a patient's pain problem can keep a dissatisfied spouse from leaving the marriage because the patient has a legitimate need for care. Treatment that improves the patient's pain may threaten to expose him or her to the greater pain of losing a spouse.

A patient reporting that pain has interfered with performance at work or that he or she is currently receiving worker's compensation due to injury resulting in pain provides an opportunity for any team member to inquire about the patient's vocational and educational experiences (Mendelson 1994). It is critical to learn what incentives or disincentives influence a patient's pain complaints and impact the motivation to return to productive employment. Patients should be asked about their work history, education, and vocational skills. A patient who has had a poor work history with multiple jobs, has not completed high school, and has limited work skills will represent a significant challenge for pain and vocational rehabilitation. Another patient who has worked for a company for many years and is injured on the job may express disappointment with the company's treatment. In this case, the patient's resentment may interfere with participation in treatment directed at returning to work. Similarly, a patient who reports attendance problems, conflicts with coworkers, or discontent with work will require vocational counseling in addition to pain management strategies (Mendelson 1994).

The issue of compensation and litigation in a patient's pain experience is very complex and requires more discussion than is possible in this chapter. Several areas should be explored in a behavioral assessment, however, including (1) how does the current level of compensation compare to the patient's previous income, (2) does improvement in pain or disability threaten the patient's level of compensation or the financial outcome of the litigation, (3) is the patient being advised by his or her attorney or family to avoid any demonstration of improvement, and (4) does the patient have a realistic opportunity to return to his or her former job or will he require vocational counseling and training (Romano et al. 1989). It is important to understand that there is no consensus in the research on the relationship of compensation, litigation, chronic pain, and treatment (Mendelson 1994). However, assessment of these factors is critical in developing an appropriate treatment plan or determining if treatment should be postponed until legal issues have been resolved.

The most commonly used measures of functional disability used by behavioral psycologists are the Chronic Illness Problem Inventory (CIPI) (Kames et al. 1984), the Sickness Impact Profile (SIP) (Bergner et al. 1981), and the Multidimensional Pain Inventory (MPI) (Kerns et al. 1985).

The CIPI is a 65-item instrument that assesses physical limitations, psychosocial functioning, health care behaviors, and marital adjustment. The CIPI appears to be useful as a screening tool that can assist in focusing an assessment and as an outcome measure to evaluate progress during treatment. The SIP is a questionnaire with 136 items and 12 categories: sleep and rest, eating, work, home management, recreation and pastimes, ambulation, mobility, body care, movement, social interaction, alertness behavior, and communication. Although the SIP is lengthy, it has good psychometric properties and is a sensitive measure of change as a function of pain treatment. The MPI attempts to evaluate the impact of patients' pain on multiple areas of their lives. It is a 56-item assessment that is composed of three sections. The first section evaluates (1) interference of pain on social, vocational, and family functioning; (2) support from a spouse or significant other; (3) severity of pain; (4) perception of life control; and (5) negative mood. The second section evaluates the patients' perception of the responses of others as being solicitous, distracting, or punishing. The third section evaluates the frequency of patients' participation in household chores, outdoor work, social activities, and activities outside of home. The MPI describes three patterns of patient responses: "dysfunctional," "interpersonally distressed," and "adaptive coper." These patient profiles are useful in determining areas of distress and dysfunction requiring specific attention in treatment.

The psychologist should also determine the nature of the patients' associated emotional distress. The most frequently encountered areas of distress reported by patients with chronic pain are depression, anxiety, and anger.

Additional problems include memory and concentration difficulties, post-traumatic stress disorders, and sleep disturbances.

Depression is the disorder most commonly associated with chronic pain. Patients describe feeling demoralized, irritable, fatigued, isolated, discouraged, and hopeless; they also report problems with sleep, appetite, sexual interest, and an inability to enjoy any pleasurable activity. Often a depressed patient expresses passive suicidal wishes such as "I sometimes hope that I will not wake up in the morning." The Beck Depression Inventory (BDI) (Beck and Speer 1987) is a particularly useful instrument for assessing the presence and severity of depression. The BDI is a brief (21 questions), self-administered instrument that assess both the cognitive-affective and neurovegetative signs of depression. If a patient does present with depression, further inquiry is necessary to determine (1) if the patient has had a previous history of depressive disorder, (2) if the patient is being prescribed sedative-hypnotics or significant amounts of opioids, and (3) if the patient is using alcohol or other substances that would create a presentation similar to depression.

Anxiety is generally suspected when patients describe jitteriness; racing thoughts; difficulty falling asleep; excessive muscle tension; difficulty concentrating; and symptoms of autonomic arousal such as palpitations, dyspnea, tachycardia, or nausea. As with depression, there are patients who report that they cannot function due to pain when, in fact, the primary cause of the patients' avoidance of activity is a generalized anxiety disorder. In other situations, the patient may have been injured in a traumatic accident, and the resulting post-traumatic stress disorder is the major factor contributing to the patient's inability to function. The State-Trait Anxiety Inventory (STAI) (Spielberger 1983) is a popular instrument for assessing both a patient's current *state* of anxiety and the patient *trait* (or characteristic experience) of anxiety. The STAI has 40 questions and can be self-administered and completed in 20 minutes.

Anger and hostility are important aspects of a patient's emotional distress in response to persistent pain. The expression of anger as hostility or defensiveness can seriously compromise the therapeutic relationship between the patient and every member of the rehabilitation team. Conversely, patients who minimize or deny anger in circumstances that would realistically elicit these feelings may be contributing to their excessive muscle tension or inappropriate use of medications to modulate this negative affect. The Symptom Checklist-90 Revised (SCL-90R) (Derogatis 1983) is a 90-item self-report checklist that measures psychological symptoms, including somatization, obsessiveness, interpersonal sensitivity, depression, anxiety, hostility, phobic anxiety, paranoia, and psychoticism. These nine subscales can be averaged and used to compute a Global Symptom Index that assesses a patient's degree of psychological distress. The SCL-90R is particularly useful as a screening tool to highlight areas of the patient's psychological functioning that require further examination. The SCL-90R takes approximately 20–30 minutes to complete. It therefore has a distinct advantage over more comprehensive psychological inventories such as the Minnesota Multiphasic Personality Inventory, which is often too time-intensive for patients with pain who have difficulty concentrating on a task.

Assessing Cognition and Coping

Patients' cognitions include beliefs, appraisals, and expectations regarding the pain diagnosis and treatment options. Their beliefs and expectations can be placed into one of three categories: (1) beliefs about the pain, (2) beliefs about the treatment, and (3) coping styles (Bradley et al. 1989, DeGood and Shutty 1992). For example, if a patient believes that referral to a psychologist suggests that her physician views her pain as being "psychological," this perception will evoke mistrust, defensiveness, and hostility. Thus, the patient may begin to exaggerate pain behavior in order to convince the physician that her pain is "real." If a patient is told by his physician that his back pain is a result of degenerative disc disease or a bulging disc, the patient may fear that any activity will cause more damage or disability. As a result, the patient may resist recommendations to engage in a physical therapy program despite the risks associated with serious deconditioning. These examples demonstrate how an individual's belief about his or her pain will influence the patient's pain perception, suffering, coping effort, and disability.

Patients routinely question why they are having pain. Therefore, it is important for team members to ask patients what they have been told about the cause of their pain and what they believe is the cause of their pain. These questions are important because patients frequently are told that their pain is due to a relatively benign disorder, but their anxiety makes them suspicious that the pain is due to a much more serious and undiagnosed problem. A common example of this misperception is the patient who suffers a soft-tissue injury causing diffuse pain that persists for several months. Because most patients are socialized to believe that pain is a symptom of an underlying disorder, it is difficult to help the patient accept the notion that pain may represent an interaction of physiology, psychology, and environmental factors (Romano et al. 1989, DeGood 1988).

It is common for patients to describe disappointment that their physician reported that there was no serious medical problem identified by the clinical examination and diagnostic testing. Patients often believe that they will receive treatment to ameliorate their pain if a specific medical problem is diagnosed. The lack of clinical findings does not reassure patients but instead impels them to seek further medical consultation. Therefore, a significant component of the psychologist's treatment is focused on assisting patients in reconceptualizing their pain problem. Many patients with chronic pain should be encouraged to see their pain as an interaction of somatic, psychological, and social factors (biopsychosocial model) rather than as a symptom of disease (medical model) (Hanson and Gerber 1990).

The psychologist's questions may also explore the patient's expectations of the consequences of pain. Many patients are prone to catastrophizing (DeGood and Shutty 1992, Turk et al. 1983).

Patients commonly believe that all rehabilitation treatment should fix their pain so that they will be able to resume life as it was before the onset of pain. They expect health care providers to have the answers and that they should merely be a passive recipient of treatment. Some patients believe that "dramatic" and invasive treatments are more likely to provide relief. Many patients would prefer surgical intervention or a series of painful nerve blocks than physical rehabilitation or lifestyle adjustment. Patients who have already been prescribed potent narcotic medications conclude that there is a serious problem if such medical intervention is warranted. Therefore, any "lesser" treatment (e.g., physical rehabilitation) will be viewed as insufficient to address their pain.

When a treatment approach is presented to a patient, there are two important beliefs that influence the patient's acceptance of the treatment. First, patients must determine if the treatment, such as relaxation exercises, is a credible intervention that will have a positive impact on their pain perception. This is the patient's *outcome expectancy* (Bandura 1977). Second, patients must decide if they are capable of effectively using the technique for their pain. This is the patient's *self-efficacy expectancy* (Bandura 1977). Some patients may respond negatively to the suggestion that moderating their reactions to stressful events will reduce their pain because this treatment is completely incongruous with their belief that their pain is caused by a pinched nerve.

There are numerous psychometric instruments designed to measure patients' beliefs about their pain and expectations about treatment. Questionnaires with particular clinical relevance and good psychometric properties include the Pain Beliefs Questionnaire (PBQ) (Gottlieb 1984, 1986); Survey of Pain Attitudes (SOPA) (Jensen et al. 1987, Jensen and Karoly 1989); Pain Beliefs and Perceptions Inventory (PBAPI) (Williams and Thorn 1989); and the Pain and Impairment Relationship Scales (PAIRS) (Riley et al. 1988). The PBQ is a 43-item questionnaire that assesses disability expectations, self-efficacy, depression, and the perceived threat of pain. Research with this instrument has demonstrated that patients who were considered treatment successes in a behaviorally oriented treatment program had demonstrated a reduction in dysfunctional cognitions as measured by this instrument. The SOPA is a 35-item self-report scale measuring pain control, solicitude, medical cure, disability, medication, and emotion. Pain beliefs measured by the SOPA appear to be related to patient outcome after behavioral treatment. The PBAPI is a 16-item questionnaire that measures patient beliefs about stability of pain, self-blame, and perceptions of pain as mysterious. The PAIRS is composed of 15 attitudinal statements to examine the patient's association of pain with disability. Patients who strongly endorse the statements that attribute impairment to pain perception have been shown to have a greater level of disability and suffering.

Coping styles reflect how patients manage their pain, disability, and distress. Coping styles include both cognitive and behavioral efforts to control or tolerate stressful circumstances such as pain. Cognitive coping strategies include distraction, self-reassuring statements, and reinterpretation of the pain sensation. Examples of behavioral coping strategies include resting and using medication or heat. Coping strategies can be viewed as either active or passive strategies (Bradley et al. 1989, DeGood and Shutty 1992). Catastrophizing as a coping strategy is associated with the highest levels of pain and distress and also appears to be a predictor of treatment failure if it is not improved (Keefe et al. 1989, Rosenstiel and Keefe 1983, Turk and Holzman 1986, Turner and Clancy 1986). The two most popular instruments used to assess patients' coping styles are the Coping Strategies Questionnaire (CSQ) and the Vanderbilt Pain Management Inventory (VPMI) (Brown and

Nicassio 1987). The CSQ assesses both cognitive and behavioral strategies including diversion of attention, reinterpretation of pain sensations, coping self-statements, ignoring pain sensations, praying or hoping, catastrophizing, increasing activity level, and increasing pain behavior. The VPMI is a 19-item self-report scale that categorizes coping strategies as either passive or active. Both of these instruments have been used in studies that have concluded that passive coping strategies and the use of catastrophizing self-statements appear to be associated with poorer outcome with respect to subjective pain intensity, disability, and depression.

When asking about patients' coping style or strategy, it is also appropriate for the team members to ask them about their use of narcotic pain medication. A number of problems are associated with patient use of narcotic pain medications. There is a risk of iatrogenic complications, such as dependency, cognitive impairment, and dysphoric mood. Many patients who are taking prescribed narcotic pain medication become convinced that this treatment validates their belief that there is a serious medical problem causing their pain. Other patients convince themselves that because they have pain they must continue taking the medication even when the medication is no longer effective in controlling the pain. Once this topic has been raised, it is easier to inquire about the patient's use of alcohol or drugs to cope with pain. Patients are generally tolerant of questions about their past use of substances including alcohol, illicit drugs, or other prescription medications if this line of questioning is shown to be relevant to understanding how the patient copes with distressing physical and emotional states.

Behavioral Treatment

The two major approaches to the behavioral treatment of chronic pain are operant-behavioral and cognitive-behavioral. These approaches conceptualize chronic pain very differently from the disease model. In the disease, or medical, model, there is an assumption that the patient's suffering is a symptom of an underlying disease or injury and that resolution of the pathology will eliminate the suffering. This model places an emphasis on diagnostic studies to identify the pathology and places the responsibility for treatment on the health care professional. The behavioral model, however, sees suffering as a behavior that results from an interaction between cognitions, emotions, behavior, environmental influences, and any nociceptive stimuli. Behavioral approaches maintain that suffering can be reduced or eliminated through a combination of patient participation in treatment and training patients to modify thoughts, feelings, and behaviors even if the nociceptive input is not eliminated (Hanson and Gerber 1990, Turk and Holzman 1986).

Operant-Behavioral Model

The operant-behavioral approach to chronic pain was introduced by Fordyce and colleagues (Fordyce et al. 1968a, 1968b, 1973; Fordyce 1976) to explain why many patients are disabled despite insufficient evidence of any significant nociceptive input or in excess of any physical impairment.

Fordyce considered pain to be an unpleasant subjective experience communicated in some form of observable behavior such as grimacing, complaining, taking medication, or laying down. These manifestations occur irrespective of pathology. Fordyce used operant conditioning principles to treat these pain behaviors. These principles predict that behaviors followed by a positive consequence or reinforcement will reoccur more frequently and that behaviors that are no longer followed by a reinforcing consequence will diminish in frequency of occurrence (Keefe and Lefebve 1994, Ott 1992). In the operant-conditioning paradigm, behavior that avoids or postpones an aversive or unpleasant consequence is considered *avoidance learning* (Fordyce 1990). This behavioral concept emphasizes the role of the environment in maintaining the patient's suffering and disability.

The principles of Fordyce's approach and their success in treatment are highlighted in one of Fordyce's patients This patient avoided physical therapy and frequently complained about his pain. Fordyce turned away whenever the patient complained of pain but did pay attention to non–pain-related behaviors. This strategy eventually reduced the patient's pain complaints, and his attendance at physical therapy improved. These changes in the patient's behaviors occurred despite the patient's statement that he knew Fordyce was intentionally ignoring his complaints of pain (Fordyce 1990).

The operant-behavioral approach to treatment emphasizes identifying target behaviors to be modified and then developing a strategy to increase, decrease, or eliminate those specified behaviors. The treatment involves the patient, all rehabilitation team members, the therapist, members of the patient's family, and third parties such as an attorney or insurance case manager (Fordyce 1976, Roberts 1986).

The initial stage of operant-behavioral treatment involves identifying target behaviors such as reducing medication intake, increasing compliance with a home exercise program, increasing patient tolerance for a specific activity or exercise, improving mood, and enhancing family communication. The desired change in behavior should be observable and measurable. If medication reduction is the goal, the specific medication, frequency, and dosage must be clearly stated in the goal. The target behaviors should include pain behaviors and well behaviors.

Once the target behaviors have been identified, the patient, the psychologist, and those close to the patient begin to monitor the behaviors to establish what cues evoke the behaviors and what the consequences are for the behaviors.

With cooperation of the patient and others, goals are established for the target behaviors. The goals must be established with consensus from the patient (Ott 1992). Patients who feel coerced to perform a specific exercise or eliminate a medication will ultimately sabotage the plan. The goals should also be realistic and achievable by the patient.

Providing the patient with continual feedback on progress in modifying the selected behaviors by each member of the rehabilitation team is critical to the success of an operant-behavioral approach. Feedback can be both a reinforcer as well as an early warning of possible problems with the treatment plan. The feedback can be in both verbal and written forms (e.g., charts, graphs). For some patients, the charting behavior itself motivates the patient to continue with their program (Keefe and Lefebve 1994, Ott 1992, Roberts 1986).

Cognitive-Behavioral Model

The cognitive-behavioral approach to chronic pain is generally attributed to Turk et al. (1983). The cognitive-behavioral model emphasizes the role of the patient's cognitions and beliefs in pain perception, affective distress, and pain behaviors. There are five basic assumptions of the cognitive-behavioral model (Turk and Rudy 1989):

1.   Individuals are active processors of information. Patients attempt to make sense of their pain through past experiences. Therefore, the anticipated consequence of a behavior is as important as the actual consequence of behavior.

2.   Thoughts can influence mood, physiology, and behavior; mood, physiology, and behavior can influence thoughts. A patient's awareness of sudden pain can trigger catastrophizing thoughts; a patient's anxious ruminations may produce disturbed sleep resulting in a depressed mood.

3.   Behavior is reciprocally determined by the individual and by the environment. This is a departure from the operant-behavioral model that emphasizes the influence of the environment on the individual.

4.   Individuals can acquire more adaptive ways of thinking, feeling, and behaving.

5.   Individuals need to be involved actively in the changing of their maladaptive thoughts, feelings, and behaviors. In contrast to the medical model, which reinforces the passive and compliant behavior of the patient, the cognitive-behavioral model maintains that patients can be instrumental in learning and utilizing adaptive strategies for coping with and managing pain (Turk and Rudy 1989).

Cognitive-behavioral treatment has six major goals: (1) to reconceptualize the patients' views of their pain problem from being overwhelming to being manageable and optimistic; (2) to shift patients' views of themselves from being passive to being resourceful and proactive; (3) to ensure that patients learn to monitor their thoughts, feelings, and behaviors during activities to highlight the connection between these factors and their pain symptoms; (4) to teach patients the necessary skills to adaptively respond to their pain problems; (5) to encourage patients to attribute their success to their efforts at utilizing these skills; and (6) to ensure that patients are able to anticipate and manage future pain problems (Holzman et al. 1986).

The cognitive-behavioral approach is composed of four overlapping phases of treatment. These phases follow a logical course of education and training but are also flexible. Patients may progress at different rates, and at times, acute problems may occur that require the psychologist to return to an earlier phase to stabilize the patient (Turk et al. 1983, Ott 1992).

Reconceptualization

The goal of the reconceptualization phase is to educate the patient on the rationale and expectations of a cognitive-behavioral approach to pain. Ideally, this process will introduce patients to the importance of their active participation in treatment and help them develop a new perspective on their pain problem. To meet the goals of this phase, it is particularly helpful to invite patients to review the information shared in the psychologist's evaluation and to use their own experiences to demonstrate the interaction between thoughts, feelings, behavior, and the pain experience. The psychologist can also discuss the gate-control theory of pain (Melzack and Wall 1965).

It is also helpful to review the triad of pain, impairment, and disability with patients. The goal of treatment is to address these three aspects of pain. Treatment will provide relief in one or more of these areas. This approach can be reassuring to the patient who may report minimal pain relief but has increased the range of motion in an extremity or has increased participation in family activities. At the conclusion of this phase, patients should have accepted that multiple factors contribute to their pain experience and that they have the ability to influence the severity of their pain and the resultant disability.

Skill Acquisition

The task of the second stage of treatment is to promote the successful use of adaptive coping strategies that the patient already possesses and to help the patient develop new coping strategies. These strategies include relaxation strategies, attention-diversion strategies, and cognitive coping strategies.

Relaxation techniques reduce excessive muscle tension, patient's attention to pain, and the emotional arousal that can amplify pain perception. They also promote a feeling of control during episodes of pain (Turk et al. 1983). In order for these techniques to be successful, it is extremely important to emphasize to patients that relaxation strategies are learned skills that require practice and utilization in the appropriate circumstances. Relaxation techniques include jacobsonian progressive muscle relaxation, autogenic relaxation, diaphragmatic breathing, and relaxation imagery.

Progressive muscle relaxation alternately tenses and then relaxes a series of muscle groups (Bernstein and Borkovec 1973, Turk and Holzman 1986, Turk et al. 1983). The purpose of having patients initially tense their muscle groups is to train them to recognize what muscle tension feels like in their body and to discriminate between tension and relaxation. Tensing muscles and then abruptly relaxing those muscles also produces a more pronounced sensation of relaxing muscles. Patients' attention is continually focused by the therapist on the sensations occurring in the muscle groups. When patients have developed confidence in identifying tension in muscles, the tensing portion of the exercise is eliminated.

Diaphragmatic breathing exercises should begin with a discussion of the anatomy of the chest and how regulating respiration and increasing the efficiency of oxygenation can induce generalized muscle relaxation and counteract the effects of autonomic arousal. Patients are shown how to slow down breathing, inflate the lungs fully, and relax the diaphragm. Patients are instructed to breathe slowly in through the nose and then to gradually exhale through the mouth. In both muscle relaxation training and diaphragmatic exercises patients are encouraged to associate a word, phrase, or image with the sensation of relaxation while practicing the exercises. Additional components of the relaxation and breathing exercises involve asking patients to routinely scan their body throughout the day to determine if they are experiencing any muscle tension or signs of autonomic arousal. If they notice any areas of tension, they should use breathing or tension-reduction strategies to create a state of relaxation or reduce the symptoms of autonomic arousal (McCaffery 1979).

Attention-diversion strategies, or distraction techniques, consist of imagery that modifies patients' perception of the pain sensations and diverts their attention away from it (Hanson and Gerber 1990, Turk et al. 1983). Patients are presented with a rationale for this approach and examples of how attention diversion can assist them in coping with their pain. They are taught how attention can influence a person's perceptions either by selecting a focus of attention or by magnifying the awareness of a sensation. Generally, patients can identify at least one example of a situation in which they were not as focused on their pain. Examples offered by patients include being engrossed in watching a movie, absorbed in a book, engaged in watching a sporting event, or involved in an emotionally arousing interaction.

Imagery training includes pleasant, transformative, or contextual change imagery (Melzack and Wall 1988, Turk et al. 1983). The use of pleasant imagery is the most commonly used strategy and an approach most patients have some familiarity with before treatment. This form of imagery relies on the patients' creating a scene in their minds that is so vivid and absorbing that it is incompatible with awareness of the pain sensations. Not all images represent relaxing or pleasant associations to all patients. It is critical that patients be asked to offer personally meaningful scenes that they associate with pleasurable and calming experiences. Transformative imagery involves teaching patients how to modify the images of the pain to be less intrusive or distressful. This involves asking patients to describe what the pain feels like. If the patient describes pain in an extremity as a "burning pain," the patient is instructed to make use of imagery such as immersing the extremity in a cool mountain stream. Imagery that changes the context of the pain requires patients to tolerate the pain sensation but to imagine that the pain is associated with a different circumstance. For example, a patient with shoulder pain could imagine that he or she has been shot in the arm while protecting hostages or that he or she is a secret agent who is wounded while escaping from government forces.

Attention-diversion strategies also include focusing patients' attention on physical surroundings, thoughts, or a scientific and detached observation of the pain sensations. A patient experiencing pain could engage in mental activity such as planning the week's activities, performing mental arithmetic, or recalling the words to a favorite song or poem. Some patients can be successful in distancing themselves from the pain sensations by analyzing the sensation as if they were conducting a scientific experiment and were being totally objective about the sensations. Although all attention diversion strategies may not be effective for all patients all of the time, it is important for all team members to remind the patient that, by developing a repertoire of techniques, there is a greater likelihood that at least one technique will provide some degree of relief. Patients must be reminded that these techniques are skills that will become more effective if the patient is willing to consistently practice them.

Cognitive coping strategies include cognitive restructuring and social skills training (Holzman et al. 1986, Turk et al. 1983). These strategies focus on the patient's thoughts and feelings about pain. Cognitive restructuring is a specific application of the reconceptualization process described earlier in the chapter. Patients are invited to consider how their thoughts and images influence their pain experience. Cognitive restructuring enlists patients in challenging their beliefs or correcting the distortions in their thinking. The psychologist does not directly offer alternatives or tell patients what to do. Instead, a collaboration is emphasized in which patients are helped to create their own alternative views and competing thoughts or images.

Skills training recognizes that interactions with others cause many patients to experience increased pain and distress due to conflicts, misperceptions, and disappointments in relationships. In those situations, patients will benefit from learning assertive communication of their needs, effective expression of their feelings, and a capacity for active listening.

Rehearsal

In the rehearsal phase of cognitive-behavioral treatment, patients integrate the skills acquired in the previous stage and practice these skills in their everyday life. Several techniques of rehearsal are used in this stage, including stress inoculation, role playing, and homework.

Stress inoculation introduces patients to a plan for problem solving during episodes of increased pain. It teaches patients how to break down episodes of increased pain into several manageable stages. Patients are asked to consider the pain episode as requiring a period of preparation, an attempt to manage the sensations, an effort to cope with thoughts and feelings at critical moments, and a period of reviewing how the episode was handled. In the preparation phase, patients recognize that there are many periods when they do not experience intense pain. During this period, patients are encouraged to recognize early signs of increasing pain and to adopt a positive attitude. This stage is followed by patients noticing an increase in the pain and confronting the pain with the relaxation and distraction techniques. There will be times, however, when the strategies do not work and a patient becomes discouraged or begins to panic. At these critical moments, the patient must make use of coping statements such as "I may not eliminate this pain completely but if I persist I know I can make myself more comfortable." Finally, after the episode resolves, the patient is expected to review how the pain episode was handled and to consider what could be done differently the next time. Patients are also told that they must credit themselves with their efforts regardless of the relative effectiveness of the strategies.

Role playing is directed at consolidating patients' coping skills. Patients identify situations in which interactions with another person consistently elicit increased distress or pain (Turk et al. 1983). The situation is then reenacted with the psychologist assuming the role of the patient while the patient plays the role of the antagonist. The psychologist then attempts to model appropriate coping strategies including assertive communication, breathing exercises, and coping self-statements. A variation on role playing is role reversal in which the patient is asked to play the psychologist and the psychologist assumes the role of a new patient. In this version of role playing, the patient has an opportunity to convince the psychologist that he or she can learn to manage pain. The patient may teach the psychologist how to use the various coping strategies that the patient has learned.

Homework is an essential component of all stages of treatment. Its use can be best illustrated by its role in the rehearsal stage of cognitive-behavioral treatment, however. At this point in the treatment, patients are asked to engage in progressively more challenging tasks and activities in their everyday life. The homework assignments are concrete, observable, and measurable and are established in a graded fashion to parallel patients' progression (Turk and Rudy 1989). An example of homework is keeping a log of relaxation practice or medication use. As patients demonstrate greater proficiency in using coping strategies such as imagery or assertiveness, the homework assignments become more difficult. An example of homework assigned later in treatment is for a patient to attend a meeting with a supervisor to negotiate accommodations for the patient's work schedule or site. The more realistic assignments the patient can complete, the more self-confident he or she will feel.

Relapse Management

In this final phase of cognitive-behavioral treatment, patients are asked to focus on the circumstances that might make them prone to relapse (Holzman et al. 1986, Turk et al. 1983). This discussion is not intended to suggest to patients that they are expected to fail. Rather, it helps them recognize that they will likely experience exacerbations of their pain or that events may occur that will challenge their coping resources. Once these high-risk situations are identified, patients are encouraged to envision and plan for how they will handle that particular situation.

During this final stage of treatment, patients are asked to review what they have learned and to compare how they were feeling and functioning at the beginning of treatment with how they are currently feeling and functioning. If the patient has been maintaining a pain diary, these records should be reviewed. Ultimately, the goal of this stage of treatment is to reinforce (1) that the patient has developed coping strategies that have been effective in reducing pain perception and improving functioning, (2) that the success of these strategies has been a function of the patient's efforts, and (3) that continued success depends on use of these strategies (Holzman et al. 1986). It is generally recommended that the final stage of treatment be long enough to allow patients to adjust to managing their pain independently. At the conclusion of the formal treatment program, arrangements for follow-up should also be made with patients.

References

Bandura A. Self-efficacy: toward a unifying theory of behavioral change. Psychol Bull 1977;84:191.

Beck AT, Speer RA. Beck Depression Inventory. New York: Harcourt Brace Jovanovich, 1987.

Bergner M, Bobbitt RA, Carter WB, Gibson BS. The Sickness Impact Profile: development and final revision of a health status measure. Med Care 1981;19:787.

Bernstein DA, Borkovec TD. Progressive Relaxation Training. Champaign, IL: Research, 1973.

Bradley LA, Anderson KO, Young LD, Williams T. Psychological Testing. In CD Tollison (ed), Handbook of Chronic Pain Management. Baltimore: Williams & Wilkins, 1989;570.

Bradley LA, Haile JM, Jaworski TM. Assessment of Psychological Status Using Interviews and Self-Report Instruments. In DC Turk, R Melzack (eds), Handbook of Pain Assessment. New York: Guilford, 1992;193.

Brown GK, Nicassio PM. The development of a questionnaire for assessment of active and passive coping strategies in chronic pain patients. Pain 1987;31:53.

Cameron R, Shepel LF. The Process of Psychological Consultation in Pain Management. In AD Holzman, DC Turk (eds), Pain Management: A Handbook of Psychological Treatment Approaches. New York: Pergamon, 1986;240.

DeGood DE. A Rationale and Format for Psychosocial Evaluation. In NT Lynch, SV Vasudevan (eds), Persistent Pain: Psychosocial Assessment and Intervention. Boston: Kluwer Academic Publishers, 1988;1.

DeGood DE, Shutty MS. Assessment of Pain Beliefs, Coping, and Self-Efficacy. In DC Turk, R Melzack (eds), Handbook of Pain Assessment. New York: Guilford, 1992;214.

Derogatis L. The SCL-90R Manual—II: Administration, Scoring, and Procedures. Baltimore: Clinical Psychometric Research, 1983.

Fordyce WE. Behavioral Methods for Chronic Pain and Illness. St. Louis: Mosby, 1976.

Fordyce WE. Learned Pain: Pain as Behavior. In JJ Bonica (ed), The Management of Pain. Philadelphia: Lea & Febiger, 1990;291.

Fordyce WE, Fowler RS, DeLateur BJ. An application of behavior modification technique to a problem of chronic pain. Behav Res Ther 1968a;6:105.

Fordyce WE, Fowler RS, Lehmann JF, DeLateur BJ. Some implications of learning in problems in chronic pain. J Chronic Dis 1968b;21:179.

Fordyce WE, Fowler RS, Lehmann JF, et al. Operant conditioning in the treatment of chronic pain. Arch Phys Med Rehabil 1973;54:399.

Gottlieb BS. Development of the Pain Beliefs Questionnaire: A Preliminary Report. Paper presented at Association for the Advancement of Behavior Therapy. Philadelphia, 1984.

Gottlieb BS. Predicting Outcome in Pain Programs: A Matter of Cognition. Paper presented at the American Psychological Association. Washington, DC, 1986.

Hanson RW, Gerber KE. Coping with Chronic Pain. New York: Guilford, 1990.

Holzman AD, Turk DC, Kerns RD. The Cognitive-Behavioral Approach to Management of Chronic Pain. In AD Holzman, DC Turk (eds), Pain Management: A Handbook of Psychological Treatment Approaches. New York: Pergamon, 1986;31.

Jensen MP, Karoly P, Huger P. The development and preliminary validation of an instrument to assess patient's attitudes toward pain. J Psychosom Res 1987;31:393.

Jensen MP, Karoly P. Revision and Cross-Validation of the Survey of Pain Attitudes (SOPA). Poster presented at the 10th Annual Meeting of the Society of Behavioral Medicine. San Francisco, 1989.

Kames LD, Naliboff BD, Heinrich RL, Schag CC. The Chronic Illness Problem Inventory: problem-oriented psychosocial assessment of patients with chronic illness. Int J Psychiatry Med 1984;14:65.

Karoly P, Jensen MP. Multimethod Assessment of Chronic Pain. Oxford: Pergamon, 1987.

Keefe FJ, Brown GK, Wallston KA, Caldwell DS. Coping with rheumatoid arthritis pain: catastrophizing as a maladaptive strategy. Pain 1989;37:51.

Keefe FJ, Lefebve JC. Behaviour Therapy. In PD Wall, R Melzack (eds), Textbook of Pain (3rd ed). London: Churchill Livingstone, 1994;1367.

Kerns RD, Turk DC, Rudy TE. The West Haven-Yale Multidimensional Pain Inventory (WHYMPI). Pain 1985;23:345.

Kerns RD, Jacob MC. Assessment of the Psychosocial Context in the Experience of Pain. In DC Turk, R Melzack (eds), Handbook of Pain Assessment. New York: Guilford, 1992;235.

McCaffery M. Nursing Management of the Patient with Pain. Philadelphia: Lippincott, 1979.

Melzack R, Wall PD. Pain mechanisms: a new theory. Science 1965;50:971.

Melzack R, Wall PD. The Challenge of Pain. London: Penguin Books, 1988.

Mendelson G. Chronic Pain and Compensation Issues. In PD Wall, R Melzack (eds), Textbook of Pain (3rd ed). London: Churchill Livingstone, 1994.

Ott BD. Behavioral Interventions in the Management of Chronic Pain. In GM Aronoff (ed), Evaluation and Treatment of Chronic Pain. Baltimore: Williams & Wilkins, 1992.

Riley JF, Ahern DK, Follick MJ. Chronic pain and functional impairment: assessing beliefs about their relationship. Arch Phys Med Rehabil 1988;59:579.

Roberts AH. The Operant Approach to the Management of Pain and Excess Disability. In AD Holzman, DC Turk (eds), Pain Management: A Handbook of Psychological Treatment Approaches. New York: Pergamon, 1986;10.

Romano JM, Turner JA, Moore JE. Psychological Evaluation. In CD Tollison (ed), Handbook of Chronic Pain Management. Baltimore: Williams & Wilkins, 1989;30.

Rosenstiel AK, Keefe FJ. The use of coping strategies in low-back pain patients: relationship to patient characteristics and current adjustment. Pain 1983;17:33.

Spielberger CD. Manual for the State-Trait Inventory (Form Y). Palo Alto: Consulting Psychologists Press, 1983.

Turk DC, Michenbaum D, Genest M. Pain and Behavioral Medicine. New York: Guilford, 1983.

Turk DC, Holzman AD. Chronic Pain: Interfaces Among Physical, Psychological, and Social Parameters. In AD Holzman, DC Turk (eds), Pain Management: A Handbook of Psychological Treatment Approaches. New York: Pergamon, 1986;1.

Turk DC, Rudy TE. A Cognitive-Behavioral Perspective on Chronic Pain: Beyond the Scalpel and Syringe. In CD Tollison (ed), Handbook of Chronic Pain Management. Baltimore: Williams & Wilkins, 1989;222.

Turner JA, Clancy S. Strategies for coping with chronic low back pain: relationship to pain and disability. Pain 1986;24:355.

Williams DA, Thorn BE. An empirical assessment of pain beliefs. Pain 1989;36:351.

10 Neuroblockade Procedures

Andrew W. Sukiennik

The best outcomes in treatment of chronic pain patients are usually the result of collaboration. Depending on the complexity of a pain syndrome, one or more professionals may be required to evaluate and treat the patient. Today, approximately one-third of the members of professional societies primarily involved in the study of pain are anesthesiologists. More than 40 years ago, Dr. John Bonica, an anesthesiologist, helped establish the concept of a multidisciplinary pain clinic. As an anesthesiologist, he recognized the usefulness of neural blockade techniques to help control pain but realized that there were limitations in this approach. Neural blockade can decrease nociception but by itself is not always sufficient in improving function. It can be argued, in fact, that nerve blocks have no place at all in treatment strategies for certain chronic pain states.

Today, pain management is a recognized subspecialty of the American Board of Anesthesiology. Completion of training in the diagnosis and management of pain in an accredited fellowship program is mandatory in order for anesthesiologists to sit for the extended qualifications examination and become certified in pain management. Nerve block procedures are taught during fellowship, along with other modalities and facets of pain management. The goal of this chapter is to introduce the physical therapist to neural blockade techniques. When nociception interferes with the execution of the therapeutic plan, the physical therapist may consider referring patients to the anesthesiologist to be evaluated for this procedure in order to facilitate the continuation of therapy. The use of neuroaugmentative procedures such as dorsal column stimulation, peripheral nerve stimulation, and subarachnoid opioid infusions are discussed, since patients may occasionally be treated with these implanted devices.

The following topics are discussed in this chapter:

1. Epidural steroid injections
2. Myofascial trigger point injections
3. Peripheral nerve blocks

4. Sympathetic nerve blockade
5. Neurolytic procedures
6. Chronic neuraxial opioid infusions
7. Spinal column stimulation; neuroaugmentation

Epidural Steroid Injections

Epidural steroid injections are considered by some to be without proven effectiveness in the treatment of back pain (Fordyce 1995). Although no double-blind, crossover, randomized study has been done, there is a body of clinical evidence that suggests a role for this procedure in pain management.

The epidural space is a potential space filled with blood, lymphatic vessels, fat, and nerves traversing from the spinal cord to exit the neural foramina. During epidural steroid injections, the epidural space is entered, with or without fluoroscopy, by a technique termed *loss of resistance*. Constant pressure is applied to the syringe's plunger as a Tuohy needle is advanced. When the tip of the needle passes into a less resistant area, loss of resistance occurs, indicating that the needle tip is within the epidural space. At this point, a corticosteroid is injected alone or with a local anesthetic, and the needle is removed. Fluoroscopy is used to place the solution at a specific level (depending on the patient's signs, symptoms, and magnetic resonance imaging findings) when the patient has a spondylitic spine and to ensure proper needle placement, since false positives occur due to needle placement.

The best indication for an epidural corticosteroid injection is nerve root compression secondary to disc herniation that does not require surgery (White et al. 1980) Nerve root compression by a disc fragment is rarely helped by this procedure and may need more invasive treatments. Other spinal pain conditions are rarely helped. One exception might be the septuagenarian who has severe spondylosis, is a poor surgical candidate, and cannot tolerate drugs. In my experience, months of relief can be obtained with a series of injections (a maximum of three) in some of these patients.

There are two parts to the theory of the mechanism of corticosteroid action in reducing pain in a radiculopathy due to disc herniation. Corticosteroid acts as a membrane stabilizer and reduces nerve root swelling, allowing for less mechanical impingement of the nerve as it passes through the intervertebral foramen. Indirectly, corticosteroids reduce cellular and humoral mediators of inflammation. It has been shown by Saal (1995) that a certain enzyme within the nucleus pulposus, obtained at time of discectomy, is 20,000 times more active than in tissue taken from an injured knee at the time of arthroscopic surgery.

The patient must not be anticoagulated before the procedure. Complications of the procedure include postdural puncture headache (1%) and permanent nerve damage (0.002%) (Abram, O'Connor 1996). The headache is postural and intensified by a sitting or standing position. If conservative measures fail to alleviate the headache, a blood patch is performed. The nerve damage requires rapid (within 4–6 hours) neurosurgical decompression. Occasionally, patients may complain of increased low back pain lasting up to 3 days after the procedure. This may be due to needle trauma to the soft tissues

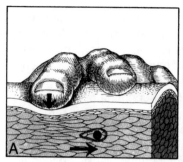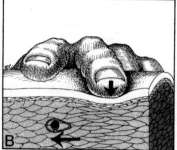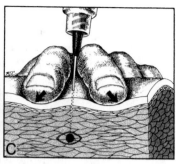

FIGURE 10.1 *Flat palpation to localize the taut band and fix the trigger point for injection. A and B. Use of alternating pressure between two fingers to confirm the location of the band. C. Positioning of the band between the fingers for injection of the trigger point that lies within the band. (Reprinted with permission from JG Travell, DG Simons. Myofascial Pain and Dysfunction: The Trigger Point Manual [Vol. I]. Baltimore: Williams & Wilkins, 1983;83.)*

or to the steroid solution itself. No clinical signs of neurologic impairment are found as a result of the procedure, but the physician should be made aware of the patient having increased blood pressure. Although there have been questions raised about the safety of steroids, an overwhelming record of safety has been seen in our clinic and by others performing this technique. Patients are usually able to resume their physical therapy the next day.

Myofascial Trigger Point Injections

Although much has been written about the diagnosis of myofascial pain disorders, their pathophysiology is still unclear. Trigger point injections used in conjunction with intensive physical therapy and stress relaxation techniques probably provide patients with the best means of managing their pain (Travell and Simons 1983). When a particularly troublesome myofascial area is refractory to physical therapy treatment, a local anesthetic injection into the trigger should be considered (Figure 10.1).

Pain is usually reduced within 5 minutes, and relief may last for more than 3 days. If needed, repeat injections can be performed twice weekly as long as they result in improved function. Some centers use a corticosteroid/local anesthetic solution, others a dry needle inserted into the muscle. Patients should resume physical therapy as soon as possible or the same day of injection.

Peripheral Nerve Blocks

Occasionally, a patient may experience such severe pain or dysfunction in a particular extremity that it is difficult or next to impossible for the patient to progress in physical therapy. For instance, a patient may have developed a frozen shoulder along with severe myofascial pain involving neck and arm musculature. To maximize soft tissue mobilization techniques, it may be necessary to reduce nociception and relax spastic musculature by injecting a weak solution of local anesthetic into the brachial plexus. Patients with a neuroma can also benefit from a combination of peripheral nerve injections and physical therapy. Some patients develop neuromas after foot surgery. This is an infrequent occurrence, but it can be quite devastating. Patients with severe complaints of neuralgic pain (e.g., shooting or electrical pain, allodynia) will inevitably avoid using their affected limb, causing deconditioning and neuromuscular imbalance. Local anesthetic blockade of the affected nerve proximal to the neuroma and around it with a corticosteroid and local anesthetic mixture usually helps to decrease pain so that the patient can more easily participate in physical therapy. When conservative methods fail, a patient may benefit from a peripheral nerve stimulator.

Nerve block procedures carry a small risk of nerve damage as a result of trauma to the nerve during needle placement, injection, or both. Currently, local anesthetic solutions used for injection allow for no longer than 10–12 hours of analgesia. New delivery technologies are being tested that may allow for a much longer duration blockade (3 days) after a single injection. The therapist must remember that proprioception may also be decreased with these injections. Avoidance of excessive ranges of motion and protection of the extremity from trauma must be monitored closely in these patients. Coordination between the therapist's schedule and the physician's must be done in order to properly carry out this combined plan of management.

Sympathetic Nerve Blockade

The diagnosis and management of reflex sympathetic dystrophy (RSD) is a controversial topic in pain management. Traditionally, whenever a cold, hot, allodynic, hyperpathic, edematous, or atrophic extremity was seen, this syndrome came to mind. In 1995, however, a task force of the International Association for the Study of Pain released a new terminology for RSD-like states in order to decrease confusion (Stanton-Hicks et al. 1995). Complex Regional Pain Syndrome (CRPS) I (RSD) and II (causalgia) are diagnoses now used to indicate that the appearance of the affected limb can be a manifestation of several disease states. Three different schools of thought still exist. The first believes that there is no evidence to support the concept that the sympathetic nervous system has anything to do with nociception. Ochoa and Verdugo (1993) cogently argue against the sympathetic model of pain. Much of Ochoa's work has looked at the function of the nociceptor (peripheral sensory organ) as a cause of CRPS (Ochoa 1986, Ochoa et al. 1989, Ochoa and Yarnitsky 1994, Ochoa and Verdugo 1993). Ochoa and others believe that the patient's "mind-brain" can also be partly (if not totally) responsible for the patient's clinical presentation. They admonish the medical community for holding on to invalid arguments and for the harm that these views have caused patients. The second group believes that experimental studies and clinical work support some role for the sympathetic nervous system in pain. Janig (1992) cites numerous experimental data that seem to implicate the sympathetic nervous system's involvement. The third group takes a moderate view. Members of this group are aware of the discrepancies in evaluation and outcomes and still subscribe to the idea of some role of the sympathetic nervous system, but with less certainty.

It is important to differentially diagnose conditions that present as CRPS. A sound evaluation of the pathophysiology of the nervous system and the psychology of the patient should be completed. A team approach in managing these patients is necessary for optimal outcome. Often patients require a hybrid program of functional restoration after their medical condition is treated.

The two most common sympathetic nerve blocks used are the cervicothoracic (stellate ganglion) and lumbar sympathetic block. The patient's skin temperature is monitored in both limbs to determine if a sympathetic block has occurred. A rise of at least 3°C signifies a successful block. The patient is told that placebo will be used at some point in the series of blocks. The patient is asked to score his or her pain on 0–10 scale after approximately 30 minutes. We have witnessed in a patient a graded response to the density of sympathetic blockade, as measured by temperature, lasting well beyond the local anesthetic or placebo effect.

Neurolytic Procedures

The use of neurolytic procedures in pain management has decreased with the increasing use of subarachnoid opioid infusions and spinal column stimulation. They are useful at times in cancer pain management and in certain benign chronic pain problems. In the elderly patient with diagnosed facet joint pain, neuroablation of the medial ramus of the posterior nerve is usually quite helpful in the few that truly suffer from this pain. A chemical or radiofrequency lesion is most often used to destroy the nerve. Some specialists use neurolysis to destroy the sympathetic innervation for months at a time. In some individuals with severe lower extremity spasticity who have lost bowel and bladder function and are wheelchair bound, subarachnoid infusion can be quite effective in reducing pain. For this procedure, the patient is placed in a sitting position, and phenol is injected into the subarachnoid space. Because phenol is denser than cerebrospinal fluid, it will bathe the cauda equina, resulting in their destruction. Peripheral nerve destruction is used less due to potential neuroma formation and deafferentation pain.

Subarachnoid Opioid Infusions

After all conservative measures fail, it may be necessary to treat a patient with subarachnoid opioid infusions to control pain. After a successful trial period of subarachnoid opioid injections, a catheter is placed in the subarachnoid space in the lumbar region and is attached to a subcutaneous pump, usually located in the abdominal region at the anterior axillary line. Morphine is often the drug used with this procedure because it travels up and down the neuraxis, exerting potent inhibitory effects on neurons located near the spinal cord's surface. Patients who undergo these procedures are usually those who cannot tolerate opioids and other medications at doses found effective to control neuropathic pain. Pain from collapsed vertebrae of an osteoporotic spine and from failed back surgery is often helped by subarachnoid morphine infusions. Paice et al. (1996) found that 61% of patients were relieved by these infusions; however, the greatest relief occurred in those who had visceral pain. Activity of daily living measures increased, and approximately half the patients noted moderate to significant improvement. Prospective studies identifying the outcomes and risks of long-term chronic opioid infusions have not been published. There are no contraindications for this technique.

Spinal Column Stimulation

Peripheral nerve stimulators are electrical devices that block nerve pain through electrical stimulation of the somatic nerve proximal to the injury. These fairly wide electrodes must be surgically placed immediately over the nerve by cutdown and exposure. A generator is placed in the extremity and tested for efficacy. The usefulness of this device lies in its ability to target only specific nerves.

Spinal column stimulation has gained in popularity with the advent of multiple-lead catheters and sophisticated microprocessor-controlled, electricity-generating devices. A percutaneously inserted catheter with the width of a plastic pen ink refill is placed behind the posterior columns of the spinal cord, within the epidural space. The position of the catheter varies with the dermatomal level of nociception. For instance, in lumbar-related radiculitis the catheter is placed so that its tip (0-electrode) lies at T10. The small electric generator is connected to the catheter and buried subcutaneously in the abdominal wall along the anterior axillary line. Sometimes, an antenna is placed subcutaneously and the generator is external with the electrical energy transmitted to the antenna underneath the skin. It is theorized that its effectiveness in controlling pain is due to release of neuropeptides that modulate pain within the spinal cord or by direct electrical stimulation of the posterior horns. This device can be used successfully for patients not helped by back surgery with associated radiculitis, plexopathies, and peripheral vascular disease (North et al. 1993). The pattern of stimulation changes with position, although ever so slightly. The patient is instructed not to participate in aggressive activities for 1 month. After this time, the device is fairly secure in its position. North et al. (1993) reported that 47% of patients are helped moderately by this procedure and that approximately 25% of these patients (10% of the sample) returned to work.

References

Abram SE, O'Connor TC. Complications associated with epidural steroid injections. Reg Anesth 1996;21:149.

Fordyce W. Back Pain in the Workplace. Seattle: IASP, 1995.

Janig W. Pathophysiological Mechanisms Operating in Reflex Sympathetic Dystrophy. In F Sicuteri, L Terenius, L Vecchiet, CA Maggi (eds), Pain Versus Man. Advances in Pain Research and Therapy (Vol 20). New York: Raven, 1992;111.

North R, Kidd D, Zahurak M, et al. Spinal cord stimulation for chronic intractable pain: experience over two decades. Neurosurgery 1993;32:384.

Ochoa JL. The newly recognized ABC syndrome: thermographic aspects. Thermology 1986;2:65.

Ochoa JL, Roberts WJ, Cline MA, et al. Two mechanical hyperalgesias in human neuropathy. Soc Neurosci Abstract 1989;15:472.

Ochoa JL, Yarnitsky D. Triple cold (CCC) syndrome: cold hyperalgesia, cold hypoesthesia, and cold skin in peripheral nerve disease. Brain 1994;117:185.

Ochoa JL, Verdugo R. Reflex Sympathetic Dystrophy: Definitions and History of the Ideas with a Critical Review of Human Studies. In P Lowe (ed), Clinical Autonomic Disorders. Little, Brown, 1993;473.

Paice J, Penn R, Shott S. Intraspinal morphine for chronic pain: a retrospective multicentered study. J Pain Symptom Manage 1996;11:71.

Saal JS. The role of inflammation in lumbar pain. Spine 1995;20:1821.

Stanton-Hicks M, Jänig W, Hassenbusch S, et al. Reflex sympathetic dystrophy: changing concepts and taxonomy. Pain 1995;63:127.

Travell JG, Simons DG (eds). Myofascial Pain and Dysfunction. The Trigger Point Manual. Baltimore: Williams & Wilkins, 1983.

White AH, Derby R, Wynne G. Epidural injections for the diagnosis and treatment of low back pain. Spine 1980;5:78.

11   Assessment and Prevention of Disability

Gerald M. Aronoff, Margaret Layden,
Ed Green, and Rosemary Goodall

This chapter reviews the assessment and prevention of disability and what
the physical therapist can do to maximize function and prevent disability in
patients with chronic pain.

Assessment of Disability

The Pain Estimate Model (Figure 11.1) is based on studies by Brena et al.
(1975) and is helpful in assessing the relationship of pain and disability in
individual patients. The findings of physical, neurologic, and radiologic
examination and laboratory studies are considered in determining a gross
pathology score and are plotted on the horizontal axis. Pain behaviors,
including pain verbalizations, activity level, medication use, and psychopathology, are plotted on the vertical axis. The four quadrants formed by
the intersecting axes represent four distinct clinical profiles and indicate
appropriate variations in treatment. Class I patients are "pain amplifiers."
Their subjective complaints and pain behaviors are disproportionate to
objective findings. These individuals frequently require more time for evaluation and treatment. These patients generally do not respond well to medical
or physical therapies if they are not accompanied by psychosocial interventions. Class II patients are "pain verbalizers," with minimal objective pathology and minimal pain behaviors. If these individuals have a relatively good
premorbid psychological profile, they can usually be expected to respond
appropriately to medical and physical therapy interventions. In the absence
of defined stressors or secondary gains, they are unlikely to have a prolonged disability disproportionate to their impairment. Class III patients are
"chronic sufferers," with significant pathology and excessive pain behavior.
These patients often have a rather poor premorbid psychological profile and

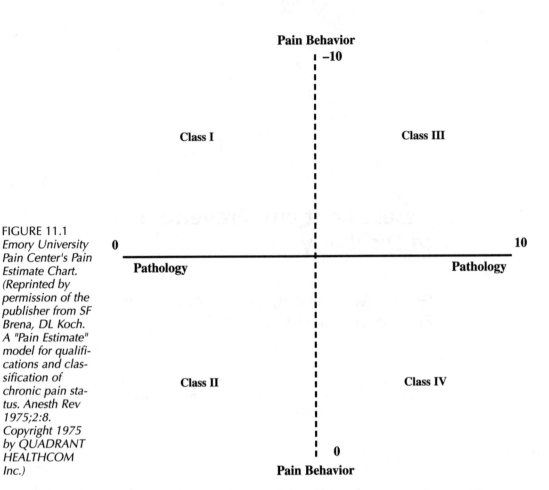

FIGURE 11.1
Emory University Pain Center's Pain Estimate Chart. (Reprinted by permission of the publisher from SF Brena, DL Koch. A "Pain Estimate" model for qualifications and classification of chronic pain status. Anesth Rev 1975;2:8. Copyright 1975 by QUADRANT HEALTHCOM Inc.)

are prone to pain symptoms and physical impairments (Blumer and Heilbronn 1982). Without psychosocial interventions, their response to treatment is generally less successful than Class II or Class IV patients. Their disability is often disproportionate to objective impairment. Class IV patients are "pain reducers," with significant objective pathology but minimal pain behaviors. These patients are highly motivated and respond appropriately or better than expected to treatment. They often view their medical problem as a challenge to be overcome and are less disabled than their impairments would suggest. Naturally, Class I and III patients are often difficult to work with because of their excessive somatizing. Even the most experienced clinicians have difficulty with these patient populations. Some of these patients are virtually untreatable without multidisciplinary treatment that includes psychotherapy. Class II patients are the least likely to develop significant disability. Although Class IV patients have objective impairments, their motivation in treatment often prevents the development of disabilities.

The results of physical therapy evaluations and functional capacity evaluations are often used to justify an impairment rating for disability determination. It is vital, therefore, that the evaluation document factors such as submaximal effort, inconsistencies in motor or sensory tests, symptom magnification, and pain behavior. Patient reports of sitting, standing, and walking tolerances must be distinguished from the therapist's observations.

Prevention of Disability

In treating patients with chronic pain, the authors favor the use of a directive return-to-work approach. Catchlove and Cohen (1982) found that when patients in a rehabilitation setting are told they are expected to return to work after completion of treatment, they are more likely to do so than when the decision is left to the patient. Furthermore, patients who were told that they were expected to return to work demonstrated the ability to remain at work and used fewer health care resources. This study demonstrates that patients will live up to expectations that they can return to a productive life. If they learn helplessness, they can become disabled unnecessarily. The belief system of clinicians treating chronic pain may be a determining variable in whether a patient is rehabilitated or remains disabled.

The Americans with Disabilities Act (ADA) (American Medical Association 1993a) is based on the belief that individuals with disabilities (including those due to chronic pain) can and should be able to return to work. Because the provisions of the ADA affect many of their patients, physical therapists should be familiar with its guidelines for returning to work. The ADA seeks to facilitate employment of qualified individuals with disabilities. A *disability* is defined in this chapter as an impairment that significantly limits an individual in one or more major activities of daily living. If a patient arrives for an appointment, it is evident that he or she is able to get out of bed, wash, dress, eat, and use transportation (possibly with assistance). This patient may have an impairment, but this does not necessarily prevent him or her from having a job. The patient may have a dysfunction of some body part and still be capable of fulfilling essential work functions. Consider the examples of a physical therapist and a typist who have both lost the third finger of the left hand. It is likely that the physical therapist could continue to do his or her job, and the typist would probably learn to use other fingers to compensate for the lost digit. Both would be considered to have an impairment but are still capable of working in the same position. They are not disabled. A concert violinist or pianist, on the other hand, may have significantly more vocational disability with such an injury.

The ADA guidelines are specifically written so that individuals with impairments are not discriminated against in the workplace. A workplace is expected to make reasonable accommodations for a person with a disability or impairment. In some cases, however, even generous accommodations will not enable the individual to perform job requirements. In this case, other types of employment should be explored. The ADA states that the employer is not required to reallocate essential job functions but that he or she can be required to make minor accommodations to allow an impaired employee to perform a particular job function. Most recommendations are comparatively inexpensive.

Therefore, chronic pain and pain-related behaviors are not necessarily impairments that prevent an individual from returning to work. Assessment of ability to function and perform activities of daily living should be done, however (American Medical Association 1993b). It has been the authors' experience that a patient who can drive to and from our pain program, actively participate throughout the 8-hour day despite complaints of pain, and return for treatment the next day is generally capable of returning to some form of work with or without accommodation. Recommendations for return to work are based on sitting, standing, and walking time; lifting capacity; and other evaluated parameters.

The physical therapist must consider whether a patient's impairments substantially limit a major life activity (e.g., sitting, standing, walking, reaching, lifting, performing manual tasks) or whether the limitations are self-imposed and are based more on cognitive distortions than actual impairment.

Although the ADA provides for physical accommodations to help a person return to work, the factors affecting a chronic pain patient's decision to return to work are complex. Several studies have been conducted on the interaction between pain-related disability, litigation, and treatment (Aronoff 1996, Brena and Chapman 1984, Ellard 1970, McGill 1968, Seres and Newman 1983). All of these studies found that to some degree psychosocial and socioeconomic variables may be more important than organic pathology in determining whether an injury results in disability. The Boeing research done by Fordyce et al. (1992) studied the relationship of industrial injuries to pain and disability. Their results indicate that mood or psychological states (as determined by the Minnesota Multiphasic Personality Inventory) may be more predictive than biomechanical or ergonomic factors in whether workers file back injury reports in many work situations. Waddell et al. (1993) found that the best predictor of the timing and likelihood of an injured individual's return to work was his or her beliefs about whether pain would increase or decrease on returning to work.

Many studies indicate that pain treatment is less successful for those receiving worker's compensation or with litigation pending (Waddell et al. 1979, Seres and Newman 1983, Aronoff et al. 1987, Leavitt et al. 1972, Aronoff 1991). Other studies, however, have reported contradictory results. Dworkin et al. (1985) found that only employment status at initial evaluation predicted treatment response in 454 chronic pain patients (employed patients had better outcomes than those not employed); neither litigation nor compensation was a significant predictor of treatment outcome. Similarly, Peck et al. (1978) and Schofferman and Wasserman (1994) found no significant effects of either litigation or representation by an attorney on the pain behaviors of patients with pending worker's compensation claims. Tollison (1993) noted an 18% higher return-to-work rate among noncompensated occupational injury patients compared with the compensated worker shortly after pain center discharge. At 6-month follow-up, there was essentially no difference in the return-to-work rate. Tollison cites the studies of Burke (1976) and Fishbain et al. (1986), who found that patients not receiving worker's compensation experience a better outcome. Trief and Stein (1985) reported that, although some clinicians would recommend withholding treatment until litigation is resolved, there have been significant behavioral

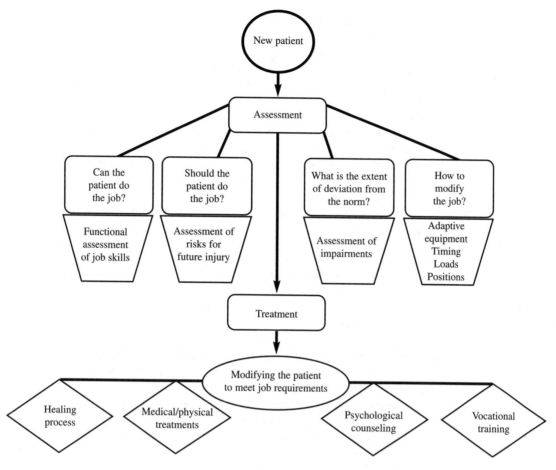

FIGURE 11.2   *Disability assessment and treatment algorithm.*

improvements in pain patients despite pending litigation. Figure 11.2 provides an algorithm of the approach to disability evaluation and treatment described in this chapter and includes the roles of psychological counseling and vocational training. The physical therapist contributes to all of the assessment steps and to the patient's physical treatment.

A detailed job description should be obtained if the patient is to return to work, and treatment should be planned accordingly. Activities and abilities the patient demonstrates in therapy that are consistent with the job description should be documented.

If the patient is resistant to functional restoration treatment, a visit to the patient's workplace may be appropriate. Mini-goals associated with work and specific measurable activities should be established.

A work site analysis is recommended if the patient is returning to work at a specific position and if the job description is not available or not specific. The site visit should include static and dynamic evaluation and assessment of the psychological environment. The static evaluation is an assessment of the patient's posture when he or she is fixed in a particular position for more than a few minutes. Any deviation from neutral position should be noted, particularly if joints must be maintained in a close-packed position. Even in relatively comfortable positions, maintained static positions should be noted so that appropriate stretching exercises may be recommended.

Maladaptive static posture may be corrected by changing the work environment. Accommodations include job restructuring (e.g., raising or lowering a platform that a person is required to load), modification of devices (e.g., providing a thicker grip for a knife or pen), and ergonomic improvements (e.g., seating support, wrist support, a springy floor covering, adaptive footwear). The patient should also make suggestions for improvements.

The dynamic evaluation assesses how the individual worker moves to accomplish certain tasks. Maintenance of neutral position, proper body mechanics, variety of movement, and the presence of a nonabrasive environment are assessed. The amount of time needed to complete a common task or the number of repetitions per minute possible for a certain task should be measured while the patient is closely observed for evidence of submaximal effort.

Maladaptive dynamic movement should be corrected by patient education, physical conditioning, or mechanical change of environment. Splinting, wearing a filter mask, altering equipment, changing procedures for a particular task, and bracketing (alternating types of tasks) are all helpful adaptations.

Measurements of heights for lifting, reaching, and climbing and of weight and force should be taken during work simulation. Having the employer videotape the job with another employee performing the patient's tasks helps the physical therapist understand the patient's job task requirements.

Determinants of psychological environment include the employer's expectations and eagerness or hesitancy about the patient's return, the changes the employer is willing to make, and the patient's attitude about his or her employer.

Remember that the patient has the most experience with his or her job. Individuals often perform extra tasks not noted on the job description or have a particular way of doing certain tasks. For example, the job description may provide for the employee to ask for help when lifting above a certain weight, but the patient has never requested this help.

The risk of returning to work should also be assessed. Objective findings may indicate that there are additional risk factors for reinjury. The risk to coworkers should also be considered. For example, if the patient is a furniture mover, there may be an increased risk that he might drop his end of the sofa causing injury to a coworker on the other end.

Goals of Rehabilitation

Chronic pain behaviors and psychopathology can contribute to and result from the suffering that accompanies chronic pain syndromes. Additional factors such as litigation, worker's compensation, and learned dependence on health care providers may also have an impact on an injured worker. Physical therapists must evaluate whether a patient's statements about inability to perform essential activities of daily living are based on objective impairment or are self-imposed due to gradually conditioned dysfunctional pain behaviors. Aronoff (1993) summarized the goals of rehabilitation this way:

> We must realize that rehabilitation is preferable to disability and improve our ability to reinstate the function and productivity of people with pain. Individualism is a process that can and must be addressed by the health care system. It remains my conviction that the individual who must endure chronic pain suffers less when his life has purpose and meaning. Gainful employment frequently serves as a distraction from pain. Rehabilitation and occupational health personnel can facilitate the return of an injured worker to employment by devising creative employment opportunities geared toward the limitation of the patient. Unfortunately, collusion between health care providers and patients sometimes results in certification of disability because of chronic pain.

The legal and judicial systems frequently become involved in the disability process. Those of us in health care should work more closely with them for the good of our patients. Individuals with legitimate painful injuries should be appropriately compensated for pain and suffering. Patients who are mercenary in their motives should be recognized and, if possible, returned to work.

References

American Medical Association. Americans with Disability Guidelines—Guide to the Evaluation of Permanent Impairment (4th ed). Chicago: American Medical Association, 1993a.

American Medical Association. Guides to the Evaluation of Permanent Impairment (4th ed). Chicago: American Medical Association, 1993b;304.

Aronoff GM. Chronic pain and the disability epidemic. Clin J Pain 1991;7:330.

Aronoff GM. Psychiatric illness, chronic pain and disability. J Disability 1993;3:63.

Aronoff GM. Pain and Disability. In SL Demeter, GBJ Anderson, GM Smith (eds), Disability Evaluation. St. Louis: Mosby, 1996;529.

Aronoff GM, McAlary PW, Witkower A, Berbell MS. Pain treatment programs: do they return workers to the workplace? A state of the art review. Spine 1987;2:123.

Blumer D, Heilbronn M. Chronic pain as a variant of depressive disease. J Nerv Ment Dis 1982;170:3686.

Brena SF, Koch DL, Moss RM. Reliability of the "Pain Estimate" model. Anesth Rev 1975;4:28.

Brena SF, Chapman SL. Pain and Litigation. In D Wall, R Melzack (eds), Textbook of Pain. New York: Churchill Livingstone, 1984;832.

Burke FD. Lumbar disk surgery: a review of a series of patients. Br J Clin Pract 1976;30:29.

Catchlove R, Cohen K. Effects of a directive return to work approach in the treatment of worker's compensation patients with chronic pain. Pain 1982;14:181.

Dworkin RH, Handlin DS, Richlin DM, et al. Unraveling the effects of compensation, litigation and employment on treatment response in chronic pain. Pain 1985;23:49.

Ellard J. Psychological reactions to compensable injury. Med J Aust 1970;2:349.

Fishbain D, Goldberg M, Mengher B. Male and female chronic pain patients categorized by DSM III psychiatric diagnostic criteria. Pain 1986;29:181.

Fordyce W, Bigos S, Battie M, Fisher L. MMPI Scale 3 as a predictor of back injury report: what does it tell us? Clin J Pain 1992;8:222.

Leavitt SS, Beyer R, Johnston TL. Monitoring the recovery process: pilot results of a systematic approach to case management. Ind Med Surg 1972;41:25.

McGill CM. Industrial back problems: a control program. J Occup Med 1968;10:174.

Peck JC, Fordyce WE, Black R. The effect of pendency of claims for compensation upon behavior indicative of pain. Wash Law Rev 1978;53:257.

Schofferman J, Wasserman S. Successful treatment of low back pain and neck pain after a motor vehicle accident despite litigation. Spine 1994;19:1007.

Seres JS, Newman RI. Negative influences of the disability compensation system: perspectives for the clinician. Semin Neurol 1983;3:4.

Tollison CD. Compensation status as a predictor of outcome in nonsurgically treated low back injury. South Med J 1993;86:1206.

Trief P, Stein N. Pending litigation and rehabilitation of chronic back pain. Arch Phys Med Rehabil 1985;66:95.

Waddell G, Kummel EG, Lotto WN, et al. Failed lumbar disc surgery following industrial injuries. J Bone Joint Surg [Am] 1979;61:201.

Waddell G, Newton M, Henderson I, et al. A Fear-Avoidance Beliefs Questionnaire (FABQ) and the role of fear-avoidance in chronic low back pain and disability. Pain 1993;52:157.

12   **Guide to Pain Treatment Facilities**

Ronald J. Kulich

The clinical focus of pain treatment facilities varies depending on the customers as well as on the bias and training of the clinicians at the facility. "Customers" include not only the patient but also the referring health care provider, employer, insurance carrier, and attorney. Because of the many different approaches to treatment offered by pain treatment facilities, it is helpful for the clinician to have certain guidelines for center classification and appropriate referral, including determining whether a pain center is multidisciplinary or unidisciplinary, determining whether the pain center's treatment approach is appropriate for the patient, and determining the center's quality of care.

The following checklist is provided for physical therapists or other clinicians who are determining the appropriate referral for a patient:

- What are the patient's problems?
- Does the patient have chronic pain syndrome?
- If the problem appears complex,
  - Is the program multidisciplinary, with full-time staff including a physical therapist and psychologist specializing in pain?
  - Does the facility have dedicated staff and space?
  - Is the staff active in patient treatment or is most treatment relegated to other in-hospital employees, residents, or trainees?
  - Are staff members active in or members of academic pain organizations?
  - Is a physical examination and medical review required on admission to the facility?
  - Are the staff employing state-of-the-art outcome measures and providing ongoing feedback to other professionals?
  - Are the staff familiar with complicating issues that may impact treatment, such as worker's compensation or disability laws?

TABLE 12.1   Chronic pain referral guide

Problem	Peripheral treatment approach	Rehabilitation/operant treatment approach	Psychologic treatment approach	Pharmacologic treatment approach	Self-help	Existence of public policy guidelines
Pain	X		X	X	X	X
Nociceptive/tissue damage	X					
Impairment	X	X	X		X	X
Perceived disability		X	X		?	X
Financial loss						X
Work disability	X					X
Medication misuse		X	X	X	?	X
Aerobic capacity		X			?	
Strength	X	X				
Range of motion	X	X				
Depression		X	X	X	X	X
Anxiety/tension		X	X	X	X	X
Sleep disorder		X	X	X	?	
Family disruption		X	X		X	
Somatization		X	X			X

Is the treatment time-limited, with specific goals for each component of treatment?

Is a structured follow-up protocol offered, particularly in cases of relapse?

What are the specific components of the relapse prevention intervention for the facility?

Types of Pain Treatment Services

A referral guide for different types of chronic pain is provided in Table 12.1.

The International Association for the Study of Pain (IASP) has identified four classifications for pain facilities. These are presented in Appendix 12.1.

The distinction between multidisciplinary and unidisciplinary approaches to treatment is important in the selection of appropriate services for a given patient. In a multidisciplinary center, a varying number of pain subspecialists work together to assess and treat complex pain patients in a coordinated fashion at a facility specifically dedicated to pain treatment. The IASP's 1991 guidelines for treatment facilities state that a pain clinic "should have access to at least three types of medical subspecialties or health care providers. Although these subspecialties are not rigidly defined, the role of physical therapy is paramount. Furthermore, if one of the physicians is not a psychiatrist, a clinical psychologist is essential." A space designated for activities, regular patient review, and interaction at multidisciplinary team meetings is also important. According to the IASP definition, the pain center should also have the capability of treating a wide range of pain disorders. The following statement summarizes the IASP (1991) guidelines:

> There is some question as to whether any pain management facilities that are not multidisciplinary should exist in a developed nation . . . the developed nations should require that any facility calling itself a pain clinic or pain center offer a multidisciplinary array of diagnostic and treatment facilities. Single modality therapy programs should be identified by the modality they utilize; e.g., "Biofeedback Clinic" rather than the term "Pain Clinic." Neurosurgeons who perform pain-relieving procedures do not call themselves a "Pain Clinic," nor should any other solitary specialist. Health care professionals who specialize in one region of the body should be identified by that region in the title; e.g., "Headache Clinic," rather than "Pain Clinic." A Multidisciplinary Pain Clinic or Center should provide comprehensive, integrated approaches to both assessment and treatment." (See Section 4, Appendix 12.1.)

Unfortunately, these recommendations for an ideal pain clinic are rarely adhered to. Although most health care providers and patients suffering from chronic pain acknowledge the multifaceted nature of the problem, most pain clinics remain unidisciplinary in nature. The trend of certifying physicians in pain management compounds the problem. Although many health care professions still hold the misconception that the single health care provider can be all things to all patients, the scientific literature and current standards of practice confirm that the solo practitioner may offer a disservice to the complex patient with chronic nonmalignant pain and disability.

Treatment objectives and content of clinical services offer another distinction between pain facilities. The referring clinician should consider these characteristics with the specific needs of the patient in mind. Many specific services can be implemented in unidisciplinary or multidisciplinary settings, although the content of some services are, by definition, multidisciplinary.

Peripheral Treatment

Peripheral (nociceptive) treatment services are commonly in unidisciplinary settings, although they are increasingly offered in multidisciplinary facilities. Peripheral approaches have the inherent assumption that the pain is treated at the site of the nociception or injury; therefore, pain centers that specialize in peripheral approaches are most appropriate for patients with trigger points, ongoing inflammatory conditions, and clear evidence of peripheral nociceptive tissue damage. Treatment objectives usually include an effort to correct structural problems or to ameliorate tissue damage or inflammation. In some cases of ongoing nociception, the objective is to block or interrupt nociceptive input to the cortex. Pain relief and reduction of impairment may be important goals, but correcting the underlying problem that is triggering nociceptive input is the critical focus of intervention. Some physical therapy approaches (see Chapter 6), use of electromyographic biofeedback (see Chapter 6), anesthesia procedures such as selective nerve blocks (see Chapter 10), and surgical ablative procedures (see Chapter 10) are all examples of peripheral (nociceptive) approaches.

Operant Treatment

The multidisciplinary rehabilitative, or operant, approach has another focus of treatment, a focus that has been classified as being "centralist" rather than "peripheral." Operant approach asserts that chronic pain is a complex phenomenon influenced by the patient's perceptual processes as well as by social and economic consequences that determine the individual's perception of pain and related disability. Pain centers that specialize in peripheral approaches are most appropriate for patients who have chronic pain but no evidence of ongoing tissue pathology. Many patients are viewed as being generally deconditioned and sometimes lacking basic coping skills that assist with a return to normal functioning. Although the operant approach does not deny the presence of nociception, disability or pain behavior is thought to be primarily reinforced by a constellation of environmental or operant factors. Hence, the patient with persistent pain engages in activity, experiences discomfort, and is "punished" for what otherwise may have been a necessary or perhaps enjoyable pursuit. The patient then engages in alternative behaviors that may foster pain relief on an intermittent basis (e.g., lying down, use of heat or pain medications, asking for assistance, stopping work) or that may terminate a negative state (e.g., pain, an undesirable job, or demands from a family member). Hence, the behavior is rewarded (negative reinforcement), and the patient engages in additional disability behavior as the reinforcement continues. Therefore, even though nociception may be present, pain behavior, functional limitations, depression, and other concomitants of pain become the primary problems facing the patient.

In distinguishing between a peripheral and centralist approach to pain, many specialists grant that there are forms of chronic pain that have an underlying central mechanism, just as patients with recurrent acute pain from underlying chronic pathologies (such as arthritis) may have long-lasting distress that results from a combination of peripheral and central causes.

Most multidisciplinary pain facilities that emphasize a centralist approach to physical rehabilitation now address treatment from a peripheral perspective as well. Areas of specific weakness, structural deficits, and tissue damage may be addressed with physical therapy interventions. Aerobic training and strengthening techniques are emphasized, however, often regardless of the site of tissue damage.

The Historical Perspective

The first multidisciplinary pain center that included rehabilitation was the University of Seattle's Multidisciplinary Pain Center, directed by John Bonica in the early 1960s. Various treatments that emphasized a structured rehabilitation approach to the problem were also being used at this time in other settings: In the early 1960s, President John F. Kennedy's physician outlined an intensive rehabilitation approach that focused on swimming and resumption of normal activity to treat Kennedy's back pain. Previous physicians had emphasized bed rest and use of invasive procedures. The centralist, rehabilitation approach was much more successful.

Almost all multidisciplinary pain rehabilitation programs in the 1970s were inpatient facilities, with intensive multidisciplinary diagnostic and treatment services provided daily for as long as 2 months (Brena 1992). The patients entering the program were usually diagnosed with chronic pain syndrome.

In 1982, the Commission on the Accreditation of Rehabilitation Facilities (CARF) began certifying multidisciplinary inpatient programs and enacting limited standardization measures. It was initially mandated that all outpatient certified programs operate on a full-time basis 5 days per week. These guidelines have changed over the years to reflect the fact that different patient populations may not require such intensive services. Also, further emphasis has been placed on adequacy of assessment and ongoing measurement of treatment outcome.

In the mid-1980s, changes in reimbursement policies and the desire for services in community hospital and rural settings caused many inpatient programs to be shortened to 2 weeks and offer fewer services. Patients increasingly sought treatment at the outpatient pain centers that were being established across the United States. Many of these centers sought CARF certification, and programs began to focus more on the occupationally injured patient. Return to work was considered a primary treatment objective for many programs and continues to be so today.

Mayer (1988) and associates developed a program that retained the same operant theoretical underpinnings of earlier rehabilitation-oriented pain centers. However, they placed an increased focus on returning to work and on supplemented services with more intensive, goal-directed conditioning. The term *functional restoration* was used to describe these services, thereby emphasizing a return to function rather than pain relief. Multidisciplinary outpatient facilities that emphasized use of "high-tech" exercise equipment were developed.

During this time, psychologist Leonard Matheson was developing purely work-oriented rehabilitation services known as *work hardening*. (Matheson 1984, Matheson et al. 1985). The approach, considered nonpsychological, focused less on functional rehabilitation for goals unrelated to work. These largely unidisciplinary programs were staffed mostly by occupational or physical therapists. Objective work goals were outlined, and patients began a daily routine of work-task simulation. The patient's hours of participation are increased until they are ready to resume normal work. Simulated work tasks are similar to actual physical job demands, and close coordination with the work site is emphasized. A staff accreditation system has been developed, largely through the efforts of Matheson and his colleagues. Unfortunately, work hardening programs have not undergone the scientific scrutiny of controlled outcome studies, and reports of effectiveness often are anecdotal. Multidisciplinary pain rehabilitation centers, functional restoration programs, and work-hardening programs have undergone significant downsizing. Costly equipment has been abandoned in favor of simpler simulation tasks and more rapid integration into the work site, with patients undergoing a graded or gradual return to work. The term *work conditioning* has been developed to better describe and market these reduced intensity efforts. Other terms have been used to describe these programs, although the concept and mode of service delivery remain essentially the same.

Functional restoration and work-hardening programs have sometimes been faulted for not admitting complex or severely disabled patients, who typically participate in traditional multidisciplinary pain rehabilitation programs. Comparatively better outcomes may occur because of the higher baseline function of patients in the former programs. Unfortunately, there are no investigations that compare facilities while taking into account the varying disability levels of patients.

Psychological Approaches

Formalized psychological treatment of pain using a scientific basis began to be used at the beginning of this century (Morris 1991). Early efforts focused on the role of hypnosis, placebo, and suggestion in the amelioration of pain, with placebo and suggestion as recognized and active components of all rehabilitation team treatments. Fordyce (1976) developed the learning theory model of operant pain behavior. This model is the basis of many multidisciplinary pain rehabilitation and functional restoration programs and is usually considered to be more rehabilitative than psychological. Pain centers that specialize in psychological approaches are most appropriate for patients with chronic pain without objective findings of ongoing tissue damage.

Results of unidisciplinary psychological and psychoeducational treatments have been reported for years, with an emphasis on time-limited group interventions (Flor et al. 1992). These are strategies that primarily focus on pain reduction and improved perceived control over pain through relaxation, distraction, or cognitive coping skills. Hypnosis and self-hypnosis often are considered as variations of relaxation training. Some psychological treatment programs focus on pain relief, whereas others focus on increasing perceived control over function despite pain (Kulich and Gottlieb 1985). Because patients with acute or chronic pain often feel disempowered, treatment involves engaging the patient in techniques that emphasize self-control. Anxiety and depression, which are often concomitants of pain, are treated, and emotional improvement is realized when the patient increases involvement in enjoyable activity and reduces anxiety about reinjury. Unidisciplinary short-term group psychosocial programs, which are less expensive than long-term multidisciplinary programs, are currently being studied most and are reported in the scientific literature. Group sessions may be held for 6–10 weeks, usually on a weekly basis. This method has been effective in treating depression associated with pain. Pain relief and patient satisfaction have been greater in these programs than in traditional individual psychotherapy. Outcome studies demonstrate that cognitive and relaxation procedures may be cost-effective, particularly for patients with a less severe level of physical and emotional dysfunction than is evident in patients with chronic pain syndrome or those patients typically seen in a multidisciplinary pain center. Some managed care organizations have embraced this as a cost-conscious approach, although attempts to screen for patients who may be better treated in more intensive rehabilitation programs have been lacking.

Pharmacologic Approaches

Pharmacologic approaches to pain treatment primarily provide pain relief or target coexisting problems such as sleep disruption, depression, and anxiety. To some extent, all treatment facilities use pharmacologic approaches. Pain medications may be over- or underprescribed to chronic pain patients so that an appropriate adjustment in pharmacology is emphasized. Analgesics can be helpful in chronic pain, and a thorough discussion is provided in Chapter 3. Oral analgesics that have been shown to be effective in alleviating mild to moderate pain, such as nonsteroidal anti-inflammatory drugs, aspirin, and acetaminophen, are usually tried first. Second-tier analgesics include oral opiates; the third-tier analgesics include alternate methods of delivery such as transdermal opioids (fentanyl), subcutaneous infusion, intravenous infusion, and other more invasive routes of delivery (Carr et al. 1994). The decision about who is treated with second- and third-tier analgesics should be made by pain rehabilitation team members, who consider why the patient's pain is not responsive to first-tier drugs and whether pharmacologic approaches make sense in the context of other treatments and psychosocial issues in a given patient. Operant and functional restoration programs often have resisted use of analgesics, viewing their use as a pain behavior. The use of analgesics has become more accepted, however, particularly when they are used on a time-contingent rather than pain-contingent basis. Opioid use for nonmalignant chronic pain is increasingly accepted in all facilities. Treatment guidelines for the use of opioids in chronic noncancer pain have been established and a report from the IASP (Schug and Large 1995) provides the most thorough review and recommendations (see Tables 3.1 and 3.2).

In addition to analgesics, other pharmacologic agents with pain-relieving properties are used to alleviate pain, including anticonvulsants and antipsychotic medications, and may be particularly helpful in neuropathic pain conditions. Most commonly, tricyclic antidepressants have been prescribed for symptoms associated with pain such as sleep disorder, depression, and anxiety, although these drugs have also been reported to demonstrate analgesic effect. More recently, the selective serotonin reuptake inhibitors (e.g., venlafaxine [Effexor], paroxetine [Paxil]) have been used due to their effectiveness with fewer side effects. Benzodiazapines have been shown to be less effective for long-term use with chronic pain, although there are exceptions. Summarizing recent investigations, Haddox (1996) commented that "most authors recognize the usefulness of these drugs for short-term indications but feel there is little benefit from using benzodiazepines in the management of chronic pain."

Self-Help Approaches

Most, if not all, pain treatment facilities find their efforts with chronic pain patients to be greatly enhanced by self-help organizations. The American

Chronic Pain Association has branches across the United States and internationally. Support groups are led by patients and focus on reinforcement of coping skills for management of pain and related symptoms. Meetings generally take place outside of medical settings in order to encourage a wellness model. Many other support organizations focus on specific types of chronic pain, including the Reflex Sympathetic Dystrophy Association; Interstitial Cystitis Foundations; the National Chronic Pain Outreach Association; Fibromyalgia Foundation; and the Jaw, Joints, and Allied Musculoskeletal Disorders Foundation. There are no outcome studies available on the benefits of participation in such groups. Although many patients may benefit from participation, some groups may unwittingly reinforce disability behavior or treatment interventions that lack proven efficacy. Increasing communication between pain specialists and the support group organizations is beginning to address this possible problem. These support organizations also are advocates for access to proper treatment (Appendix II).

Factors Influencing Quality of Care

Economic conditions and public policy influence return-to-work rates, reduction of pain-related suffering, and pain relief. Clinicians treating chronic pain should familiarize themselves with state and federal laws governing occupational and liability claims, as well as documentation standards for assessment of impairment and disability. The Americans with Disabilities Act (ADA) offers some protection to individuals suffering from chronic pain (for a discussion of the ADA, see Chapter 11). Public policy studies have shown that modifications in worker compensation and health care delivery systems for chronic pain can result in reduced costs and more rapid return-to-work rates.

Although malingering, or conscious feigning of symptoms, is rare, success with a given treatment intervention is often affected by issues of job satisfaction, fears of financial ruin, anger at others who may have "caused" the patient's problem, or despair because the employer "failed to call or make contacts" after the worker's injury. An effective treatment plan must involve all individuals who have an impact on the patient's treatment, including the attorney, insurance adjuster, rehabilitation nurse, and employer.

To provide standards for service and associated fees for multidisciplinary facilities specifically in the area of pain treatment, CARF developed a certification program in the early 1980s. Standards for work services, industry-based programs, and other related facilities have also been formulated. Since the certification has been offered, the majority of programs seeking certification have been rehabilitation-based. Because of the complexity and costs of the services required by the guidelines, insurers did not wholeheartedly endorse the certification standards, and recent modifications have been made to certify scaled-down facilities. Although standards have developed from a consensus of clinicians in the pain field, studies demonstrating better outcomes for pain management are lacking.

Several directories are available that list information about pain treatment facilities. The first organization to offer a facilities directory was the American Society of Anesthesiologists in 1977. The American Pain Society and the American Academy of Pain Medicine offer directories containing information provided voluntarily by the pain centers listed. Similarly, Oryx Press published *Directory of Pain Treatment Centers in the United States and Canada* in 1989 (Muir 1989). Although the compilers of these directories acknowledge limitations, the existing directories have been disappointing at best, and their publication may be a disservice because of the inaccuracies and exaggerations of those listing their services.

Efforts to certify clinicians have increased since the late 1980s. The concept of certification in pain medicine was first proposed in 1983 by the American Society of Algology, which has since been renamed the American Academy of Pain Medicine. This group requires an examination, and certification is restricted to physicians with specialty training in certain areas. The American Academy of Pain Management (AAPM) was also formed in order to offer certification. The initial "grandfathering" of many pain specialists and the policy of including nonphysicians as members caused much initial controversy. The AAPM now also offers a certification examination. Specialty exams also are available in single-discipline medical societies, such as the American Society of Regional Anesthesia. Similar certification is available in dentistry, with a focus on craniomandibular disorders and pain. Studies do not show that certified providers are necessarily better, and it has been argued that certification can obscure the multidisciplinary model. Currently, there is no requirement that certified practitioners adhere to the 1991 IASP facilities guidelines, and unidisciplinary pain clinics staffed by a single certified practitioner appear to be the norm rather than the exception.

Several academic pain societies focus primarily on communication among pain specialists, encouragement of pain research and education, and dissemination of information. The IASP has members in more than 60 countries. The American Pain Society (APS) is one of 19 national chapters in the IASP with members in each state. The APS hosts a well-attended annual meeting, and membership is open to all pain specialists regardless of discipline. Regional academic and educational societies are also active, including the New England Pain Association, Eastern Pain Society, Philadelphia Pain Society, Western Pain Society, and Southern Pain Society. Other more specialized societies such as the American Association for the Study of Headache also exist. As with any field, membership and participation in academic societies does not ensure that the clinician or facility delivers the optimum clinical care. One should, however, question the standard of care in facilities with staff who fail to participate in educational efforts offered by multidisciplinary societies.

The Future of Pain Treatment Facilities

Many issues create obstacles for successful outcomes in pain treatment, regardless of the type of treatment facility. It is unlikely that patients suffering from chronic pain and pain-related disability will ever be a viable political force in the health care arena. Although it is easy for the general population to identify with the suffering of a cancer patient or a patient with medically complicated diseases, a diagnosis of chronic pain syndrome fails to raise concern from the general population. A pain patient is typically blamed for his or her plight, and organized health care efforts often complicate the problem by relabeling the patient's disorder as a psychiatric disorder. This can reduce costs for the insurance carrier, since psychiatric services have lower reimbursement rates than other services. Even health care providers are often cynical and reluctant to treat patients with chronic pain and disability. Few physical therapists have sought to specialize in this area.

Although some pessimism is warranted, some promising changes can be expected in the next 10–15 years. Multidisciplinary inpatient services will probably be restricted to patients who have unstable adjunct medication conditions that cannot be treated on an outpatient basis. Their treatment will probably be brief, with rapid transition to an outpatient pain facility. Many inpatient programs are now closing their doors; others are transforming themselves to meet the needs of a population with significant medical illness.

Pain treatment facilities will need to address return-to-work issues, which will continue to be determined by economic and public policy factors independent of any particular clinical intervention. With increasing changes in worker compensation laws and recognition that returning to work is often beneficial to many patients, periods of work-related disability are currently decreasing. In turn, more aggressive use of the ADA for patients who suffer from persistent pain and pain-related limitations can be expected. Requirements for modified work duty and accommodations are increasing. The clinician treating the patient with pain should reinforce these changes and accommodations for modified work duty.

Invasive procedures will likely continue to be a focus of treatment at many clinics, although methods for screening and use of objective quality of life scales and functional indicators will probably replace current informal outcome measures such as pain rating scales. Expensive procedures such as spinal column stimulation will likely be performed by multidisciplinary specialty teams rather than in unidisciplinary pain clinics.

Psychological and physical therapy interventions will continue to be increasingly used, in part because of their comparatively low cost.

The immediate future of pharmacologic treatment of chronic pain is clear. Although more specifically targeted medications will continue to be developed, opioids will still be important in the treatment of chronic nonmalignant pain. Health care providers are increasingly acceptant of opioid use for chronic nonmalignant pain, despite a decidedly slower positive response from state regulators. Therefore, analgesic use will be a part of behavioral therapies in pain treatment facilities in the future.

The future of formal functional restoration and outpatient pain rehabilitation programs may be less clear. These programs now treat the most intractable cases, and functional outcome results have been promising. However, patient satisfaction might be achieved with less cost using unidisciplinary efforts such as opioid maintenance or psychological group treatments. If a sufficient population continues to view pain from a centralist perspective and sees functional rehabilitation as important, these programs will continue to be used widely.

References

Brena SF, Sanders SH. Are pain clinics in crisis? Problems and strategies for prosperity. APS Bull 1992;2:1.

Carr DB, Jacox AK, Payne R. Management of Cancer Pain. Clinical Practice Guidelines. Rockville, MD: Agency for Health Care Policy and Research, Publication No. 94-0592. U.S. Dept. of Health and Human Services, 1994.

Flor H, Fydrich T, Turk DC. Efficacy of multidisciplinary pain treatment centers: a meta-analytic review. Pain 1992;49:221.

Fordyce WE. Behavioral Methods for Chronic Pain and Illness. St. Louis: Mosby, 1976.

Haddox JD. Coanalgesic Agents. In PP Raj (ed), Pain Medication: A Comprehensive Review. St. Louis: Mosby–Year Book, 1996;142.

International Association for the Study of Pain. Task Force Guidelines for Desirable Characteristics for Pain Treatment Facilities. Seattle: IASP, 1991.

Kulich RJ, Gottlieb BA. Cognitive Functioning Approach for Chronic Pain Management. In D Upper, S Ross (eds), Handbook of Behavioral Group Therapy. New York: Plenum, 1985;489.

Matheson LN. Work Capacity Evaluation: Interdisciplinary Approach to Industrial Rehabilitation. Anaheim, CA: Employment and Rehabilitation Institute of California, 1984.

Matheson LN, Dempster Ogden L, Violette K, Schultz K. Work hardening: occupational therapy in industrial rehabilitation. Am J Occup Ther 1985;39:314.

Mayer TG, Gatchel RJ. Functional Restoration for Spinal Disorders: The Sports Medicine Approach. Philadelphia: Lea & Febiger, 1988.

Morris DB. The Culture of Pain. Los Angeles: University of California Press, 1991.

Muir RG (ed). Directory of Pain Treatment Centers in the United States and Canada. Phoenix: Oryx, 1989.

Schug SA, Large RG. Opioids for chronic noncancer pain. Pain Clin Updates 1995;3:3.

Pain Facilities Classifications

The International Association for the Study of Pain has identified four classifications for pain facilities:

   1.   *Modality-oriented clinic.* This is a health care facility that offers a specific type of treatment and does not provide comprehensive assessment or management. Examples include a nerve block clinic, acupuncture clinic, or a biofeedback clinic. Such a facility may have one or more health care providers with different professional training; because of its limited treatment options and the lack of an integrated, comprehensive approach, it does not qualify for the term *multidisciplinary.*

   2.   *Pain clinic.* A health care delivery facility focusing on the diagnosis and management of patients with chronic pain. A pain clinic may specialize in specific diagnoses or in pains related to a specific part of the body. A pain clinic may be large or small but it should never be a label for an isolated solo practitioner. A single physician functioning within a complex health care institution that offers appropriate consultative and therapeutic services could qualify as a pain clinic, if chronic pain patients were suitably assessed and managed. The absence of interdisciplinary assessment and management distinguishes this type of facility from a multidisciplinary pain center or clinic. Pain clinics can, and should be encouraged to, carry out research, but it is not a required characteristic of this type of facility.

   3.   *Multidisciplinary pain clinic.* A health care delivery facility staffed by physicians of different specialties and other non-physician health care providers who specialize in the diagnosis and management of patients with chronic pain. This type of facility differs from a multidisciplinary pain center only because it does not include research and teaching activities in its regular programs. A multidisciplinary pain clinic may have diagnostic and treatment facilities that are outpatient, inpatient, or both.

   4.   *Multidisciplinary pain center.* An organization of health care providers and basic scientists that includes research, teaching and patient care related to acute and chronic pain. This is the largest and most complex of the pain treatment facilities and ideally would exist as a component of a medical school or teaching hospital. Clinical programs must be supervised by an appropriately trained and licensed clinical director. A wide array of health care specialists is required, such as physicians, psychologists, nurses, physical therapists, occupational therapists, vocational counselors, social workers, and other specialized health care providers.

The many disciplines of health care providers required are a function of the varieties of patients seen and the health care resources of the community. The members of the treatment team must communicate with each other on a regular basis, both about specific patients and about overall development. Health care services in a multidisciplinary pain clinic must be integrated and based upon multidisciplinary assessment and management of the patient. Inpatient and outpatient programs are offered in such a facility.

Reprinted with permission from the International Association for the Study of Pain. Task Force Guidelines for Desirable Characteristics for Pain Treatment Facilities. Seattle: IASP, 1991.

Appendixes

Pain Curriculum for Students in Occupational Therapy or Physical Therapy

Introduction

A. *Overview of roles and responsibilities of occupational therapists and physical therapists.* Pain is a common problem for many of the clients/patients seen by occupational therapists and physical therapists. For these clients/patients, the primary therapeutic objectives are reduction of pain and associated disability, promotion of optimal function in everyday living, and development of meaningful family and social relationships. Promotion of health and well-being through prevention of pain and disability or handicap resulting from pain is a fundamental concern. It is essential that occupational therapists and physical therapists take a holistic and collaborative view of the needs of the client/patient with pain. Therapists should be able to recognize the numerous misconceptions that prevail about pain and people with pain and be able to refute and challenge their existence.

The professions of occupational therapy and physical therapy vary in their underlying theoretical foundations and in their overall approach to pain.

Occupational therapists are primarily concerned with the psychosocial and environmental factors that contribute to pain and the impact of pain on the individual's everyday life. Their roles and responsibilities include the following:

1. Assessment of the impact of pain on occupational performance in the areas of self-care, paid and unpaid work, interests and leisure pursuits, customary habits and routines, and family relationships. Assessment will include evaluation of psychosocial and environmental factors aggravating pain in the home and workplace.

2. In collaboration with the client/patient, development of an occupational therapy program to increase self-esteem, restore self-efficacy, and promote optimal occupational function despite pain. Intervention strategies may include assistive devices and adaptive equipment; purposeful and productive occupations and activities; and vocational rehabilitation or work hardening to improve endurance and work skills and reestablish roles, habits, and rou-

tines of everyday life. Education about pain and supportive individual, family, or group counseling are utilized as needed.

3. Liaison and referral within an interdisciplinary team approach.

Physical therapists apply a wide range of physical and behavioral treatments to reduce pain and prevent dysfunction. Their roles and responsibilities include the following:

1. Assessment of the primary and secondary chemical (infection and inflammation), biomechanical (stress and strain), and behavioral factors that contribute to pain, the pain activity cycle, and overall function.

2. In collaboration with the client/patient, development of a physical therapy program directed at modification of the effect of primary and secondary contributors to pain, promotion of tissue healing, and reduction of the factors that may lead to the recurrence of pain and dysfunction. Intervention may include education; exercise; manual therapy; movement facilitation techniques; and application of electro/physical agents based on thermal, mechanical, electrical, or phototherapeutic modalities. Education is focused on understanding pain and on improved posture, body mechanics, and gait. Exercise is directed toward the strengthening of specific muscle groups as well as counteracting the effects of generalized deconditioning. Movement is used as a mechanism to control and decrease pain and to increase mobility.

3. Liaison and referral within an interdisciplinary team approach.

Cognitive-behavioral strategies and supportive/educational approaches for pain management may be implemented by occupational and physical therapists to reduce pain and improve function and overall quality of life. Therapists from either profession have a common commitment to person-centered care, the promotion of health and well-being, and the prevention of long-term disability and handicap resulting from pain. Family education is an integral component of therapeutic programs.

To carry out professional responsibilities for clients with pain, occupational therapists and physical therapists must have an understanding of the physiologic basis and the psychological and environmental components of pain and their impact on pain experience across the life span. Therapists should be familiar with pain assessment and measurement approaches and should be able to implement a broad variety of management strategies from their specific professional orientations. While neither occupational therapists nor physical therapists are responsible for pharmacologic management, they should have sufficient knowledge about pharmacologic agents and their side effects to act as advocates for optimal pharmacologic management and to support proper use of medication by clients/patients.

B. *Overview of the interdisciplinary pain curriculum for students in occupational therapy or physical therapy.* This pain curriculum is designed as an interdisciplinary course of study to support and encourage professional collaboration. The focus of the course is on the pain experience of clients/patients and the physiologic, psychosocial, and environmental components of that experience, with an application of profession-specific theoretical frameworks to assess and manage pain and the impact of pain on everyday life. In this respect, this course presents new knowledge that will be applicable to students in either occupational therapy or physical therapy. However, in some educational programs, it may not be feasible or practical to offer this course in an interdisciplinary framework.

Inclusion of specific management strategies, as detailed in this curriculum, may depend on whether these strategies have been previously examined in other course work. Review of interventions rather than detailed instruction of each management strategy is expected in this course. Course instructors should modify management strategies where necessary if this curriculum is presented as a profession-specific course.

Students should be familiar with the theoretical models behind interventions as well as the empirical evidence of effectiveness of any management strategies. Course instructors are encouraged to adopt a critical appraisal perspective as a basis for decision making when reviewing the benefits and limitations of interventions.

Occupational therapy and physical therapy programs have different clinical areas of priority for student education. A suggested list of common pain problems for discussion according to definition, prevalence, clinical features, and possible interventions is included. The relevance of these pain problems within the curriculum should be decided by individual course instructors. All pain terminology and definitions used in this course should be consistent with Merskey and Bogduk (1994), *Classification of Chronic Pain: Descriptions of Chronic Pain Syndromes and Definition of Pain Terms.*

Considerable variation exists from country to country in the academic structure of professional programs for occupational therapy or physical therapy and in the professional expectations of an entry-level therapist. Faculty in occupational therapy and physical therapy programs should incorporate the specific content of this pain curriculum within their programs using whatever structural and educational approaches would be the most appropriate to meet local professional and program needs. However, this curriculum is designed to be most appropriate for students who have previously completed courses in anatomy, physiology, kinesiology or movement, and the majority of their professional therapeutics courses. In a traditional curriculum format, completion of this curriculum as constructed would require two semesters in a senior year and would be the approximate equivalent of a four– to six–credit hour course.

Course Objectives

Upon completion of this course, the occupational therapy or physical therapy student will

1. Understand the current theories of the anatomic, physiologic, and psychological bases of pain and pain relief.
2. Recognize how age, gender, family, culture, spirituality, and the environment contribute to the pain experience and must be considered in assessment and management of pain.
3. Be able to assess the pain experience and resulting therapeutic needs for an individual according to an occupational therapy or physical therapy framework.
4. Recognize the differences between acute and chronic pain and their implications for assessment and management of pain.
5. Emphasize performance of a comprehensive evaluation and treatment in the acute pain phase to prevent the onset of chronicity.
6. Be familiar with the reliability, validity, benefits, and limitations of self-report, behavioral, and physiologic measures to assess and measure pain, pain experience, and impact of pain on everyday life.
7. Use a person-centered perspective to formulate collaborative intervention strategies consistent with an occupational therapy or physical therapy perspective.
8. Adopt a critical appraisal perspective toward the use of assessment and intervention strategies and outcome measures.
9. Understand the prevention of pain problems in the home and workplace within a framework of health promotion and illness prevention.
10. Be familiar with the roles and responsibilities of other health care professionals in the area of pain management and the merits of interdisciplinary collaboration.
11. Recognize the changing nature of knowledge about underlying pain mechanisms and the importance of ongoing pain education.

Course Outline

I. Introduction
   A. Definition of pain as a multidimensional experience
   B. The epidemiology of pain as a public health problem with social, ethical, and economic considerations
   C. Barriers to pain assessment and management
   D. Role of occupational therapy and physical therapy in pain care (complementary roles)
II. Nature of pain
   A. Historical theories
      1. Descartes' theory of pain
      2. Gate control theory of pain

B. Physiologic basis of pain
 1. Peripheral and central mechanisms (including nociceptive events, ascending and descending pathways, effects of inflammation and tissue damage on nociceptors, nerve trauma and entrapment, central and peripheral sensitization)
 2. Biochemical and biomechanical nociception
 3. Sympathetic nervous system mechanisms in pain
 4. Tonic and phasic pain
 5. Referred pain (visceral and somatic pain)
 6. Physiologic and pathologic effects of unrelieved pain
 7. Trigger point mechanisms (e.g., myofascial pain)
 8. Postural components (home and work)
C. Distinction among acute, recurrent, and chronic pains
 1. Definitions and classifications of acute and chronic pains
 2. Impact on physiology of pain
 3. Impact on psychological response to pain
 4. Specific pain definitions including pain threshold, pain tolerance, and pain endurance
D. Psychological and behavioral components of pain experience and relationship to acute or chronic nature of pain
 1. Anxiety, fear, crisis reactions, stress
 2. Impact on spirituality and meaningfulness, hope and hopelessness
 3. Psychological effect of unrelieved pain on perceptions of control and self-efficacy
 4. Depression, wish to die, suicidal risks
 5. Impact of persistent pain on habits, roles, occupational performance, and future quality of life
 6. Personality and gender influences on pain experience
E. Environmental components of pain experience
 1. Family and social influences
 2. Ethnic and cultural considerations
F. Interaction of physiologic basis of pain with psychological and environmental components and their impact on pain perception and pain response
III. Pain across the life span (physiologic and psychosocial factors, implications for assessment, measurement, and intervention)
 A. Pain in infancy, childhood, and adolescence
 B. Pain in the elderly
IV. Assessment and measurement of pain
 A. Application of professional models to assessment of pain (e.g., in occupational therapy, the models of human occupation and occupational performance; in physical therapy, the orthopedic model, the acute pain model, and movement theory)
 B. World Health Organization model of impairment, disability, and handicap
 C. Utility, reliability, and validity of pain measures

D. Self-report measures as the gold standard of measurement for pain intensity, location, quality, temporal variation, chronology of pain, and factors that increase or decrease pain

E. Behavioral and physiologic measures

F. Benefits and limitations of measurement strategies for acute, recurrent, or chronic pain

G. Assessment of pain impact on daily life and quality of life
    1. Using daily diary recording of pain, activity level (including self-care, work, leisure activities, exercise)
    2. Changes in routines, roles, and skills

H. Meaning of pain behavior considering age of the individual, nature of pain, and contextual characteristics of the pain

I. Assessment and measurement of pain when the client has communication problems due to age, language, or physical/cognitive difficulties

J. Outcome measures

V. Management of pain and prevention of negative consequences of pain on everyday life occupations/activities

A. Person-centered intervention through collaborative goals using concepts and strategies from clinical reasoning to understand the experience and needs of a person with pain

B. Principles of critical research appraisal and application to clinical decision making

C. Principles of a therapeutic milieu to reduce pain and promote optimal function
    1. Trust and honesty
    2. Control and predictability
    3. Anticipating when pain may occur
    4. Using baseline and daily measures of pain and activity
    5. Developing a daily routine to support readjustment of habits and roles according to individual capacity and life situation
    6. Modification of physical and psychosocial factors that promote pain or negative consequences of pain on daily life
    7. Involvement of family members and significant others
    8. Encouragement of active over passive participation
    9. Communication and team process

D. Using an interdisciplinary team approach
    1. Roles and responsibilities of the health care team

E. Consideration of management strategies according to nature of pain (acute, recurrent, or chronic) and the client's statement of needs

F. Group approaches for education, support, and encouragement

G. Cognitive-behavioral interventions
    1. Setting short- and long-term goals
    2. Developing a daily routine
    3. Pacing of activities
    4. Coping strategies and appraisals
    5. Distraction
    6. Relaxation

      7. Visual imagery
      8. Play and art
      9. Use of meaningful occupations/activities
H. Operant strategies to support effective coping strategies
I. Physical interventions
      1. Movement to control pain
      2. Exercise to correct posture and improve strength
      3. Movement and exercise to improve self-esteem, restore self-efficacy, normalize body awareness, and promote optimal function
      4. Heat and cold
      5. Massage
      6. Mobilizations/manipulation
      7. Transcutaneous electrical nerve stimulation and other electrical protocols
      8. Biofeedback
      9. Laser
    10. Acupuncture
    11. Spray and stretch
    12. Biomechanical therapies
    13. Other interventions (ultrasound, rolfing, shiatsu, pulsed electromagnetic fields, McKenzie's techniques, Alexander techniques, trager, muscle energies, myofascial release and craniosacral techniques, mobilization of the nervous system)
J. Assistive devices and adaptive equipment
      1. Benefits and limitations
K. Reintegration into work (paid and unpaid employment)
      1. Work assessment, work hardening
      2. Application of ergonomic principles
      3. Reducing pain-producing hazards
      4. Work simplification
      5. Using groups to support reintegration to work
      6. Litigation and compensation and possible medicolegal implications for clients/patients and therapists
L. Back care
      1. Reducing hazards to good back care
      2. Posture in standing, sitting, and sleeping
      3. Strategies for bending, lifting, and reaching
      4. Building exercise and relaxation into daily life
M. Sleep
      1. Alternatives to medication
      2. Creating a sleep environment for restorative sleep
      3. Readjusting the biological clock
      4. Sleep problems and relationship to somaticovisceral pain
N. Role of pharmacologic approaches
      1. Principles of administration
      2. Nonsteroidal ani-inflammatory drugs, opioids, adjunctive medications, and other alternatives
      3. Modes of administration

4. Side effects
5. Tolerance, physical dependence, psychological dependence, and drug-seeking behavior
6. Addiction risks
7. Patient-controlled analgesia
8. Role of occupational therapy and physical therapy in supporting optimal pharmacologic strategies
O. Nutrition and diet
P. Intimacy and sexuality
Q. Placebo effect of management strategies
VI. Common pain problems (definition, prevalence, clinical features, possible interventions)
A. Migraine and headache
B. Back and neck pain
C. Musculoskeletal pains (arthritis, fibromyalgia, myofascial pain, reflex sympathetic dystrophy, temporomandibular dysfunction)
D. Neuralgias
E. Pain associated with burns
F. Pain associated with progressive disease, terminal illness (cancer), palliative care
G. Pain and psychiatric illness
H. Pain in acquired immunodeficiency syndrome
I. Pain due to health care procedures
VII. Service delivery
A. Traditional pain management model, multidisciplinary pain treatment clinics and facilities, modality-specific practice
B. Ethical and legal standards of pain management

Reprinted with permission from the International Association for the Study of Pain. Ad Hoc Subcommittee for Occupational Therapy/Physical Therapy Curriculum. Pain Curriculum for Students in Occupational Therapy or Physical Therapy. IASP Newsletter. 1994;November/December:3.

Support Groups

AIDS Action Council
1875 Connecticut Avenue, Suite 700
Washington, DC 20009
(202) 986-1300

American Cancer Society
1599 Clifton Road, NE
Atlanta, GA 30329
(404) 320-3333

American Chronic Pain Association
P.O. Box 850
Rockin, CA 95677
(916) 632-0922

American Pain Society
4700 W. Lake Avenue
Glenview, IL 60025
(708) 375-4715
e-mail: aps@dial.cic.net

American Spinal Injury Association
345 East Superior Street, Room 1436
Chicago, IL 60611
(312) 908-3425, (312) 908-6207

Arachnoiditis Information and Support Network
P.O. Box 1166
Baldwin, MO 63022
(314) 394-5741

Arthritis Foundation
1314 Spring Street, NW
Atlanta, GA 30309-2998
(404) 872-7100

Back Pain Association of America
P.O. Box 135
Pasadena, MD 21122-0135
(410) 253-3633

Cancer Care Inc.
(New York only)
1180 Avenue of the Americas
New York, NY 10036
(212) 221-3300

Candlelighters Childhood Cancer Foundation
7910 Woodmont Avenue, Suite 460
Bethesda, MD 20814
(301) 657-8401

Endometriosis Association
5885 North 7th Place
Milwaukee, WI 53223
(414) 355-2200

International Association for the Study of Pain
909 NE 43rd Street, Suite 306
Seattle, WA 98105
(206) 547-6409
e-mail: IASP@locke.hs.washington.edu

Interstitial Cystitis Association
P.O. Box 1553
Madison Square Station
New York, NY 10159
(212) 979-6057

National Arthritis, Musculoskeletal and Skin Disease Information
9000 Rockville Pike, Box AMS
Bethesda, MD 20892
(301) 495-4484

National Association for Sickle Cell Disease
3345 Wilshire Boulevard, Suite 1106
Los Angeles, CA 90010-1880
(213) 736-5455

National Chronic Pain Outreach Association
7979 Old Georgetown Road, Suite 100
Bethesda, MD 20814-2429
(301) 652-4948

National Coalition for Cancer Survivorship
1010 Wayne Avenue NW, 5th Floor
Silver Spring, MD 20910
(505) 764-9956

National Headache Foundation
428 West St. James Place
Chicago, IL 60614
(312) 388-6399

National Multiple Sclerosis Society
30 West 26th Street, 9th Floor
New York, NY 10016
(212) 986-3240

Reflex Sympathetic Dystrophy Association
P.O. Box 821
Haddenfield, NJ 08033
(609) 795-8845

Resource Center for State Cancer Pain Initiatives
University of Wisconsin-Madison Medical School
Medical Sciences Center Room 3675
1300 University Avenue
Madison, WI 53706

Trigeminal Neuralgia Association
P.O. Box 340
Barnegat Light, NH 08006
(609) 361-1014

Varicella Zoster Virus Research Foundation
(Shingles)
40 East 72nd Street
New York, NY 10021
(212) 472-3181

Washington Intractable Chronic Pain Advocacy
2308 NE 94th Street
Vancouver, WA 98665
(360) 574-0467

Y-Me National Organization for Breast Cancer
212 West Van Buren Street, 4th Floor
Chicago, IL 60607
(312) 986-8338

Index